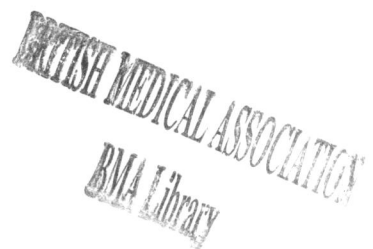

Determining Health
Expectancies

Determining Health Expectancies

Edited by

Jean-Marie Robine
INSERM, Equipe Démographie et Santé, Parc Euromédecine, Montpellier, France

Carol Jagger
Department of Epidemiology and Public Health, University of Leicester, UK

Colin D. Mathers
Epidemiology and Burden of Disease, World Health Organization,
Geneva, Switzerland

Eileen M. Crimmins
Andrus Gerontology Center, University of Southern California, Los Angeles, USA

Richard M. Suzman
Behavioral and Social Research, National Institute on Aging, Bethesda, USA

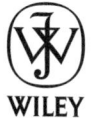

WILEY

Other Wiley Editorial Offices

John Wiley & Sons Inc., 111 River Street, Hoboken, NJ 07030, USA

Jossey-Bass, 989 Market Street, San Francisco, CA 94103-1741, USA

Wiley-VCH Verlag GmbH, Boschstr. 12, D-69469 Weinheim, Germany

John Wiley & Sons Australia Ltd, 33 Park Road, Milton, Queensland 4064, Australia

John Wiley & Sons (Asia) Pte Ltd, 2 Clementi Loop #02-01, Jin Xing Distripark, Singapore
129809

John Wiley & Sons Canada Ltd, 22 Worcester Road, Etobicoke, Ontario, Canada
M9W 1L1

Wiley also publishes its books in a variety of electronic formats. Some content that
appears in print may not be available in electronic books.

Library of Congress Cataloging-in-Publication Data

Determining health expectancies / edited by Jean-Marie Robine ... [et al.].
      p.cm.
   Includes bibliographical references and index.
   ISBN 0-470-84397-7 (alk. paper)
      1. Health expectancy.   2. Health status indicators.   3. World health.   I. Robine,
Jean-Marie.
   RA407 .D47 2002
   614.4′2–dc21   2002031130

British Library Cataloguing in Publication Data

A catalogue record for this book is available from the British Library

ISBN 0 470 84397 7

Typeset by Dobbie Typesetting Ltd, Tavistock, Devon
Printed and bound in Great Britain by T.J. International, Padstow, Cornwall
This book is printed on acid-free paper responsibly manufactured from sustainable forestry
in which at least two trees are planted for each one used for paper production.

Contents

PART II   THE RELEVANCE OF HEALTH EXPECTANCIES

PART III   MEASUREMENT, COLLECTION AND CALCULATION PROBLEMS

List of Contributors

EMILY M. AGREE

Johns Hopkins University, Dept of Population Dynamics, School of Hygiene and Public Health, 615 North Wolfe Street, 21205-2179 Baltimore, MD, USA
Email: eagree@sph.jhu.edu

MADHAVI BAJEKAL

National Centre for Social Research, London EC1V 0AX, UK
Email: m.bajekal@natcen.ac.uk

JAN J. BARENDREGT

Erasmus MC, Dept of Public Health, PO Box 1738, 3000 DR Rotterdam, The Netherlands
Email: barendregt@mgz.fgg.eur.nl

ANDREW BEBBINGTON

University of Kent, Personal Social Services Research Unit, Cornwallis Building, Canterbury CT2 7NF, Kent, UK
Email: a.c.bebbington@ukc.ac.uk

JEAN-MARIE BERTHELOT

Statistics Canada, Health Analysis and Measurement Group, R.H. Coats Building, 24-P, K1A 0T6 Ottawa, Ontario, Canada
Email: berthel@statcan.ca

HENDRIEK BOSHUIZEN

National Institute for Public Health and the Environment, Computerization and Methodological Consultancy Unit, PO Box 1, 3720 BA Bilthoven, The Netherlands
Email: Hendriek.Boshuizen@rivm.nl

VITTORIA BURATTA

ISTAT, DIREZIONE CENTRALE PERE Indagini Sulle Istitutson: Sociali, Via Liegi, 13, 00198 Rome, Italy
Email: buratta@istat.it

EMMANUELLE CAMBOIS   *INSERM, Equipe démographie et santé, Centre Val d'Aurelle, Parc Euromédecine, 34298 Montpellier Cedex 5, France*
Email: cambois@valdorel.fnclcc.fr

EILEEN CRIMMINS   *Andrus Gerontology Center, University of Southern California, 90089-0191 Los Angeles, California, USA*
Email: crimmin@usc.edu

PETER DAVIS   *Christchurch School of Medicine and Health Sciences, University of Otago, PO Box 4345, Christchurch, New Zealand*
Email: Peter.Davis@chmeds.ac.nz

DORLY J.H. DEEG   *Faculty of Medicine/LASA, Vrije Universiteit, Van der Boechorststraat 7, room H-036, 1081 BT Amsterdam, The Netherlands*
Email: djh.deeg.emgo@med.vu.nl

VIVIANA EGIDI   *ISTAT, Dipartimento delle Statistiche Sociali, via A. Rava' 150, 00142 Rome, Italy*
Email: egidi@istat.it

PATRICK GRAHAM   *Department of Public Health and General Practice, Christchurch School of Medicine and Health Sciences, PO Box 4345, Christchurch, New Zealand*
Email: patrick.graham@chmeds.ac.nz

ROBERTO HAM-CHANDE   *El Colegio de la Frontera Norte, Department of Population Studies, Abelardo Rodriguez 2925 – Zona Rio, 22320 Tijuana, BC, Mexico*
Email: rham@colef.mx

MARK D. HAYWARD   *The Pennsylvania State University, Population Research Institute, 501 Oswald Tower, University Park, PA 16802-6210, USA*
Email: hayward@pop.psu.edu

CAROL JAGGER   *University of Leicester, Dept Epidemiology and Public Health, 22–28 Princess Road West, Leicester LE1 6TP, UK*
Email: cxj@le.ac.uk

SUTTHICHAI JITAPUNKUL *Department of Medicine, Faculty of Medicine, Chulongkorn University, Bangkok 10330, Thailand*
Email: jsutthic@chula.ac.th

SARAH B. LADITKA — *Center for Health and Aging, State University of New York Institute of Technology, Box 3050, Utica, New York 13504-3050, USA*
Email: laditks@sunyit.edu

VICKI L. LAMB — *Center for Demographic Studies, Duke University, Box 90408, Durham, NC 27708-0408, USA*
Email: vlamb@cds.duke.edu

ALAN D. LOPEZ — *Evidence and Information for Policy, World Health Organization, 20, Via Appia, CH 1211 Geneva 27, Switzerland*
Email: lopeza@who.int

COLIN D. MATHERS — *Epidemiology and Burden of Disease, World Health Organization, Geneva, Switzerland*
Email: mathersc@who.int

FRANCE MESLÉ — *INED, Institut National d'Etudes Démographiques, 133 Boulevard Davout, 75980 Paris Cedex 20, France*
Email: mesle@ined.fr

JEAN-PIERRE MICHEL — *Institutions Universitaires de Gériatrie, Route de Mon-Idée CH-1226 Thonex-Genève, Switzerland*
Email: Jean-Pierre.michel@hcuge.ch

CHRISTOPHER J.L. MURRAY — *Evidence and Information for Policy, World Health Organization (WHO), 20 Avenue Appia, 1211 Geneva 27, Switzerland*
Email: murrayc@who.int

MARGARETA MUTAFOVA — *Medical Academy, Department of Social Medecine, Belo More Str, 8, 1527 Sofia, Bulgaria*
Email: m_mutafova@cybernet.bg

GEORGE C. MYERS — Deceased

WILMA J. NUSSELDER — *Erasmus MC, Department of Public Health, University Medical Centre Rotterdam, PO Box 1738, 3000 DR Rotterdam, The Netherlands*
Email: nusselder@mgz.fgg.eur.nl

ROM J.M. PERENBOOM — *TNO Prevention and Health, Division Public Health, PO Box 2215, 2301 CE Leiden, The Netherlands*
Email: RJM.Perenboom@pg.tno.nl

YVES PÉRON   *Université de Montréal, Département de*
                            Démographie, C.P. 6128, Succursale A, H3G 3J7,
                            Montréal, Québec, Canada
                            Email: perony@magellan.umontreal.ca

CATHERINE POLGE   *INSERM EMI 99/30, Hôpital La Colombière*
                            Pavillon Calixte Cavalier 42, 39, Avenue Charles
                            Flahault BP 34493, 34093 Montpellier, France
                            Email: polge@montp.inserm.fr

XIAOCHUN QIAO   *Institute of Population Research, The People's*
                            University of China, Department of Demography,
                            175 Haidian Road, 100872 Beijing, China
                            E-mail: qiaoxch@hyper.netchina.co.cn

KAREN RITCHIE   *INSERM EMI 99/30, Hôpital La Colombière,*
                            Pavillon Calixte Cavalier 42, 39, Avenue Charles
                            Flahault BP 34493, 34093 Montpellier, France
                            Email: ritchie@montp.inserm.fr

JEAN-MARIE ROBINE   *INSERM, Equipe démographie et santé, Centre Val*
                            d'Aurelle, Parc Euromédecine, 34298 Montpellier
                            Cedex 5, France
                            Email: robine@valdorel.fnclcc.fr

ISABELLE ROMIEU   *INSERM, Equipe démographie et santé, Centre Val*
                            d'Aurelle, Parc Euromédecine, 34298 Montpellier
                            Cedex 5, France
                            Email: iromieu@valdorel.fnclcc.fr

RITU SADANA   *Global Programme on Evidence for Health Policy,*
                            World Health Organization (WHO), 20 Avenue
                            Appia, 1211 Geneva 27, Switzerland
                            Email: sadanar@who.int

YASUHIKO SAITO   *Nihon University, Center for Information*
                            Networking, 4-25 Nakatomi-Minami,
                            359 Saitama-ken Tokorozawa-shi, Japan
                            Email: yasuhik@mls.cin.nihon-u.ac.jp

JOSHUA A. SALOMON   *Global Programme on Evidence for Health Policy,*
                            World Health Organization (WHO), 20 Avenue
                            Appia, 1211 Geneva 27, Switzerland
                            Email: salomonj@who.int

RICHARD SUZMAN   *National Institute on Aging, Behavioral and Social*
                            Research, 7201 Wisconsin Avenue, Gateway

Building 2C-234, 20892 Bethesda MD, USA
Email: suzmanr@gw.nia.nih.gov

JACQUES VALLIN
INED, Institut National d'Etudes Démographiques, 133 Boulevard Davout, 75980 Paris Cedex 20, France
Email: vallin@ined.fr

HERMAN VAN OYEN
Scientific Institute of Public Health, Unit of Epidemiology, Juliette Wytsmanstraat, 14, 1050 Brussels, Belgium
Email: vanoyen@iph.fgov.be

LOIS M. VERBRUGGE
University of Michigan, Institute of Gerontology, 300 North Ingalls, 48109-2007 Ann Arbor, Michigan, USA
Email: verbrugg@umich.edu

List of abbreviations

ADL	Activities of Daily Living
DALE	Disability-Adjusted Life Expectancy
DALY	Disability-Adjusted Life Year
DemLE	Dementia-free Life Expectancy
DFLE	Disability-Free Life Expectancy
DSM	Diagnostic and Statistical Manual of Mental Disorders
EC	European Community
GBD	Global Burden of Disease
GDP	Gross Domestic Product
GHQ	General Health Questionnaire
GNP	Gross National Product
HALE	Health-Adjusted Life Expectancy
HE	Health Expectancy
HLE	Healthy Life Expectancy
HSE	Health State Expectancy
HUI	Health Utility Index
IADL	Instrumental Activities of Daily Living
ICD	International Classification of Diseases
ICIDH	International Classification of Impairments, Disabilities and Handicaps
LE	Life Expectancy
LED	Life Expectancy with Disability
MHI	Mental Health Index
OECD	Organization for Economic Cooperation and Development
PYLL	Potential Years of Life Lost
QALY	Quality-Adjusted Life Years
REVES	Réseau Espérance de Vie en Santé/International Network on Health Expectancy and the Disability Process
SES	Socio-Economic Status
SMPH	Summary Measure of Population Health
UN	United Nations
UNFPA	United Nations Population Fund
WHO	World Health Organization
YLD	Years Lived with Disability
YLL	Years of Life Lost

Introduction

JEAN-MARIE ROBINE, CAROL JAGGER[1], COLIN D. MATHERS[2],
EILEEN M. CRIMMINS[3], RICHARD M. SUZMAN[4] and YVES PÉRON[5]

INSERM, Montpellier, France, [1]University of Leicester, UK, [2]World Health
Organization, Switzerland, [3]University of Southern California, USA,
[4]National Institute on Aging, USA, [5]Université de Montréal, Canada

The impetus for the creation of the International Network on Health Expectancy and the Disability Process, the French acronym for which was REVES (Réseau Espérance de Vie en Santé), came in the 1970s and 1980s. During this time life expectancy was increasing in the developed world and these countries were beginning to see substantially greater numbers of older people. The common view that old age brought a greater demand for health and social care warranted evidence of whether these new populations of elderly would be healthier, and therefore make fewer demands than previous cohorts, or whether they were simply successes of medical advances, being kept alive longer but with poorer health. Scenarios of the compressions and expansion of morbidity, as well as the intermediate ones, such as the dynamic equilibrium theory, were drawn up (Gruenberg, 1977; Kramer, 1980; Fries, 1980, 1989; Manton, 1882).

In 1964, Sanders first developed the idea of a population health indicator bringing together data on both quantity – through mortality – and quality of life – usually disability – (Sanders, 1964) with the first explicit method of calculation by Sullivan in 1971 (Sullivan, 1971a, 1971b). However, in the years following, the evidence for compression or expansion of morbidity was unclear, with some reports favouring one and some another, even in the same country. The first estimates of disability-free life expectancy (DFLE), called 'expectation of healthy life' and defined as 'free of bed-disability and institutionalization', were made for the United States in 1969 and showed that DFLE had increased slightly from 1958 to 1966 for both genders whilst life expectancy (LE) over the same period had appeared to stagnate (US Department of Health, 1969). In 1974, another calculation based on Japanese

Determining Health Expectancies. Edited by J-M. Robine, C. Jagger, C.D. Mathers, E.M. Crimmins and R.M. Suzman.
© 2003 John Wiley & Sons, Ltd

data from 1966 to 1970 showed a slightly more rapid increase in LE than in DFLE (The Council of National Living, 1974). In these calculations, DFLE corresponded to the 'average healthy life span' and was defined as 'free from functional loss due to disease' and was the first example of a calculation of years of healthy life lost from injury and disease.

At the annual meeting of the American Public Health Association in 1979, a paper examined the trend in the health of Americans from 1964 to 1974. The calculations clearly showed that 'although overall life expectancy has increased over this decade, almost all of this increase was years of disability' (McKinlay and McKinlay, 1979; McKinlay *et al*, 1983). In 1980, a series of calculations with the US data spanning from 1966 to 1976 distinguished, for the first time, the levels of disability. Over this decade, LE increased by 2.2 years while DFLE only rose by 0.6 year. These alarming results were linked to an increase of both mild and severe forms of disability (Colvez, 1980, 1992; Colvez and Blanchet, 1983).

The first book totally devoted to health expectancies, *Healthfulness of Life*, was published in Canada in 1983 by Wilkins and Adams. Using the 1978–1979 data of the Canadian Health Survey, they computed DFLE for 1978 and then used the 1950–1951 data of the Canadian Sickness Survey to produce an estimate of DFLE for the past. Despite conceptual and methodological differences between the two surveys which limited comparisons, 'the importance of knowing (...) whether healthfulness increased or decreased as LE rose from 1951 to 1978 was sufficient to justify at least attempting to make such comparisons' (Wilkins and Adams, 1983a). Here, too, most of the increase in life expectancy was in years with disability (Wilkins and Adams, 1983b, 1987). In 1994, a short but valid series of health expectancies were published for Canada with the repetition in 1991 of the 1986 Health and Activity Limitation Survey – HALS (Wilkins *et al*, 1994). In 1983, another Canadian book devoted to health expectancies, *Durée ou qualité de la vie?*, presented a few previously unpublished calculations by Colvez based on the 1962 and 1965 US National Health Interview Survey (NHIS) data (Dillard, 1983).

In 1988, Bebbington published the first series of expectation of life without disability in England and Wales for the years 1976, 1981 and 1985. His conclusions were as pessimistic as the American or Canadian ones: most of the increase in LE was in years with chronic disability. However, this author emphasized that during the previous decade a significant improvement both in LE and in DFLE had taken place for older people (Bebbington, 1988). This series has since been regularly updated (Bebbington, 1991, 1992; Bone *et al*, 1995; Bebbington and Darton, 1996).

Immediately prior to the first REVES meeting in 1989, further results for the US were published for the decade beginning in 1970. The conclusion was similar to others: 'Over the decade 1970–80, life expectancy at birth increased in the United States by about three years for both males and females. Most of this increase was in years with disability' (Crimmins *et al*, 1989; Crimmins,

1992). This work differed from previous studies in that greater importance was attached to the validity and quality of the data. Calculations were restricted to the census years when accurate estimation of the institutionalized population was possible and to a period of time without major change in the NHIS data collection (such major changes occurred between 1957 and 1958 and between 1981 and 1982). The same authors were also able to reproduce the calculation of DFLE made by Sullivan for the year 1965 (Sullivan, 1971b), for 1970 and 1980 (Crimmins *et al*, 1989), and then for 1990 (Crimmins *et al*, 1997), and observed that 'looking only at bed disability, most of the increase in LE at birth between 1970 and 1980 was in non-disabled or healthy years'. Also in 1989 a previous series from 1964 to 1974 was updated with a calculation for 1985 (MacKinlay *et al*, 1989) but without attention to the changes that had occurred in the NHIS design. Interestingly, they noticed a major decrease in average life free of disability.

These early calculations, prior to the creation of REVES, highlight the difficulties of monitoring DFLE consistently both within countries over time and between countries. In this context, it is easy to understand why one of the main goals of the REVES network in 1989 was to know if the increase in LE was accompanied by an increase in DFLE. When REVES was created, 11 papers dealing with this topic had been published (Colvez and Blanchet, 1981; Wilson, 1981; Feldman, 1983; Verbrugge, 1984; Wilson and Drury, 1984; Newachek *et al*, 1984; Verbrugge and Madans, 1985; Palmore, 1986; Newachek *et al*, 1986; Chirikos, 1986; Robine and Brunelle, 1986). Even if most of the authors had underlined that no evidence existed for an increase of disability among the elderly (Verbrugge, 1989), taken all together these studies gave the general impression that disability was increasing.

At the time of its creation in 1989, the REVES network was made up of 10 invited teams coming from Canada, France, the Netherlands, Switzerland, the United States and the United Kingdom. The first three meetings continued with these teams but in 1991, at the fourth meeting in Leiden in the Netherlands, the network was opened up to any researchers interested in health expectancy and disability. From 48 participants and 6 countries represented at the first meeting in Quebec in 1989, REVES now includes amongst its membership some 150 scientists from 30 countries and at every meeting new scientists and policy makers are welcomed to the network.

The role of REVES has developed much over the decade. The extension of the name to include the disability process, at the Geneva meeting in 1990, highlighted the need to be able to differentiate levels of disability for comparability and to explain potential changes over time in the distribution of severity. Issues such as the interpretation of time series of health expectancies and the promotion of health expectancy for planning public policy and public health programmes have always been in the forefront. However, over the years, REVES has paid more attention to improving the quality and comparability of the available data, and in particular promoting the use of standardized and new methods for both data collection and calculation of health expectancies. In this context REVES members have conducted three workshops – in association with Nihon University, Peking University and IUSSP (International Union for the Scientific Study of Population) – to disseminate methods to researchers and policy makers in developing countries. The first two workshops, Tokyo (1999) and Beijing (2001), concentrated on the basic method of health expectancy calculation, the Sullivan method, requiring only cross-sectional data on the prevalence of health states. The most recent workshop in Tokyo (2002) focused on advanced methods using long-itudinal data.

A considerable strength of REVES is the wide range of scientists and policy makers it attracts, from disciplines including: demography, epidemiology, gerontology, sociology, psychology, public health, health policy, health economics, medicine, biology, and statistics, and it has developed strong links with international agencies such as the UN, WHO, OECD and Eurostat. More geographically close sub-networks have also been spawned, to encourage and support more local research, including Asia-REVES and Euro-REVES. Much of the passage of information is via the REVES web pages (www.reves.net).

This book presents essentially the first decade of work of REVES, with almost annual meetings from 1989. The first section provides the background to health expectancies and how they evolved. The second section concentrates on the use of health expectancies to describe social and geographical inequalities in health as well as the contributions to ill-health from different diseases and conditions. The third section is focused around the problems involved in comparability of health expectancies: the measurement of disability, collection of data and method of calculation employed. This section also includes a description and critique of other forms of health expectancies (health-adjusted life expectancy and disability-adjusted life expectancy). The final section provides an up-to-date description of health expectancies in different regions of the world. In the preparation of this book and in the work of REVES as a whole, we have concluded that the language we use is of paramount importance, particularly in the context of an international network with researchers from a variety of disciplines. We have tried to make as explicit as possible the underlying concepts of health measurement, the definitions of disability and health, and the way in which we have merged and weighted different health dimensions. It is only in this way that we can have truly comparable health expectancies to answer the important question of whether we are living longer, healthier lives.

REFERENCES

Bebbington, A.C. (1988) 'The expectation of life without disability in England and Wales', *Social Science and Medicine* 27, 321–326.

Bebbington, A.C. (1991) 'The expectation of life without disability in England and Wales, 1976–1988', *Population Trends* 66, 26–29.

Bebbington, A.C. (1992) 'Expectation of life without disability measured from the OPCS disability surveys', in Robine, J-M., Blanchet, M. and Dowd, J.E. (eds) *Health Expectancy*. London: HMSO.

Bebbington, A.C. and Darton, R.A. (1996) *Healthy Life Expectancy in England and Wales: Recent Evidence*. London: PSSRU.

Bone, M.R., Bebbington, A.C., Jagger, C., Morgan, K. and Nicolaas, G. (1995) *Health Expectancy and its Uses*. London: HMSO.

Chirikos, T.N. (1986) 'Accounting for the historical rise in work-disability prevalence', *Milbank Quarterly* 64(2), 271–301.

Colvez, A. (1980) *Evolution de l'état de santé au cours de la dernière décennie: Peut-on continuer à parler d'amélioration?* Quebec: Ministère des Affaires Sociales (Services des Etudes Epidémiologiques; document dactylographié).

Colvez, A. (1992) 'Changes in disability-free life expectancy in the USA between 1966 and 1976', in Robine, J-M., Blanchet, M. and Dowd, J.E. (eds) *Health Expectancy*. London: HMSO.

Colvez, A. and Blanchet, M. (1981) 'Disability trends in the United States population 1966–76: analysis of reported causes', *American Journal of Public Health* 71(5), 464–471.

Colvez, A. and Blanchet, M. (1983) 'Potential gains in life expectancy free of disability: a tool for health planning', *International Journal of Epidemiology* 12, 224–229.

Crimmins, E.M., Saito, Y. and Ingegneri, D. (1989) 'Changes in life expectancy and disability-free life expectancy in the United States', *Population and Development Review* 15, 235–267.

Crimmins, E.M., Saito, Y. and Ingegneri, D. (1992) 'Changes in life expectancy and disability-free life expectancy in the United States', in Robine, J-M., Blanchet, M. and Dowd, J.E. (eds) *Health Expectancy*. London: HMSO.

Crimmins, E.M., Saito, Y. and Ingegneri, D. (1997) 'Trends in disability-free life expectancy in the United States, 1970–90', *Population and Development Review* 23, 555–572.

Dillard, S. (1983) *Durée ou qualité de la vie?* Montreal: Les Publications du Québec. (Conseil des Affaires Sociales et de la Famille; collection: La santé des Québécois).

Feldman, J.J. (1983) 'Work ability of the aged under conditions of improving mortality', *Milbank Memorial Fund Quarterly/Health and Society* 61(3), 430–444.

Fries, J. F. (1980) 'Aging, natural death, and the compression of morbidity', *New England Journal of Medicine* 303, 130–135.

Fries, J.F. (1989) 'The compression of morbidity: near or far?', *Milbank Quarterly* 67, 208–232.

Gruenberg, E.M. (1977) 'The failures of success', *Milbank Memorial Fund Quarterly/Health and Society* 55, 3–24.

Kramer, M. (1980) 'The rising pandemic of mental disorders and associated chronic diseases and disabilities', *Acta Psychiatrica Scandinavica* 62, 382–397.

Manton, K.G. (1982) 'Changing concepts of morbidity and mortality in the elderly population', *Milbank Memorial Fund Quarterly/Health and Society* 60, 183–244.

McKinlay, J.B., McKinlay, S.M., Jennings, S. and Grant, K. (1983) 'Mortality, morbidity, and the inverse care law', in Greer, A.L. and Greer, S. (eds) *Cities and Sickness*. Beverly Hills: Sage.

McKinlay, J.B., McKinlay, S.M. and Beaglehole, R. (1989) 'A review of the evidence concerning the impact of medical measures on recent mortality and morbidity in the United States', *International Journal of Health Services* 19, 181–208.

McKinlay, S.M. and McKinlay, J.B. (1979) 'Examining trends in the nation's health', American Public Health Association annual meeting, New York.

Newacheck, P.W., Budetti, P.P. and McManus, P. (1984) 'Trends in childhood disability', *American Journal of Public Health* 74(3), 232–236.

Newacheck, P.W., Budetti, P.P. and Halfon, N. (1986) 'Trends in activity-limiting chronic conditions among children', *American Journal of Public Health* 76(2), 178–184.

Palmore, E.B. (1986) 'Trends in the health of the aged', *The Gerontologist* 26(3), 298–302.

Robine, J.M. and Brunelle, Y. (1986) *La hausse de l'invalidité*. Quebec: Les Publications du Québec.

Sanders, B.S. (1964) 'Measuring community health levels', *American Journal of Public Health* 54(7), 1063–1070.

Sullivan, D.F. (1971a) 'A single index of mortality and morbidity', *HSMHA Health Reports* 86, 347–354.

Sullivan, D.F. (1971b) *Disability Components for an Index of Health*. Rockville, MD: National Center for Health Statistics (Vital and Health Statistics; series 2; no 42).

The Council of National Living (1974) *Social Indicators of Japan*. Tokyo: The Council of National Living, Research Committee.

US Department of Health, Education, and Welfare (1969) *Toward a Social Report*. Washington, DC: US Department of Health, Education, and Welfare.

Verbrugge, L.M. (1984) 'Longer life but worsening health? Trends in health and mortality of middle-aged and older persons', *Milbank Memorial Fund Quarterly/Health and Society* 62(3), 475–519.

Verbrugge, L.M. (1989) 'Recent, present, and future health of American adults', *Annual Reviews in Public Health* 10, 333–361.

Verbrugge, L.M. and Madans, J.H. (1985) 'Social roles and health trends of American women', *Milbank Memorial Fund Quarterly/Health and Society* 63(4), 691–735.

Wilkins, R. and Adams, O.B. (1983a) *Healthfulness of Life*. Montreal: The Institute for Research on Public Policy.

Wilkins, R. and Adams, O.B. (1983b) 'Health expectancy in Canada, late 1970s: demographic, regional and social dimensions', *American Journal of Public Health* 73(9), 1073–1080.

Wilkins, R. and Adams, O.B. (1987) 'Changes in the healthfulness of life of the elderly population: an empirical approach', *Revue d'Epidémiologie et de Santé Publique* 35, 225–235.

Wilkins, R., Chen, J. and Ng, E. (1994) 'Changes in health expectancy in Canada from 1986 to 1991', in Mathers, C.D., McCallum, J. and Robine, J.M. (eds) *Advances in Health Expectancies*. Canberra: Australian Institute of Health and Welfare, AGPS.

Wilson, R.W. (1981) 'Do health indicators indicate health?' *American Journal of Public Health* 71(5), 461–463.

Wilson, R.W. and Drury, T.F. (1984) 'Interpreting trends in illness and disability: health statistics and health status', *Annual Reviews in Public Health* 5, 83–106.

PART I

The Main Trends in the Evolution of the Population's Health Status

Introduction

JEAN-MARIE ROBINE

INSERM, Montpellier, France

During the last decade of the 20th century, the increase of the oldest-old population attracted significant attention (Suzman *et al*, 1994). Some feared that the combination of low mortality with the increasing size of birth cohorts, especially the baby-boom cohorts, would dramatically increase the size of the oldest-old population of the future. The most critical point in evaluating the meaning of a growing and longer-lived older population was uncertainty about the level of health of this population and the associated costs. People feared not only an increase in the costs associated with medical care but also increased costs associated with high levels of disability and dependency of these oldest old persons.

Since the mid-1980s three conflicting theories about the relationship between mortality and population health have been put forward. For Gruenberg and Kramer the observed decline in mortality rates among the oldest old was due to the decrease in the fatality rate of chronic conditions leading to a significant increase in the prevalence of disability, dementia and co-morbidity among these new survivors (Gruenberg, 1977, 1980; Kramer, 1980). At the same time, Fries and Crapo proposed the exact opposite theory, that the natural limit to human life expectancy would prevent future gains in term of years of life but that the postponement of the onset of chronic diseases to more advanced ages would lead to a compression of the period of morbidity (Fries, 1980; Fries and Crapo, 1981). Between these two extremes, Manton introduced the theory of dynamic equilibrium acknowledging a possible slowing down in the pace of progression of chronic diseases leading to an increase in the prevalence of light and moderate (but not severe) disability as mortality falls among the oldest old (Manton, 1982). Although the three theories offered three possible visions of the future, the first one, the pandemic of disability, was both the most feared and the most foreseen at the beginning of the 1990s.

Determining Health Expectancies. Edited by J-M. Robine, C. Jagger, C.D. Mathers, E.M. Crimmins and R.M. Suzman.
© 2003 John Wiley & Sons, Ltd

In this context, there was a growing interest from policy makers and various public authorities in global health indicators that take into account both the quantity and the quality of life, such as disability-free life expectancy proposed by Sullivan as early as 1971 (Sullivan, 1971), or active life expectancy proposed by Katz and his colleagues in 1983 (Katz et al, 1983). But chronological series that allowed these demo-epidemiological changes to be monitored were still rare. Some calculations brought good news such as parallel increases in life expectancy and disability-free life expectancy, for instance in France. In 1997 several international agencies, including the G7 who gathered in Denver and the World Health Organization, recommended the calculation of various heath expectancies, including active life expectancy, to improve the relevance of health indicators and monitor the world health situation (G7, 1997; WHO, 1997).

At the end of the 1990s, the interest in the calculation of health expectancies was boosted by accumulation of new data on the oldest old and on human longevity. Firstly the number of centenarians was shown to be doubling every 10 years in low mortality countries since the end of World War II. Secondly, in several countries, female life expectancy at birth was approaching the value of 85 years, presented by Fries as the natural limit (Fries, 1980), and there did not appear to be any slowing down in the annual pace of increase of this life expectancy. These empirical data raised new questions about the length of human life and the shape of the survival curve. Again a crucial point was to know whether the compression of morbidity foreseen by Fries or the dynamic equilibrium anticipated by Manton could occur in such a context. What is the likelihood of a limit to the increase in the number of extremely old persons, frail and disabled, if human life span is not limited per se?

The four chapters of this first section examine these issues – which formed the background framework of the development of the health expectancies – from a historical and theoretical point of view. France Meslé and Jacques Vallin from the National Institute of Demographic Studies in France (INED) describe how life expectancy increased during the last decades of the 20th century in low mortality countries and discuss the impacts of this increase on the shape of the survival curve and its 'rectangularization'. Behind this odd word stands a measure of the heterogeneity/homogeneity of individual life duration. In the second chapter Wilma Nusselder from Erasmus University in the Netherlands describes in detail the occurrence of the compression of morbidity in low mortality countries. In the third chapter George Myers, Vicki Lamb and Emily Agree from Duke University and Johns Hopkins University in the United States put these new demo-epidemiologic facts in perspective and introduce the functional transition (disability) which explains how the occurrence (incidence), the level (prevalence) and the severity of disability change with the mortality changes associated with the demographic and epidemiologic transitions. Finally, Jean-Marie Robine, Isabelle Romieu and

Jean-Pierre Michel from the National Institute of Health and Medical Research in France (INSERM) and from the University of Geneva introduce and discuss the various chronological series of health expectancies. Thus together these four chapters present the context and the relevance of the health expectancy indicators to be examined in greater detail in the following sections.

REFERENCES

Fries, J.F. (1980) 'Aging, natural death, and the compression of morbidity', *New England Journal of Medicine* 303, 130–135.

Fries, J.F. and Crapo, L.M. (1981) *Vitality and Aging*. San Francisco: WH Freeman and Company.

Gruenberg, E.M. (1977) 'The failures of success', *Milbank Memorial Fund Quarterly/ Health and Society* 55, 3–24.

Gruenberg, E.M. (1980) 'Epidemiology of senile dementia', in *Epidemiology of Aging*. Washington, DC: US Department of Health and Human Services.

G7 (1997) *Final communiqué*, Denver, 22 June.

Katz, S., Branch, L.G., Branson, M.H., Papsidero, J.A., Beck, J.C. and Greer, D.S. (1983) 'Active life expectancy', *New England Journal of Medicine* 309, 1218–1224.

Kramer, M. (1980) 'The rising pandemic of mental disorders and associated chronic diseases and disabilities', *Acta Psychiatrica Scandinavica* 62(Suppl. 285), 282–297.

Manton, K.G. (1982) 'Changing concepts of morbidity and mortality in the elderly population', *Milbank Memorial Fund Quarterly/Health and Society* 60, 183–244.

Sullivan, D.F. (1971) 'A single index of mortality and morbidity', *HSMHA Health Reports* 86, 347–354.

Suzman, R.M., Willis, D.P. and Manton, K.G. (eds) (1994) *The Oldest Old*. New York: Oxford University Press.

World Health Organization (1997) *Conquering Suffering, Enriching Humanity. The World Health Report 1997*. Geneva: World Health Organization.

1

Increase in Life Expectancy and Concentration of Ages at Death

FRANCE MESLÉ and JACQUES VALLIN
INED, Paris, France

In two centuries, life expectancy in most of the northern countries has risen from 30 to nearly 80 years. More recently, southern countries have followed and most have life expectancies close to northern countries. Though some populations have experienced or are currently experiencing major setbacks in the historic march towards improved health (former USSR countries, sub-Saharan Africa), it does appear that the move towards improved health and longer life is becoming more general. The most controversial question today is whether this move is reaching what some consider to be the fixed limit of human longevity. One indicator of this limit could be the process by which the survival curve has become increasingly rectangular over the last two centuries, but this rectangularisation could simply be temporary, leading to a renewed increase in the age of death if it were found that the limit of longevity was not immutable. It is therefore important to measure this rectangularisation process accurately in order to be able to detect any changes in the pattern. Various authors have suggested a range of indicators. We prefer to use two of these here, one suggested by John Wilmoth and Shiro Horiuchi and the other by Väinö Kannisto, to trace the development of the phenomenon in France since the mid-18th century.

THREE CENTURIES OF IMPROVED LIFE EXPECTANCY IN FRANCE

In France, we can use various historical reconstructions to trace the increase in life expectancy at birth since the mid-18th century. INED has recently

Determining Health Expectancies. Edited by J-M. Robine, C. Jagger, C.D. Mathers, E.M. Crimmins and R.M. Suzman.

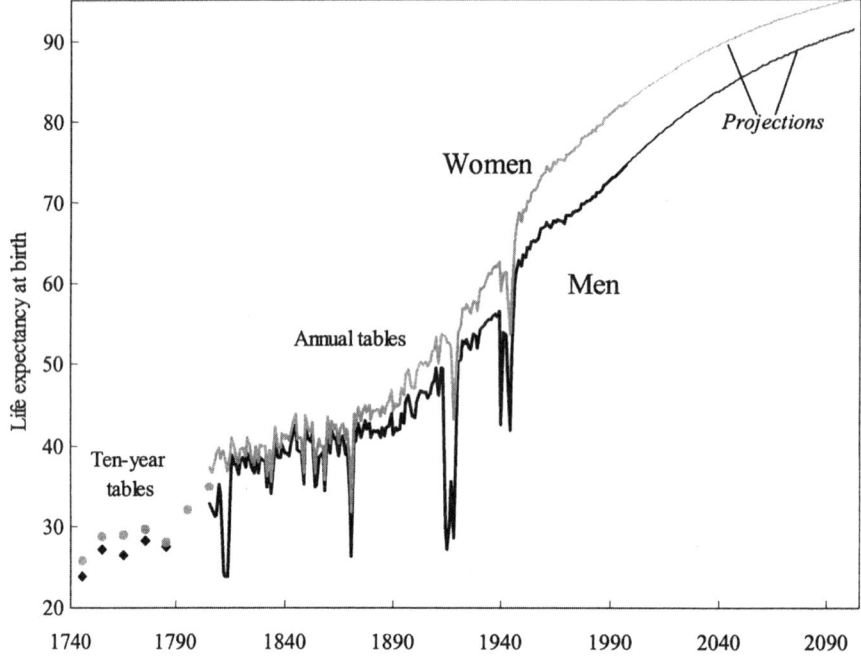

Figure 1.1. Life expectancy at birth in France: annual increase from 1806 to 1997, 10-year estimates for the 18th century and extrapolations for the 21st century

published a reference volume containing annual life tables by year of age for the 19th and 20th centuries along with extrapolated tables for the whole of the 21st century (Vallin and Meslé, 2001). The book also contains complete life tables for every cohort between 1806 and 1996. While the results reflect long periods of time, the underlying data differ for different time periods. Those for the 20th century are based on detailed, regular death statistics; those for the 19th century are mainly based on reconstructions using incomplete data; and projections for the 21st century are based on an extension of recent trends in mortality by age below 105 years combined with a constant life expectancy at the age of 105. They nevertheless provide an overall consistency that gives an accurate picture of the history of French mortality using both longitudinal and cross-sectional indicators. They can also be supplemented, though in more summary fashion, using Louis Henry's well-known survey of 18th century parish registers, from which a series of abridged life tables by 10-year period were drawn up, going from 1740–1749 to 1820–1829 (Blayo, 1975).

While in 1740–1749 life expectancy at birth barely reached 25 years (23.8 for men and 25.7 for women), by 2000 it was almost 80 years (75.2 for men and

82.7 for women)[1] and, if trends in mortality by age over the last 15 years continue, it could exceed 90 years by the end of the century (91.3 for men and 95.0 for women in 2102). Such tremendous progress has not been without its ups and downs, as Figure 1.1 shows for the period in which annual monitoring is possible. Some periods have been more favourable than others. For example, the late 18th century saw a very rapid initial phase of progress that spanned roughly the period between the 1780s and the 1820s (taking out the effects of the imperial wars for men). On the other hand, the mid-19th century saw less progress and even some stagnation until the early results of the Pasteur revolution starting in the 1890s. The latter opened the way to the great period of rapid progress that reached its height with the distribution of antibiotics after the Second World War. There was another slowdown in the 1960s as the benefits of the fight against infectious diseases expired, but the cardiovascular revolution in the 1970s brought another considerable increase in life expectancy.

Meanwhile, the great fluctuations of the past have disappeared, whether caused, especially for men, by military activity (Napoleonic wars, war of 1870 and the Paris Commune, First and Second World Wars) or by the last great epidemics (cholera in the 19th century, influenza in the 20th). Since 1970, after the last great flu epidemic of 1968–1969, annual fluctuations in life expectancy have been extremely subtle.

Taking account of the strength of this development, current life expectancy combined with the risk of death by age for a given year has increasingly diverged from that of the cohort born that year (Figure 1.2).[2] As regards measuring the degree of rectangularisation of the survival curve, it would therefore be useful to explore period survival curves as well as those for real cohorts.

Period life expectancy is obviously much more sensitive to the effects of short-term accidents than cohort life expectancy. However, cohort life expectancy is not totally free of annual fluctuation. It is particularly sensitive to fluctuations in infant mortality, which explains not only most of the fluctuations seen in the cohorts born during the 19th century but also the quite significant declines (for both sexes) for the cohorts born in 1911 and during the First and Second World Wars. For men, it is also very sensitive to the losses sustained in the First World War, to the extent that, for all cohorts born between 1882 and 1899, cohort life expectancy is lower than that for the year of birth, in spite of the huge progress in health care that these cohorts enjoyed before they died. For example, the male cohort born in 1895, which suffered the heaviest losses in the 1914–1918 war, had a life expectancy of only 37.6

---

[1] Provisional figures (Prioux, 2001).
[2] Figure 1.2 only begins in 1806 insofar as the 10-year figures available for the 18th century do not give us an accurate picture of the survival of cohorts.

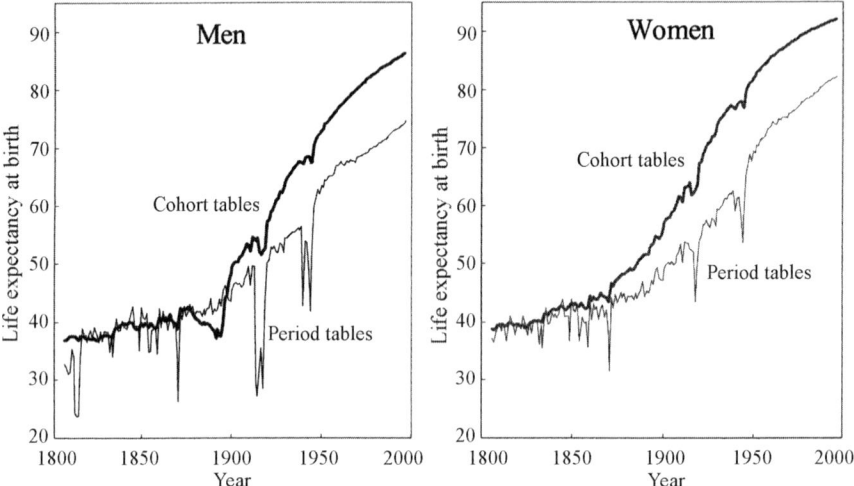

Figure 1.2. Development since 1806 of life expectancy at birth by calendar year and by cohort (for cohorts, figures are allocated to the year of birth)

years, while the table for its year of birth gave it a life expectancy of 42.7 years. On the other hand, women of the same cohort had a life expectancy of 53.4 years, while, when they were born, the period table gave them only 46.2 years.

Apart from these accidents of history, the most significant factor has been that, since the late 19th century, improved health has gradually created a divergence between period life expectancy and cohort life expectancy. As long as period and cohort life expectancy depended mainly on infant mortality and, in addition, progress in health was slow, the two indicators virtually coincided, except that the period indicator fluctuated more than the cohort indicator. This situation prevailed until the 1860s in women and even up to the 1880s in men, but, since then, the gap between the two indicators has widened. Just before the Second World War, when life expectancy for 1939 was only 56.5 years for men and 62.6 years for women, life expectancy for the cohort born that year may be estimated[3] at 67.4 and 77.0 years, respectively. Thanks to the improved health care seen in its lifetime, this cohort is likely to gain 10.9 years of life expectancy for men and up to 15.4 years for women compared to the results that would have been obtained if conditions in its year of birth had been maintained. Similarly, if the results of the projection for the 21st century are realised, men born in 1996 could enjoy a life expectancy of 86.3 years, i.e. 12.1 years more

---

[3] As this cohort is now only just over 60, its life expectancy can only be estimated by projecting the risk of death beyond that age.

than the 74.2 years given in the life table for the same year. Women would gain a little less this time (92.1 years, instead of 82.1 years).

Initially, therefore, improved health has meant that the life expectancy for cohorts has increased more rapidly than period life expectancy and, in France, men are still in this first phase. On the other hand, in the second phase that French women seem to have entered already, increases in the life expectancy of cohorts are likely to come much more slowly than increases in period life expectancy if the latter is destined to reach its ceiling below a maximum. This makes it even more interesting to examine the development of the rectangularisation of the survival curve both longitudinally and cross-sectionally.

RECTANGULARISATION INDICATORS

A large number of indicators have been suggested for measuring the degree of rectangularisation of a survival curve (Table 1.1) and several reviews have already been made of these; we shall not repeat them here. Let us simply look at the main conclusions of the reviews carried out by John Wilmoth and Shiro Horiuchi (1999) and by Jean-Marie Robine (2001).

The first two authors listed 10 indicators, which they describe as follows:

1. *Fixed rectangle.* In a standard plot of survival curve, imagine a rectangle with a height of 1 and a right boundary at (say) age 100. The measure equals the proportion of this rectangle that lies below the survival curve. As the curve becomes more rectangular, this quantity increases.
2. *Moving rectangle.* Suppose that the right boundary in this rectangle changes, depending on survival probabilities at the oldest ages. Suppose, for example, that the right boundary always equals the age at which 1/1000 of the original cohort is still alive. Again, the measure equals the proportion of the rectangle that lies below the survival curve.
3. *Fastest decline.* This measure equals the (negative) slope of the survival curve at its point of fastest decline in the adult age range. As the survival curve becomes more rectangular, this value increases.
4. *Sharpest corner.* This measure equals the (negative) second derivative of the survival curve at the point where it turns downward most quickly in the adult age range. As the survival curve becomes more rectangular, this value increases.
5. *Quickest plateau.* This measure equals the second derivative of the survival curve at the point where it levels off most quickly at very high ages. As the survival curve becomes more rectangular, this value increases.
6. *Prolate index.* This measure, proposed by Eakin and Witten (1995), is a sophisticated means of measuring the steepness of the slope of the survival curve at older ages.

Table 1.1. Main indicators suggested for measuring dispersion of length of life and the rectangular nature of the survival curve (drawn up by Jean-Marie Robine, 2001)

1. Indicators listed by Wilmoth and Horiuchi (1999)
Fixed rectangle
Moving rectangle
Fastest decline
Sharpest corner
Quickest plateau
Prolate index (Eakin and Witten, 1995)
Interquartile range
Standard deviation
Gini coefficient
Keyfitz's *H* (Keyfitz and Golini, 1975)

2. Other indicators listed by Robine (2001)
Coefficient of variation (Nusselder and Mackenbach, 1996)
Numerator of Keyfitz's *H* (Nusselder and Mackenbach, 1996)
Age of various centiles of the life span (Manton and Stallard, 1996)
Standard deviation of the age at death above the mode (Kannisto, 2000)
Standard deviation of the age at death in the highest quartile (Kannisto, 2000)
Shortest age interval in which a given proportion of deaths take place (Kannisto, 2000)

7. *Interquartile range.* This measure equals the distance between the lower and the upper quartiles of the distribution of ages at death in a life table. As age at death becomes less variable, this measure decreases.

8. *Standard deviation.* This measure equals the standard deviation of the distribution of ages at death in a life table. As age at death becomes less variable, this measure decreases.

9. *Gini coefficient.* This measure reflects the degree of inequality in age at death in a life table population. This value decreases as age at death becomes less variable.[4]

10. *Keyfitz's H.*[5] This quantity was developed to approximate the dynamic relationship between the force of mortality by age and life expectancy at birth. It also expresses the 'degree of concavity' in the survival curve (thus the opposite of rectangularity) and the increasing concentration of deaths at older ages.[6] As deaths become more concentrated, the value of Keyfitz's *H* declines.

---

[4] A recent study by Shkolnikov *et al* (2001) focused on calculating this indicator using different types of life tables.

[5] Presented for the first time in an article by Nathan Keyfitz and Antonio Golini (1975) and taken up by the former in *Applied Mathematical Demography* (Keyfitz, 1977).

[6] Some authors refer to *H* as a measure of 'entropy' in the life table (Demetrius, 1976).

Having explored the various results obtained for these indicators using Swedish, Japanese and American data and compared them in a correlation study, John Wilmoth and Shiro Horiuchi conclude:

> The interquartile range (IQR) has a twofold appeal as a single measure of variability in the life table. First, it is very simple to calculate because it equals the difference between the ages where the survival curve, $S(x)$, crosses 0.25 and 0.75. Second, being the length of the span of ages containing the middle 50% of deaths, it possesses a simple interpretation. On the basis of the correlations [...], the IQR would not be our first choice. Nevertheless, its convenience and its clear meaning make it an optimal measure for the kinds of analyses we wish to pursue.
>
> The most important argument in favour of the IQR is that it is one of only two measures considered here which are expressed in units of years of age. The standard deviation shares this advantage, but it is more difficult to compute and is less strongly correlated with almost all of the other measures.

Jean-Marie Robine (2001) took up this list and added six other indicators numbered below, following those listed by John Wilmoth and Shiro Horiuchi.

11. *Coefficient of variation.* This indicator suggested by Nusselder and Mackenbach (1996) is simply the standard deviation of the distributions of deaths by age in relation to the mean. This indicator decreases as the survival curve becomes more rectangular.

12. *Numerator of Keyfitz's H.* Also suggested by Nusselder and Mackenbach (1996), this indicator takes up that of Keyfitz, leaving out division by life expectancy. It decreases as the survival curve becomes more rectangular.

13. *Age of various centiles of the life span.* Manton and Stallard (1996) use the highly parallel increase in ages at the 25th, 50th, 75th, 95th, 99th, 99.5th, 99.9th and 99.99th centiles of deaths after the age of 65 to calculate the narrowing of the gap between ages at death.

14. *Standard deviation of the age at death above the mode.* This indicator decreases as the survival curve becomes more rectangular (Kannisto, 2000).

15. *Standard deviation of the age at death in the highest quartile.* As for the preceding indicator, this indicator decreases as the survival curve becomes more rectangular (Kannisto, 2000).

16. *Shortest age interval of deaths.* The value of this indicator is supplied by the size of the smallest intervals of ages adding up to a given proportion of deaths (Kannisto, 2000). The author is particularly interested in intervals C10, C25, C50, C90, which add up to 10, 25, 50 or 90% of deaths, respectively. All these indicators obviously decrease as the survival curve becomes more rectangular, with the exception of cases where they encompass infant mortality.

The last indicator is similar to the IQR in the sense that it is expressed in years of age, but it attempts to be more accurate in identifying the smallest age interval in which the particular percentage of deaths is concentrated. Thus, Kannisto's C50 closely resembles the IQR, recommended by John Wilmoth and Shiro Horiuchi, but differs in the fact that it is not directly linked to quartiles for the distribution of ages at death. Although the calculation is less immediate, we believe that the C50 should give a more accurate account of the concentration of ages at death in the sense that it identifies the minimum age interval. On the other hand, it has the disadvantage of not answering the question that is asked when infant and child mortality is too high. We shall therefore use French data to try and find a solution to overcome this problem and take full advantage of Väinö Kannisto's indicators.

RECTANGULARISATION OF THE FRENCH SURVIVAL CURVE

The French survival curve has become increasingly rectangular over the last two-and-a-half centuries and a projection of recent trends in mortality by age suggests that the phenomenon will continue. Figure 1.3 illustrates the case for women only, but compares the situation observed cross-sectionally through the period tables with the view offered by the cohort tables. We have represented, cross-sectionally from 1806 (first complete table), a survival curve every 20 years, to which we have added the curve for 1996, the year of birth of the most recent cohort for which we have calculated a life table. Prior to this, we have also shown the first survival curve available for the 18th century and, thereafter, the survival curve obtained for 2102, which ends our projection. Longitudinally, the first cohort represented is the one born in 1806, due to lack of detailed data for the 18th century, and, as in our cross-sectional representation, we have displayed the successive cohorts every 20 years of births. If we leave out mortality after the age of 100, we may consider that the last survival curve based on real data is that of the cohort born in 1896. For later cohorts, the curve increasingly relies on a growing fraction of projected survival rates up to the 1996 cohort, for which only survival to the age of one year really relies on actual data.

A comparison between the two graphs in Figure 1.3 shows that the phase in which the life expectancy of cohorts increases more rapidly than that of their years of birth is accompanied here by a more rapid rectangularisation of the survival curve. Thus, while the curves for the year 1806 and the 1806 cohort are quite similar, a hundred years later, the curve for the cohort born in 1906 is already much more rectangular than the curve for the year 1906. This continues up to recent years but, taking account of the observation made concerning life expectancy, we can imagine that it might have been reversed

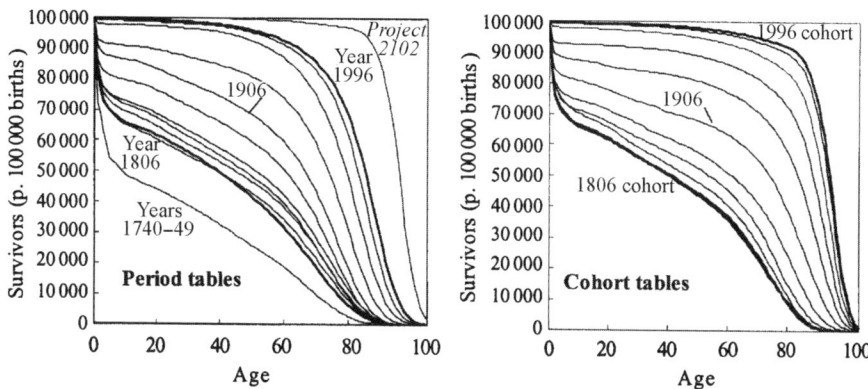

Figure 1.3. Development in 20-year bands of the survival curve for French women since 1806, projected to 2102: period tables and cohort tables

thereafter if the projection had been carried on to obtain a survival curve for the cohort born in 2102, maintaining the assumption of a fixed limit to life expectancy of 105 years.

ADVANTAGES AND SHORTCOMINGS OF IQR AND C50

Looking first at the cross-sectional data, let us try and see how the interquartile interval proposed by John Wilmoth and Shiro Horiuchi and Kannisto's C50[7] expresses this rectangularisation movement (Figure 1.4).

Both the interquartile interval and Kannisto's C50 declined rapidly in the first half of the 20th century, clearly reflecting the strength of the survival curve rectangularisation phenomenon observed during this period. However, Figure 1.4 shows the superiority of Kannisto's C50 over the IQR in the sense that the latter overestimates the speed of rectangularisation by measuring the concentration of deaths over too wide an age interval when rectangularisation is still relatively modest. This evidently stems from the fact that IQR, unlike C50, does not necessarily identify the smallest age interval adding up to 50% of deaths. On the other hand, both C50 and IQR are unable to account for the survival curve rectangularisation that was already occurring in the 18th and

---

[7] To measure Kannisto's C50 correctly from a complete life table by year of age, one must be able to place both the lower and upper limits accurately within the year of age concerned. The difficulty stems from the fact that the minimum interval required is mobile, which means that the adjustment within the first age cannot be made independently of the adjustment made to the second. One cannot therefore carry out simple adjustments to the margin as in the case of interquartile intervals. To avoid this problem, we therefore began by interpolating survival curves by hundredths of years of age before setting the minimum interval accurate to within a hundredth of a year.

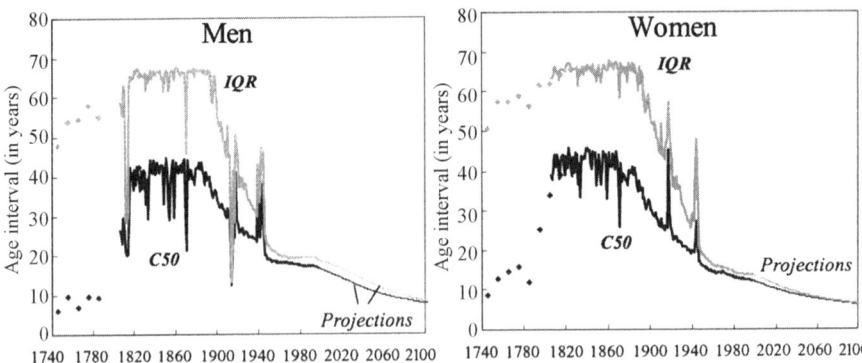

Figure 1.4. Changes in the interquartile interval and Kannisto's C50 since the 18th century in France and projections to 2102

19th centuries. Not only are these two indicators virtually stable apart from annual fluctuations from 1820 to 1880, but they also increase very considerably from 1740 to 1820 and this latter phenomenon is even more apparent with Kannisto's C50 than with IQR.

This disadvantage evidently stems from the major role played by the fall in infant and child mortality in the early increase in life expectancy. In the case of IQR, as long as infant and child mortality is very high, the second quartile starts at a very early age and IQR is relatively short. Thus, from 1740 to 1820, IQR rose as infant mortality decreased. We then come to a period in which the interquartile interval relates to a relatively flat portion of the survival curve with a slope that hardly varied in the 19th century, hence the plateau observed at a fairly high level between 1820 and 1900. In the case of C50, the influence of infant mortality is even stronger as the search for the smallest possible age interval means that infant mortality is included as soon as it exceeds a certain threshold and, the higher the infant mortality, the smaller the C50 that includes it, as can be seen in the tables for the 18th century. This phenomenon is seen more clearly in Figure 1.5, which shows the changes in the lower and upper limits of C50. From 1740 to 1820, the lower limit remains constant at age 0 and one can see the upper limit rise quite rapidly, particularly from 1780 to 1820 with the first major drop in infant mortality. Thereafter, during the whole of the 19th century, the lower limit often remains at age 0, jumping occasionally, depending on strong fluctuations in infant and child mortality to a much higher age close to 40.

The attraction for infant mortality shown by both C50 and IQR tends to divert the attention towards the part of the mortality curve that has nothing to do with the phenomena that they are supposed to measure, since what interests us about the rectangularisation of the survival curve is the change in mortality

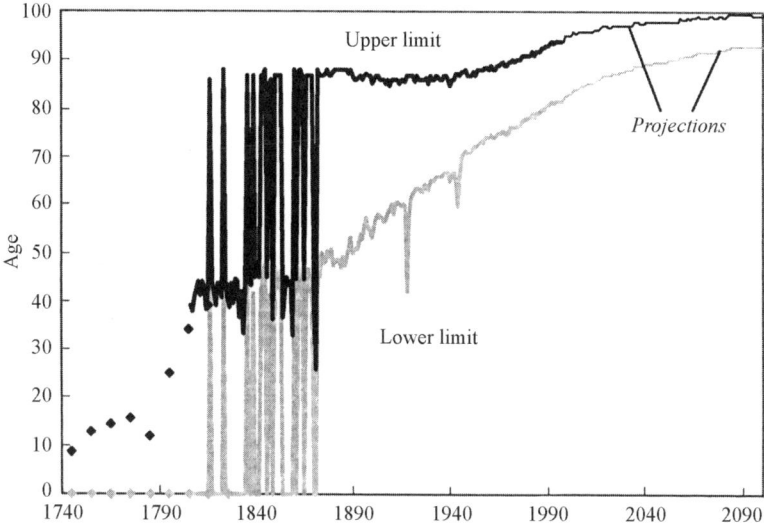

Figure 1.5. Changes in lower and upper limits of Kannisto's C50 for women since the 18th century in France and projections to 2102

at ages where the risk of death increases with age. We believe that it is possible to compensate for this disadvantage by applying a very simple correction to Väinö Kannisto's indicator. All that is required is to limit the search for the smallest age interval adding up to a given proportion of deaths from the table at ages higher than 10 years, an age at which, generally, the lowest point of a mortality curve is seen.

This new indicator, which we call $_{10}C10$, $_{10}C25$, $_{10}C50$, $_{10}C90$, using the symbols suggested by Kannisto, helps us to follow the rectangularisation of the survival curve for a much longer period. Thus, the value of $_{10}C50$ decreased considerably in the second half of the 18th century and continued to decrease, though much more slowly, during the 19th century. Figure 1.6, which compares its evolution to those of Kannisto's C50 and IQR, clearly illustrates the advantage of this indicator over the other two. It also shows that the advantage over C50 is only seen when mortality under the age of 10 is sufficiently high as to require a lower limit below this age. In all other cases, $_{10}C50$ is equal to Kannisto's C50 in its construction.

However, $_{10}C50$ is not itself totally independent of the level of infant and child mortality. On the one hand, in certain cases, where more than 50% of deaths occur before the age of 10, it simply does not exist. But this is hardly a disadvantage as, throughout the corresponding period in France's history of progress in health care, it only occurs once in the life table for 1740–1749, a period in which, as we know, France suffered severe food shortages. We can

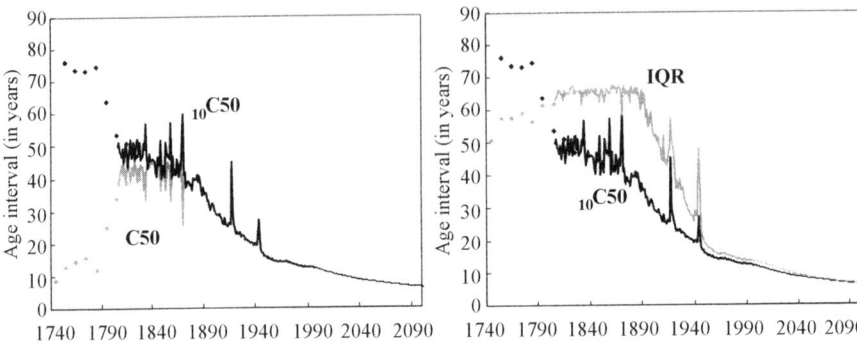

Figure 1.6. Changes in France since the 18th century and projections to 2102 for $_{10}$C50 compared to Kannisto's C50 and an interquartile interval, for women

therefore say that, if we are interested in the highest concentration of 50% of deaths, this indicator allows us to follow the process of rectangularisation in its entirety. This is obviously not the case for $_{10}$C90, which is incalculable once mortality prior to the age of 10 adds up to over 10% of deaths, which was the case in France up to the Second World War.

On the other hand, it is interesting to note the difference in sensitivity to infant mortality between $_{10}$C50 and Kannisto's C50. We can see in Figure 1.6 that, during the 19th century, the two indicators' fluctuations are almost symmetrically opposed. Once C50's lower limit is age 0, any peak in infant mortality causes the interval to narrow, as more deaths are concentrated in the early years. On the contrary, the same peaks in infant mortality produce a widening of $_{10}$C50 as the increased proportion of infant and child deaths produces an equivalent reduction in deaths after the age of 10, all things being equal elsewhere, and requires a broader age interval to encompass 50% of deaths. This phenomenon is particularly visible in 1834 with the cholera epidemic and in 1871 with the Paris Commune. This difference again argues in favour of $_{10}$C50 in the sense that, while C50 ends up escaping from the effect of infant and child mortality, it then behaves exactly like $_{10}$C50. This occurs, for example, in the infant mortality crises of 1918 (Spanish 'flu) and 1944–1945 (bombings and food crisis).

In addition, Figure 1.7 confirms the superiority of this improved version of Kannisto's indicator over the interquartile interval by illustrating the change in limits for each of the two intervals. We can see that the main problem with the interquartile interval is that it is very strongly conditioned by the weight of infant mortality in the first quartile, which forces the lower limit of the interval to remain very close to 0 as long as infant mortality is high. In fact, for women, the minimum age for the interval remained under 5 until 1895. The strong effect of infant mortality not only led to an underestimation of the

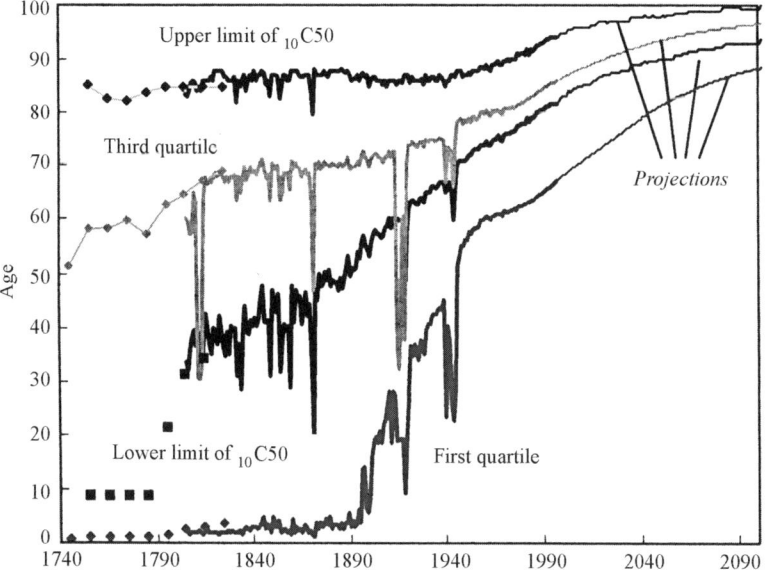

Figure 1.7. Changes in France since the 18th century and projections to 2102 of the lower and upper limits of $_{10}C50$ and the interquartile interval, for women

concentration of mortality in adult age groups but also meant that it was not possible to place this concentration accurately at the ages at which it was actually occurring, as the upper interval limit was being pulled downwards.

However, we should acknowledge that our modified version of Kannisto's indicator only takes account of one aspect of the rectangularisation of the survival curve, which we could call 'adult rectangularisation' as it is exempt from the effects of infant mortality. We could consider that there are two survival curve rectangularisation modes, the adult mode on the right and infant rectangularisation on the left, which can be seen if we go back in time to periods where levels of infant mortality were very high. Thus, at the start of progress towards better health care, we can see derectangularisation on the infant side, with erosion of the left angle of the survival curve, even though, using $_{10}C50$, we can also see very early on the beginnings of adult rectangularisation.

DEVELOPMENT OF THE RECTANGULARISATION OF THE FRENCH SURVIVAL CURVE

In two-and-a-half centuries, the smallest age interval concentrating 50% of deaths (beyond the age of 10) fell from 87 years in 1750–1759[8] to less than 17

---

[8] For 1740–1749, this indicator does not exist, as over 50% of deaths occurred before the age of 10.

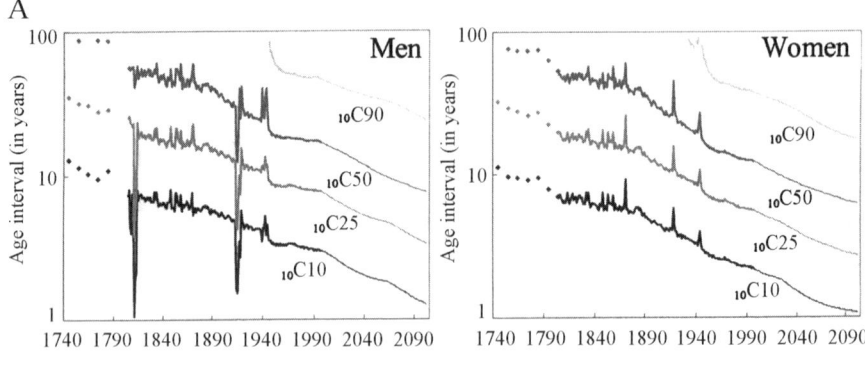

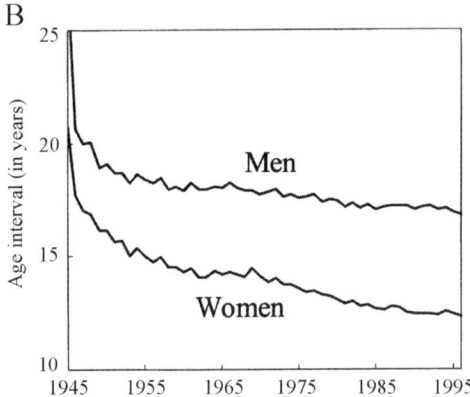

Figure 1.8. A. Changes in France since the 18th century and projections to 2102 of minimum intervals adding up to 10, 25, 50 or 90% of deaths from the life table. B. Changes in $_{10}$C50 since the Second World War

years in 1997 in men and from 76 to 12 years in women. If the future evolution in mortality follows recent trends, it could decrease to 7.6 and 6.2 years, respectively, in 2102 (Figure 1.8).

This massive movement in the concentration of ages of death has not taken place evenly over time. On the contrary, it has been marked by strong fluctuations and a few long-lasting plateaux. However, we can see very clearly in Figure 1.8A that the overall trend and, to a lesser extent, annual fluctuations are very easy to read whatever proportion of deaths is used to measure their concentration, with the exception of course of $_{10}$C90, where we have already stated that it can only be calculated after the 1940s. We can therefore examine in greater detail just one of these indicators, for example $_{10}$C50, which repeats the C50 recommended by Kannisto.

Concerning fluctuations in women, there is little to add to what we have already stated above. However, it is interesting to note here that, for men, infant mortality is not the only cause of major fluctuations. The effect of wartime losses has to be added; these are particularly visible in $_{10}C10$ and $_{10}C25$ but also affect $_{10}C50$. In contrast to infant mortality crises, these losses cause a sharp fall in the figures for the concentration of ages at death as they create an exceptional way of dying amongst the young adult age groups that is clearly higher and more concentrated than later, traditional ways. Such is the case particularly for the worst years of the 1914–1918 and Napoleonic wars.

The overall trend towards a concentration of adult ages of death has accelerated twice: once at the end of the 18th century and again during the long period between the end of the 19th century and the 1950s, and the projection used here suggests a third acceleration. On the other hand, the greater part of the 19th century and, especially in men, the 1960s were marked by stagnation.

The first acceleration observed between 1780 and 1820 is directly linked to the rapid decline in infant and child mortality during this period; the consequence of this decline was to favour the concentration of deaths in the adult age groups by greatly increasing the probability of surviving to the age of 10. This is therefore an indirect form of adult rectangularisation. We know that the rest of the 19th century, up to the 1890s, was a period of relative stagnation in life expectancy and we can deduce that, apart from fluctuations, the indicator for the concentration of ages of death remained relatively stable. On the other hand, the figures drop sharply, as one would expect, during the era of great progress in life expectancy that began at the end of the 19th century with the Pasteur revolution.

What occurred from the late 1950s onwards requires further reflection and Figure 1.8B attempts to help us by offering a close-up view of the evolution of $_{10}C50$ over the period 1945–1997. Initially, the trend towards concentration weakens and the indicator ends up by actually stagnating completely during the 1960s. This phenomenon must be attributed to a slowing in the progress of life expectancy combined with a decreasing return on the decrease in infectious mortality and the rise in man-made diseases. However, the resumption in the increase of life expectancy that followed successes in the treatment of cardiovascular diseases in the 1970s did not lead to as great a reduction of $_{10}C50$ as one would have imagined. In other words, the extension of ages at death brought on by the more and more marked drop in mortality at high ages during this period is not entirely the product of a concentration of deaths in an increasingly narrowing age band, but is also linked to a shift in the death curve's mode towards higher and higher ages. Can we consider this phenomenon as being the precursor of a re-expansion of ages at death, which could ultimately lead to an increase in $_{10}C50$? It is obviously far too soon to judge. Moreover, an extrapolation of recent trends would tend to suggest, on the contrary, that a new acceleration on the rectangularisation of the survival curve is imminent (Figure 1.8).

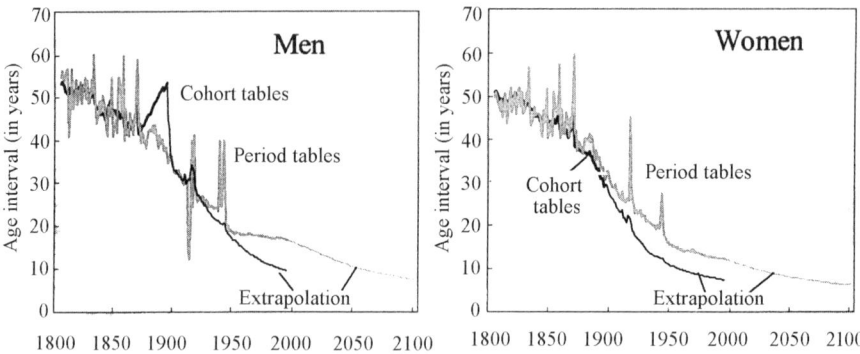

Figure 1.9. Changes since 1806 and projection to 2102 of $_{10}C50$ calculated cross-sectionally: comparison with the same indicator calculated by cohort (the cohorts are positioned on the graph according to year of birth)

However, we must question the validity of this projection from the point of view that interests us here. If we accept, due to lack of observable data beyond this age, that a life expectancy at age 105 is immutable, we eliminate any possibility of an upward expansion of ages at death and indeed lay the foundation for their increased concentration.

Comparison of changes in $_{10}C50$ measured from period tables with those obtained for cohort tables (Figure 1.9) confirms the difference already seen during examination of survival curves in Figure 1.3. Up to the end of the 19th century for women and even up to the 1930s for men, there were hardly any other differences between the $_{10}C50$ in a period table and the $_{10}C50$ in a table for the cohort born that year apart from those caused by annual fluctuations, as cohort indicators were obviously less sensitive than period indicators. However, we should note the noteworthy exception caused in men by the First World War. While, in the period table, the war caused the slaughter of a large number of young adult age groups, creating, as we stated above, a sharp fall in $_{10}C50$, it only affected a much smaller age interval for each cohort; this was not enough to attract the lower limit of the indicator, and indeed caused the latter to broaden around the traditional model for ages at death, as has already been stated for infant mortality. Thus, from 1870 to 1895, for those cohorts most badly affected by the war, the $_{10}C50$ increased strongly and then fell back again for succeeding cohorts.

From the 1890s for women and the 1930s for men, the $_{10}C50$ for each year falls less rapidly than for the cohort born in the same year. It is true that, for men, this phenomenon occurs during a period when the cohort indicator already relies to a considerable extent on the extrapolation of mortality to great ages. On the other hand, the phenomenon is already well established in women though the influence of extrapolation on cohort curves is still very weak. The divergence is therefore, at least partially, very real. As long as the concentration of adult ages at death remains mainly due to the indirect effect of the decline in infant mortality, there should be virtually no difference between the indicator for one year and the indicator for the cohort born that year. On the other hand, as it comes to depend more and more on an increase in life expectancy at age 60, as has been the case for women since 1950 and for men since 1970, the cohorts born 60 years earlier gradually acquire the potential to survive to much greater ages than the age allotted to them in the life table for their year of birth and their $_{10}C50$ decreases more rapidly.

SOME INTERNATIONAL COMPARISONS

To place this study of the French situation in an international context, we have also calculated $_{10}C50$ for three other countries for which we had a full series of life tables dating back to the end of the 19th Century: Italy,[9] Japan[10] and Switzerland[11] (Figure 1.10). The Italian and Swiss tables are all annual and can therefore be directly compared with French tables. The Japanese tables are only annual from the end of the Second World War. The oldest tables were calculated annually over five-year periods centred on the reference year. This explains the absence of fluctuations throughout the period before 1945 and the apparent small effect of the terrible earthquake of 1923.

The most surprising element in Figure 1.10 is the extraordinary convergence of the $_{10}C50$s and their virtual coincidence from the 1960s onwards. Over the previous hundred years, Japan, Italy and France closed the gap with Switzerland, which was ahead of the other three countries in terms of controlling infant and infectious mortality. The rapid reduction in Japanese $_{10}C50$ after the Second World War is particularly spectacular. Though this radical fall straightens out considerably at the start of the 1960s, it nevertheless continues, though at a much slower pace, while the indicator stagnates in the other three countries, to the extent that, in recent years, the $_{10}C50$ has been at its lowest in Japan.

CONCLUSION

Two conclusions can be drawn from this chapter. The first, we feel, is that, of all the indicators suggested, Kannisto's C (especially the C50) is the one that

---

[9] Tables kindly sent by Graziella Caselli, director of the Department of Demography at the University of Rome.
[10] Nanjo and Kobayashi, 1985; Statistics and Information Department, 1995.
[11] Calot *et al*, 1998.

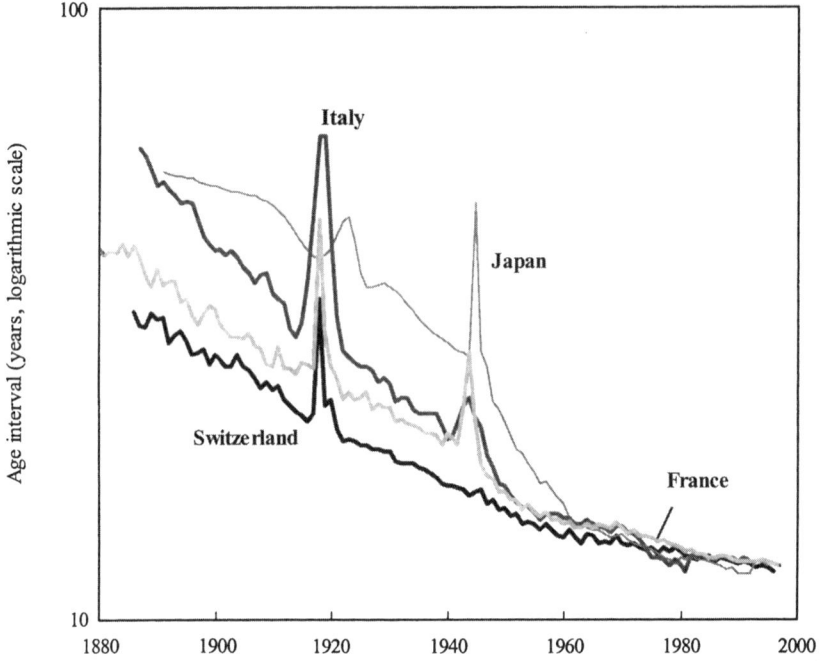

Figure 1.10. Changes in $_{10}C50$ since the end of the 19th century in four developed countries, for women

best shows up the rectangularisation of the survival curve, as long as infant mortality is at a sufficiently low level to no longer disturb the value. It can, however, be improved by limiting its field to mortality beyond the age of 10 in the form of the $_{10}C50$ as we have suggested here.

The second is that, since the 18th century, in three centuries of improvements in health, rectangularisation has continued to become more pronounced (apart from certain temporary ups and downs that have considerably upset its evolution), and this obviously goes hand in hand with a constant increase in the modal age at death: we continue to die later within an increasingly narrow age interval. This can be seen clearly in the French data and the brief international comparison made at the end of the chapter clearly shows that the situation in France is far from exceptional.

There is therefore nothing at present to help us detect any indication of an imminent shift in the span of age at death. On the contrary, within the framework of a constant life expectancy at age 105, the mortality projections obtained by extrapolating recent downward trends in mortality rates by age over a century suggest the possibility of a new rapid rectangularisation phase, with the $_{10}C50$ for French women falling from almost 12 years in 1997 to

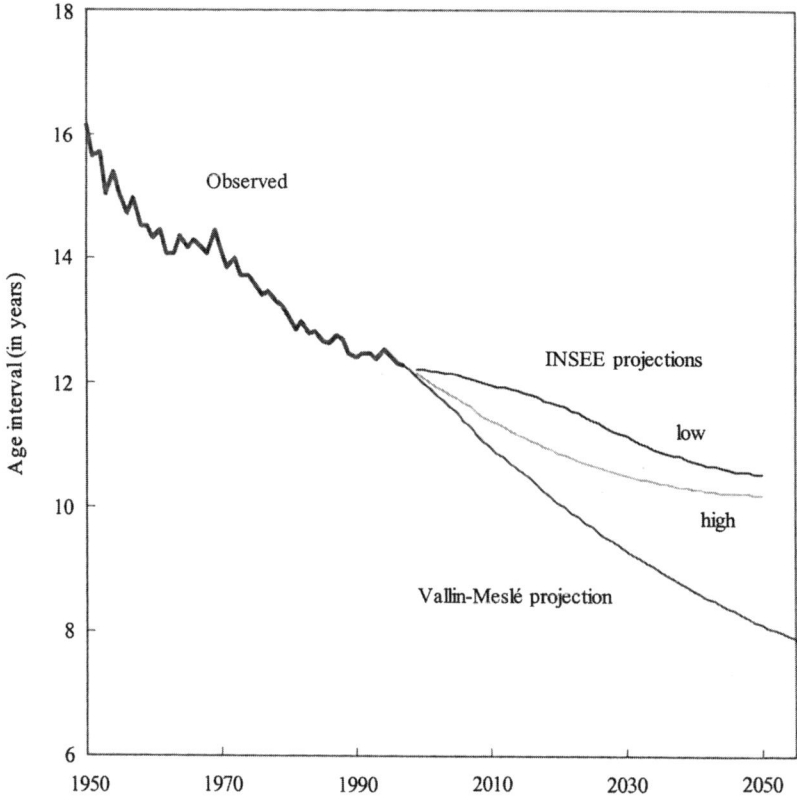

Figure 1.11. Recent changes and projection of $_{10}C50$ to 2050 according to three hypotheses concerning the rate of decline in mortality

approximately 6 years in 2102. But this is only a projection and other hypotheses can be imagined. For example, this is what INSEE (French National Institute of Statistics) did in choosing to surround its central hypothesis for projections to 2050 (very close to our own) with two other hypotheses, one (named 'low mortality') assuming an acceleration in the decline in mortality at the highest ages[12] and the other, on the contrary, assuming a deceleration in the decline at all ages (named 'high mortality'). Paradoxically, for the next fifty years, each of these hypotheses points to a slower rectangularisation than our own projection (Figure 1.11).

---

[12] The hypothesis chosen by INSEE for 'low mortality' consists of extending beyond the age of 75 the same rate of decline in mortality as that observed between 65 and 74 years over the last thirty years (Brutel, 2001). In addition, from the age of 100, it assumes that, from the start of the projection, mortality rates no longer increase with age.

This paradox is highly interesting. We were naturally expecting an accelerated decline in mortality at very old ages to slow the process of rectangularisation to the extent that the chosen hypothesis moves the mortality curve by age considerably to the right. However, we see here that a very similar result can be obtained if the decline in mortality (at any age this time) slows down. But it is even more interesting to note here that in neither case does any kind of trend reversal occur for the $_{10}$C50. We should, however, emphasise that INSEE's 'low mortality' hypothesis considerably twists Gompertz' law of exponential increase of mortality with age as it goes so far as to opt for mortality independent of age beyond 100 years and takes the projection of a decline in mortality by age up to 115 years, whereas we stopped at 105 years. In other words, even with a hypothesis fortified by a re-expansion of ages at death beyond 100 years, rectangularisation may still continue for a long time and we are without a doubt a long way from seeing it assert itself through indicators such as C50. In fact, if we are to observe any future expansion in ages at death, we must use indicators that focus exclusively on old ages (beyond 100 years), for which mortality measurements rapidly become impossible due to lack of data of sufficient quality. This confirms the urgent need to set up a reliable and sufficiently large database on mortality at very old ages.

REFERENCES

Blayo, Y. (1975) 'La mortalité en France de 1740 à 1829', *Population* 30, no. spécial, 123–143.

Brutel, C. (2001) 'Projections de population à l'horizon 2050: un vieillissement inéluctable', *INSEE première* 762, 1–4.

Calot, G., Confesson, A., Sardon, J-P., Baranzini E., Cotter, S. and Wanner, P. (1998) *Deux siècles d'histoire démographique suisse. Album graphique de la période 1860–2050*. Berne: Office fédéral de la statistique et Observatoire démographique européen.

Demetrius, L. (1976) 'Measures of variability in age-structured populations', *Journal of Theoretical Biology* 63, 397–404.

Eakin, T. and Witten, M. (1995) 'How square is the survival curve of a given species?', *Experimental Gerontology* 30(1), 33–64.

Kannisto, V. (2000) 'Measuring the compression of mortality', *Demographic Research* 3(6), 1–24.

Keyfitz, N. (1977) *Applied Mathematical Demography*. New York: John Wiley. (Re-edited in 1985 by Springer-Verlag, New York.)

Keyfitz, N. and Golini, A. (1975) 'Mortality comparisons: the male-female ratio', *Genus* 31(1–4), 1–34.

Manton, K.G. and Stallard, E. (1996) 'Longevity in the United States: age and sex-specific evidence on life span limits from mortality patterns 1960–1990', *Journal of Gerontology: Biological Science* 51A(5), B362–B375.

Nanjo, Z. and Kobayashi, K. (1985) *Cohort life tables based on annual life tables for the Japanese nationals covering the years 1891–1982*. Tokyo: Nihon University, Population Research Institute (NUPRI Research Paper Series, 23).

Nusselder, W.J. and Mackenbach J.P. (1996) 'Rectangularisation of survival curve in the Netherlands, 1950–1992', *Gerontologist* 36(6), 773–781.

Prioux, F. (2001) 'L'évolution démographique récente en France', *Population* 56(4), 571–610.

Robine, J.M. (2001) 'Redefining the stages of the epidemiological transition by a study of the dispersion of life spans: the case of France', *Population, An English Selection* 13(1), 173–194.

Shkolnikov, V.M., Andreev, E.M. and Begun, A.Z. (2001) *Gini coefficient as a life table function: Computation from discrete data, decomposition of differences and empirical examples.* Rostock: MPIDR (Working Paper WP-2001-017).

Statistics and Information Department (1995) *The 18th Life Tables.* Tokyo: Minister's Secretariat, Ministry of Health and Welfare.

Vallin, J. and Meslé, F. (2001) *Tables de mortalité françaises pour les XIXe et XXe siècles et projections pour le XXIe.* Paris: INED (Données statistiques, no. 4-2001).

Wilmoth, J. and Horiuchi, S. (1999) 'Rectangularisation revisited: variability of age at death within human populations', *Demography* 36(4), 475–495.

2

Compression of Morbidity

WILMA J. NUSSELDER
Erasmus MC, Rotterdam, The Netherlands

INTRODUCTION

Traditionally, a decline in mortality was considered to reflect a decline in morbidity in the population. Nowadays, in low mortality countries where improvements in life expectancy are mainly caused by mortality reductions from chronic diseases at older ages, serious doubts exist as to whether longer life means better health for the surviving population. It has been increasingly recognised that a consequence of these mortality reductions might be that the burden of morbidity in the population expands. Nevertheless, a more optimistic view is prevalent, which anticipates that by adopting healthier life styles, the onset of chronic diseases and related disability can be postponed or even prevented, so lifetime spent with chronic diseases and related disability reduces (Fries, 1980, 1983, 1989, 1993). Whether additional years are spent with morbidity and disability or whether increases in life expectancy are accompanied by decreases in years with morbidity – that is, with a compression of morbidity – has been a major focus of the Network on Health Expectancy (REVES). This question is important as today the aim of science and medicine is more to reduce the number of years that people spend diseased or disabled rather than to lengthen life (Greengross et al, 1997).

Since Haan (1989) introduced Fries' work on compression of morbidity in the Network and discussed the complex relation between mortality, morbidity and population health at the first REVES meeting in Quebec, this topic has received much attention. Besides trend studies of changes in health expectancy over time, aiming to assess whether compression of morbidity is actually occurring, substantial work has been done to define operationally compression of morbidity and to measure this process. In addition, characterising and understanding the dynamics underlying changes in population health in

Determining Health Expectancies. Edited by J-M. Robine, C. Jagger, C.D. Mathers, E.M. Crimmins and R.M. Suzman.

general, and compression of morbidity in particular, have become increasingly important research aims within REVES. Before paying attention to these issues, we discuss the compression-of-morbidity hypothesis and alternative views on the association between morbidity, mortality and population health, because points raised in this debate have found their expression in research in this field. The outcomes of trend studies of changes in health expectancies over time are described in a separate chapter (Chapter 4).

COMPRESSION OF MORBIDITY AND ALTERNATIVE VIEWS OF THE ASSOCIATION BETWEEN MORBIDITY, MORTALITY AND POPULATION HEALTH

There is no unequivocal association between the length of life of populations and their state of health. This is clearly illustrated by comparing health expectancies between racial groups in the United States. For Asians, longer life is associated with fewer years lived in poor health, whereas in Native Americans relatively longer lives are accompanied by an extended period of morbidity. Blacks live the fewest years, and a high proportion of these years is spent with a chronic health problem. Hispanics also live fewer years, yet the period spent with a health problem is relatively compressed (Hayward and Heron, 1999). The finding that women live longer but spend more years in poor health than men, while higher socioeconomic groups live longer but spend fewer years in poor health than lower socioeconomic groups (Robine and Ritchie, 1991), also demonstrates the complexity of the relationship between morbidity, mortality and population health.

The survival-curve model, originally introduced by the WHO in 1984 (World Health Organization, 1984), enables a direct assessment of the consequences of increased longevity for population health and can be used to describe and visualise the possible associations between morbidity, mortality and population health (Figure 2.1). The model captures the dynamics of mortality, disability and morbidity in a relatively standardised way. It consists of three survival curves, the mortality curve, the disability curve and the morbidity curve, which represent the proportion of individuals in a cohort who can expect to survive, to survive without disability and to survive without morbidity.

The area below the mortality curve presents total life expectancy, while the area below the disability and morbidity curve represent life expectancy without disability and morbidity, respectively. Examples of life expectancy without morbidity are life expectancy without hip fracture history (Herrmann *et al*, 1996) or heart disease-free life expectancy (Barendregt and Bonneux, 1995). Life expectancy without disability includes life expectancy without ADL disability, labelled as active life expectancy (Katz *et al*, 1983). Besides, other definitions of disability have been used to calculate disability-free life

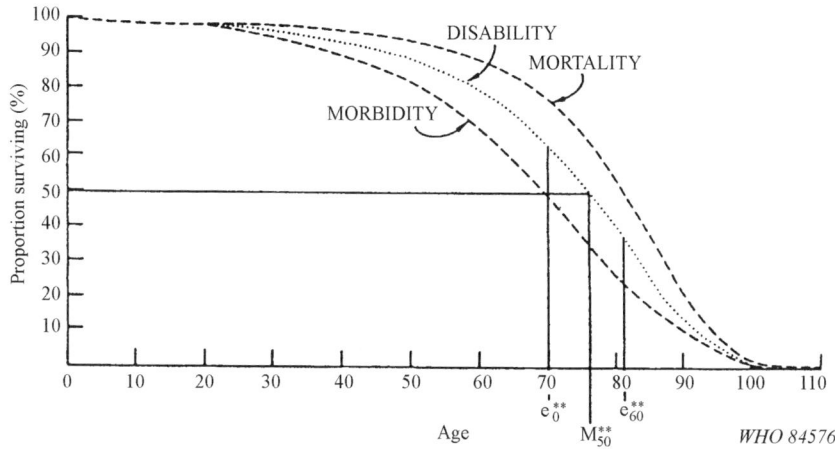

e_0^{**} and e_{60}^{**} are the number of years of autonomous life expected at birth and at age 60, respectively.
M_{50}^{**} is the age to which 50% of females could expect to survive without loss of autonomy.

Figure 2.1. Observed mortality and hypothetical morbidity and disability survival curves for females in the United States. From World Health Organization (1984). Reproduced with permission

expectancy (see Chapter 12). The area between the disability and mortality curves is life expectancy with disability. The survival curves are determined by age-specific mortality, disability and morbidity rates and are, together with total life expectancy and life expectancy with(out) disability and morbidity, derived from a life-table model. Changes in these mortality, disability and morbidity rates may alter the different survival curves and thus total life expectancy and life expectancy with and without disability and morbidity. These survival curves need not necessarily move in the same direction and to the same extent. Three different views exist of the association between changes in these curves and their effect on the length of life and the length of lifetime spent with and without morbidity and disability.

THREE DIFFERENT HYPOTHESES

The Compression-of-morbidity Hypothesis

The compression-of-morbidity hypothesis (Fries, 1980, 1983, 1989, 1993) states that the length of human life is fixed, that life expectancy is reaching this limit, that chronic diseases and related disability can be postponed to older ages by changes in life style, and that the physiological (e.g. serum cholesterol) and psychological (e.g. memory) markers of the ageing process can be modified.

Fries argues that there is a natural limit to the life span (i.e. the genetically endowed limit to life for a single individual if free of all exogenous risk factors). A linear decline in organ reserve with increasing age parallels the decline in the ability to restore homeostasis. Eventually, the smallest perturbation prevents homeostasis being restored and causes 'natural death', which may even occur without diseases. Chronic diseases can be postponed or even prevented by adopting a healthy life style, such as avoiding overweight, quitting smoking and doing exercise. As a result, the number of years with morbidity can be compressed between the increasing age at onset of morbidity and the fixed mean age at death. Expressed in terms of the survival curves of the WHO model, this hypothesis states that the mortality curve does not change substantially, whereas the morbidity and disability curves move outwards. As a result the area between the mortality and morbidity/disability curve (i.e. life expectancy with morbidity/disability) decreases.

The Expansion-of-morbidity Hypothesis

The expansion-of-morbidity hypothesis anticipates that mortality reductions produce more years with morbidity and related disability (Gruenberg, 1977; Kramer, 1980; Olshansky et al, 1991; Verbrugge, 1984). Mortality reductions might produce this expansion in two ways. First, the increased survival of persons with chronic conditions due to medical interventions might prolong the lives of the seriously chronically ill. In Figure 2.1, the mortality curve moves outwards, whereas the other curves remain unchanged. In addition, increased survival might push the saved population into the oldest-old ages where the risks of non-fatal diseases of ageing are high. Hence, declining mortality from fatal diseases produces a population with high risks of chronic morbidity and related disability and thus leads to a shift in the distribution of causes of disability from fatal to non-fatal diseases associated with old age. This second mechanism cannot be easily illustrated with the WHO model, although it is taken into account in the life-table model by default.

The Dynamic-equilibrium Hypothesis

The intermediate hypothesis, the 'dynamic-equilibrium' hypothesis (Manton, 1982), also states that increased survival produces an increase in years with morbidity. However, according to this hypothesis, the years with *severe* morbidity and disability remain relatively constant, because medical interventions or life style changes reduce the rate of progression of chronic diseases. When disability is interpreted as severe morbidity, this hypothesis states that the area between the mortality and morbidity curves increases, because the mortality curve moves faster outwards than the morbidity curve. The area between the disability (here: severe morbidity) and mortality curves does not increase according to this hypothesis.

DIFFERENT MECHANISMS

Although the debate on which hypothesis is most likely to occur in reality has still not been solved completely, it shows the possible mechanisms that affect population health. Firstly, the debate has made clear that whether or not a longer life is accompanied by additional years without morbidity and disability largely depends on the phase in the disease process where changes in morbidity and mortality occur (Crimmins and Ingegneri, 1993; Manton, 1982). If mortality declines only because people do not develop the disease any more, develop the disease later in life, or recover from the disease, the mortality reduction is accompanied by an increase in years without morbidity and disability. On the other hand, if mortality declines among persons who already have the disease, if the disease progression is reduced or if only death is delayed, then the mortality reduction is not accompanied by an increase in years without morbidity, but only by additional years spent in poor health. Secondly, proponents of the expansion-of-morbidity hypothesis (Olshansky *et al*, 1991; Verbrugge, 1984) have convincingly argued that an additional mechanism may affect the duration in poor health when life expectancy increases. That is, reductions in morbidity and mortality (irrespective of the phase of the disease process where they occur) may increase the number of persons who survive to advanced ages (where the risks of chronic diseases and related disability are high). As a result, the time spent with disability expands. In fact, in this line of reasoning, changes in mortality and morbidity affect the distribution of the population (in this case by age, and age is strongly associated with disease and disability), which – in turn – affects future morbidity and mortality.

Other, more complex, mechanisms operating indirectly through changes in the population distribution may explain why a longer life does not necessarily mean better health of the living population. The first relates to mortality selection. Due to lower mortality, frailer and weaker persons become a relatively more numerous group in the population, and as a result future mortality and morbidity in the population may increase (Alter and Riley, 1989; Deeg, 1997; Manton, 1982). The second relates to the risk-factor distribution of the population. Since chronic diseases can share common risk factors or since one disease can act as a risk factor for a second disease, lower case-fatality of one chronic disease may imply higher susceptibility to morbidity and further mortality. On the other hand, morbidity at one point in the life course might also have negative consequences for morbidity and mortality later in life. Damage from illness or injury may increase the susceptibility to disease and mortality later in life (Alter and Riley, 1989). Alternatively, experiencing greater mortality risks might exhaust resources to escape the hardships that killed their age peers and thus leave little resilience to avoid adverse health (Deeg, 1997).

In summary, the relationship between morbidity, mortality and population health is complex, and different mechanisms, with sometimes opposite effects on the lifetime spent in good or poor health, have been suggested in literature.

ASSESSMENT OF COMPRESSION OF MORBIDITY

Since there is no unequivocal association between the length of life and population health, a longer life may imply either an expansion or a compression of morbidity. Compression of morbidity, in the presence of an increasing life expectancy, is generally considered a favourable development of population health, as it implies that years in poor health are being replaced by years in good health. The combination of a compression of morbidity and increased longevity means that both disability-free and total life expectancy increase and that the increase in disability-free life expectancy exceeds that in total life expectancy. As a result the period in poor health is being compressed. A compression of morbidity without an increase in life expectancy should not necessarily be considered a favourable development. When it is due to a dramatic increase in premature mortality, nobody will evaluate a decline in the time spent in poor health in a positive sense. However, in general, compression of morbidity without a decline in total life expectancy is considered as favourable, and has stimulated public health policy and research to devote special attention to this issue. It is obvious that an unambiguous definition and tools to assess compression of morbidity are indispensable for progressing towards this goal. These issues have received high priority within REVES.

DEFINITION OF COMPRESSION OF MORBIDITY

When using the term 'compression of morbidity', Fries, the inventor of the compression-of-morbidity hypothesis, referred to the compression of morbidity into the shorter span between the increasing age at onset of morbidity and the fixed occurrence of death (Fries, 1980). Morbidity can be caused by chronic diseases and ageing and is used interchangeably with disability in Fries' work. Compression refers to a decrease in the number of years spent with disability. In the situation originally described by Fries, wherein the age at death is fixed, the increase in the period without disability equals the decrease in the period with disability. Delaying the onset of disability, so that people may expect to live longer in a state of good health, was sometimes considered as compression of morbidity (Robine and Ritchie, 1991). In more recent work (Fries, 1983, 1984, 1993), Fries used a more comprehensive definition of compression of morbidity, stating that the average age of onset of significant permanent infirmity may increase more rapidly than does life expectancy, thus shortening both the proportion of life spent infirm and the absolute length of the infirm period.

Disability-free Life Expectancy and Compression of Morbidity

The relationship over time between total life expectancy and disability-free life expectancy can be used to assess whether compression of morbidity occurs. When total life expectancy is fixed, a longer life without disability can be considered as compression of morbidity. It is obvious that according to the more recent definition of Fries, an increase in the number of years in good health does not automatically imply a compression of the period with disability. Several studies have shown that when life expectancy increases, a gain in disability-free life expectancy may be accompanied by an increase in years with disability (Mathers, 1994; Robine and Ritchie, 1991; Wilkins *et al*, 1994). In the presence of an increasing life expectancy, which is observed in most low morbidity countries, an increase in disability-free life expectancy may be accompanied by a constant, an increasing or a decreasing life expectancy with disability. Thus, in this context, an increase in disability-free life expectancy only means that not *all* years gained are equivalent to extra years with disability. It may well imply an increased burden of disability for both individuals and society as whole.

Considering changes in disability-free life expectancy, while disregarding changes in life expectancy with disability, may give a too optimistic assessment of changes in population health. Therefore, REVES proposed to consider the evolution of the 'complete' health expectancy, including the time spent in both the 'healthy' and 'unhealthy' states. This reflects the recommendation of the Network to use the term 'health expectancy' as a generic term to refer to the expected duration in specific health states, including both 'healthy' and 'unhealthy' states (Mathers *et al*, 1994). Based on the complete health expectancy, compression of morbidity can be measured in two ways, depending on whether a dichotomous set or a larger set of discrete states is distinguished, and on whether a summary measure is calculated by applying weights to the expected years in the various states.

Classifying Changes in Life Expectancy With and Without Disability in Terms of Compression of Morbidity

When only two health states are distinguished, or when a dichotomy based on several health states is made, changes in health expectancy can be classified in terms of compression (and expansion) of morbidity. Robine and Mathers (1993) proposed such a classification, based on the magnitude of changes in life expectancy with and without disability and the proportion of life without disability. A distinction was made between absolute compression, relative compression, relative expansion and absolute expansion of morbidity. A decrease in life expectancy with disability was classified as absolute compression of morbidity and a decrease in disability-free life expectancy as absolute expansion of morbidity. A decrease in the proportion of life with disability, in combination with an increase in the number of years with disability, was labelled as relative compression of morbidity. Finally, a decrease in the proportion of life free of disability, in combination with an increase in the number of years free of disability, was classified as relative expansion of morbidity.

In further research it turned out that the classification did not fit each situation well. The classification proved useful when total life expectancy was constant or increasing, but not when it was decreasing. Scenario calculations by Nusselder (Nusselder, 1997) showed that a decline in life expectancy without disability occurred when mortality rates increased. On the basis of the above-mentioned classification, this situation should be labelled as absolute expansion. But one may well wonder why the same situation should not be classified as absolute compression, as life expectancy with disability was declining as well. To overcome this problem, Nusselder has adjusted the classification (Nusselder, 1997). In this adjusted classification, in distinguishing between absolute compression and absolute expansion of morbidity, the change in the number of years with disability (or the difference between total life expectancy and life expectancy without disability) is decisive. A decline in the number of years with disability points to absolute compression and an increase to absolute expansion. Distinguishing only between absolute compression and expansion of morbidity may, however, sometimes be too crude. For example, it might be useful to distinguish between a situation of slight absolute expansion of morbidity being accompanied by a substantial gain in years without disability, as opposed to a situation of substantial increase in years with disability being accompanied by only a slight increase in disability-free life expectancy. The change in the percentage of life with disability provides information on the distribution between years with and without disability in the gained years as compared to the baseline situation. Therefore, as in the original classification, relative definitions of compression and expansion of morbidity are used. To determine whether relative expansion occurs, the change in the percentage of life with disability is considered, with an increase of this percentage indicating relative expansion of morbidity. Any particular situation can be classified as a combination of absolute compression or expansion, and relative compression or expansion. In the adjusted classification, compression and expansion are complementary to each other (i.e. absolute compression implies the absence of absolute expansion). Although the original classification can be used in most situations, the adjusted classification fits *any* situation and is more transparent.

Classifying Changes in Weighted Health Expectancies in Terms of Compression of Morbidity

Sometimes, a summary measure is calculated by applying weights to the expected years in the various states. These states can be either disease or disability states (or states based on other generic health measures). In the first case, the weighting includes a translation from the burden of disease to the burden of disability, taking into account that diseases differ in their severity of disability. Weighted health expectancies are known as health-adjusted life expectancies (HALE) or disability-adjusted life expectancies (DALE) and are described in more detail in Chapters 12 and 13. In current research practice, the DALE is based on disease states. Based on this indicator, absolute compression of morbidity is defined as a reduction in the difference between total life expectancy and DALE, i.e. a reduction in life expectancy with disability (Barendregt and Bonneux, 1998). Relative compression of morbidity is defined as a decline in the ratio of life expectancy with disability and total life expectancy (i.e. the percentage of life with disability). As in the revised classification for the situation with two states, compression and expansion of morbidity are complementary to each other.

THE LIFE TABLE AS MEASUREMENT TOOL OF COMPRESSION OF MORBIDITY

The value of disability-free life expectancy and life expectancy with disability can be obtained from a life table which includes both mortality and morbidity data. Time or duration is the common denominator in which mortality and morbidity are expressed. By including both mortality and morbidity data in the life table, the consequences of changes in mortality and morbidity in different phases of the disease process, as postulated in the compression versus expansion debate, are taken into account. In addition, changes in the population distribution induced by these changes are handled by default. This means that the side effect of increased survival, which pushes persons into the oldest-old ages with high risks of disability, is taken into account in the life table.

The Sullivan Method Versus the Multistate Life-table Method

Two different types of life tables are used to calculate health expectancy: the prevalence-rate life-table model (commonly known as the Sullivan method) and the multistate life table. The Sullivan method is based on the prevalence of disability, whereas the multistate method is based on transition rates between the disability states and to the dead state. Health expectancy can be calculated with the Sullivan method from readily available data on the prevalence of disability and a standard life table. The multistate life-table model is much more demanding in terms of data requirements, as longitudinal surveys or registers are needed to obtain transition rates (for more information on these two methods, see Chapter 11). Debate is still going on within REVES as to whether health expectancy indicators based on the prevalence of disability (i.e. the Sullivan method) provide an unbiased estimate of time trends in health expectancy. Barendregt *et al* (1994) have shown that the Sullivan method can produce misleading results when survival changes. This is because the Sullivan method integrates prevalence data on morbidity (stock data) in a life table on mortality (flow data). Only when the mortality and morbidity rates have been constant for a long period of time will an equilibrium situation emerge in which the Sullivan method provides an unbiased estimate. Mathers and Robine (1997a and 1997b) do not agree with this view, postulating that in realistic scenarios the use of the Sullivan method or the multistate life-table method will produce roughly the same results. The outcome of this debate is of particular importance if the purpose of studying trends is to assess whether compression or expansion of morbidity is occurring because the focus is on *changes* in total life expectancy, life expectancy with disability and life expectancy without disability (Barendregt *et al*, 1997). When using the Sullivan method for this purpose one runs a risk of confounding biases produced by the Sullivan method with real changes in health states. In addition, a deviation from the 'real' value has a larger impact on the number of years with disability than on disability-free life expectancy. It is exactly the number of years with disability that is decisive in assessing whether or not compression occurs. A small reduction in the number of years caused by the prevalence reaching its equilibrium values may be easily interpreted wrongly as compression of morbidity. This implies that, until this debate has been solved, one should be careful in interpreting the outcomes of the Sullivan method in terms of compression of morbidity.

DYNAMICS UNDERLYING CHANGES IN HEALTH EXPECTANCY

Fries and others (Fries, 1980, 1983, 1989; Michel and Robine, 1992; Michel *et al*, 1993; Verbrugge and Jette, 1994) have put great emphasis on the potential modifiability of the ageing and disablement process. Increasing evidence exists that although on average functioning declines as persons age, improvements in functioning do occur (Crimmins and Saito, 1993; Manton, 1988; Verbrugge *et al*, 1994). It has been shown that while age is a very strong determinant of disability, in addition to chronological age and (age-related) chronic diseases, health behaviours, socio-demographic factors and psychosocial factors affect the risk of disability (see, for example, Fried and Guralnik, 1997; Guralnik and Kaplan, 1989; Kaplan, 1992; Rogers *et al*, 1992; Strawbridge *et al*, 1993; Verbrugge and Balaban, 1989).

Assuming that (age-specific) disability can be reduced, which would be a favourable development as such, the question arises whether as a consequence of this decline a compression of morbidity is likely to occur. It is obvious that if disability were completely independent of mortality, compression of morbidity is likely to happen. However, this condition is not fulfilled, for at least two reasons. Firstly, because disability and mortality share common underlying diseases and non-disease risk factors (Breslow and Breslow, 1993; Kaplan, 1992) and secondly, because disability itself is a risk factor for mortality (McCallum and Shadbolt, 1994; Mulhorn, 1995; Rogers, 1993). As a result, persons with disability have higher mortality risks than those without disability; see, for example, Jagger and Clarke (1988), Mulhorn (1995) and Rogers (1993). This means that persons without or with less disability can expect to live longer. Rogers, for instance, showed that persons aged 55 without any limitations in daily activities have a life expectancy of 28.1 years as compared to 25.5 years for the average population of that age (Rogers, 1993). Given the presence of this association between disability and mortality, the effect of changing disability on health expectancy, and thus on compression of morbidity, is complex.

Within REVES, several studies have examined the consequences of changes in disability and mortality for health expectancy. The results of these studies have been, or can be, interpreted in terms of compression of morbidity. Three groups of studies can be distinguished. The first group examined the effects of overall changes in disability and mortality on health expectancy. The second group focused on the consequences of changes in specific diseases for health expectancy, through their impact on morbidity and/or mortality, whereas the third group assessed the effect of changes in modifiable risk factors. By examining the consequences of changes in overall mortality and disability patterns (first group), diseases (second group) and risk factors (third group), these studies provided insight into the conditions which are favourable or unfavourable for a compression of morbidity to occur. Such information can be used as a reference frame to evaluate the effect on compression of morbidity of autonomous or induced changes in mortality and morbidity, whether or not through changes in diseases or risk factors. This is of direct importance for setting priorities for public health policy and, in the end, might help to clarify the debate as to whether compression of morbidity occurs or is likely to occur in the near future.

IMPACT OF CHANGES IN OVERALL MORTALITY AND DISABILITY

The increasing availability of longitudinal studies has provided researchers with data on mortality and disability dynamics. Based on repeated measurements of disability and vital status, transition rates between disability states and to mortality can be derived (Crimmins *et al*, 1994; Guralnik *et al*, 1993; Nusselder, 1997; Nusselder *et al*, 1996a). To date, no time series of these transition rates are available which allow for comparisons over time. Nevertheless, transition rates for one period (e.g. two years) can be, and have been, used to obtain a better understanding of the association between changes in morbidity and disability on the one hand, and changes in health expectancy on the other hand. We report the results of two studies, presented within REVES, which simulated changes in these transition rates and examined the consequences of these changes for health expectancy. By using a multistate life-table model, the transitions between the disability states and from each of these states to death were explicitly modelled. These transition rates determine total mortality – and thus total life expectancy – and health expectancy.

Crimmins and colleagues (Crimmins *et al*, 1994) used a multistate life-table model with four living states (i.e. no functioning problems, some functioning problems, unable to provide independent living and unable to provide personal care) for the US population aged 70 and over. In addition to these disability states, they also used a dichotomous categorisation by defining having disability as being unable to provide independent living or to provide personal care. The life-table simulations showed that decreasing incidence and progression rates of disability (i.e. decreasing the chances of getting worse) while keeping state-specific mortality rates and improvement rates (i.e. the chances of getting better) constant, produces an increase in total life expectancy and in disability-free life expectancy, and a reduction in the number of years and proportion of life with disability (Table 2.1).

The same direction of the effects, although smaller, was found when improvement rates (i.e. the chances of getting better) were increased. These findings were supported by a Dutch study of Nusselder *et al* (Nusselder, 1997; Nusselder *et al*, 1996a). The latter study simulated changes in transition rates using a two-state life table (i.e. non-disabled and disabled), which also included younger age groups (age 30 and over). The interpretation is as follows: due to improvements in disability rates, more people maintain and/or regain their health. As a result, the period without disability extends at the expense of that with disability. The rise in total life expectancy as well when disability rates improve is caused by the decrease in the proportion of persons with disability, who are exposed to higher mortality risks. Because the increase in disability-free life expectancy exceeds that of total life expectancy a compression of the period with disability (in an absolute and a relative sense) occurs.

Similar simulations suggested that reducing mortality rates (from one or more states), while keeping the disability rates constant, increases life expectancy in all states and the proportion of life with disability (Crimmins *et al*, 1994; Nusselder, 1997; Nusselder *et al*, 1996a). Increased survival of non-disabled persons (e.g. by improved acute care units) pushes more persons into the oldest-old age groups, where the risks of becoming disabled are high. Increased

Table 2.1. Life expectancy at age 70 for both sexes, by health status

	(1) Total	(2) No functioning problems	(3) Some functioning problems	(4) Unable to provide independent living	(5) Unable to provide personal care	(1) Proportion life expectancy dependent (4) + (5)
A Baseline	12.16	3.91	5.36	0.70	2.18	0.24
B Change mortality						
Increase 36.8%	10.32	3.64	4.72	0.53	1.42	0.19
Decrease 36.8%	15.38	4.25	6.22	1.01	3.91	0.32
Increase 50% (only dependent)	11.16	3.87	5.22	0.58	1.48	0.18
Decrease 50% (only dependent)	14.61	3.98	5.59	0.96	4.09	0.35
C Change getting worse						
Increase 36.8%	11.32	3.06	5.02	0.70	2.54	0.29
Decrease 36.8%	13.32	5.33	5.62	0.67	1.70	0.18
D Change getting better						
Increase 36.8%	12.50	4.47	5.27	0.69	2.08	0.22
Decrease 36.8%	11.77	3.31	5.43	0.73	2.30	0.26
E Combined change						
36.8% change toward healthier life	17.22	6.72	6.47	1.02	3.01	0.23
50% change toward healthier life	20.27	8.44	6.99	1.26	3.58	0.24
36.8% change toward worsening health	9.28	2.45	4.49	0.57	1.77	0.25

Source: Crimmins *et al* (1994).

survival of disabled persons (e.g. by better treatment of the chronically ill) extends the lives of persons with disability. Thus, mortality reductions (irrespective in which state) produce an increase in the duration and the proportion of life spent with disability. This increase is larger when reductions are concentrated in the disabled state(s) (and when reductions are larger). This consequence of mortality reductions might be important, considering that particular interventions may affect not only disability rates, but also status-specific mortality rates. For instance, medical treatment might increase the chances of regaining function and increase survival at the same time. In addition, improvements in disability can take place in the presence of mortality declines. It was shown that changing both mortality and disability rates towards better health (for instance, lower incidence, lower progression, higher recurrence and lower state-specific mortality rates) by the same percentages at all ages increases not only total life expectancy and life expectancy without disability at age 70, but also life expectancy with disability (Crimmins *et al*, 1994; Nusselder, 1997; Nusselder *et al*, 1996a).

Further analysis by Nusselder (Nusselder, 1997) focusing on the effect of changing disability rates in the presence of moderate mortality reductions (by 20%) pointed at two findings that are important for compression of morbidity. First, simulations suggested that the effect of changing all transition rates by an equal percentage towards better health differs by age. Nusselder and co-workers found that reducing state-specific mortality rates and incidence rates of disability, and increasing recovery rates from disability by 20% at all ages, produces a reduced life expectancy with disability at age 30, by −0.6 year in men and −0.3 year in women, but causes an increase in life expectancy with disability at age 70 by 0.2 and 0.4 years, respectively. In-depth analysis of the age-specific consequences of this scenario indicated that the reduction of years with disability (due to lower incidence and higher recovery rates) occurs – on average – at younger ages than the accumulation of disability (mainly due to mortality reductions) (Nusselder, 1997). Second, it was shown that with moderate declines (by 20%) in mortality rates at all ages among both disabled and non-disabled persons, at least equal proportional improvements in both incidence and recovery rates would be needed to achieve absolute compression of morbidity at age 30. For an improvement to occur in either incidence or recovery rates, improvements of at least 30% and 50%, respectively, would be required. It was also shown that greater improvements at all ages would be needed to achieve absolute compression of morbidity at age 70.

IMPACT OF SPECIFIC DISEASES

Diseases as causes of death have been studied for a long time and cause-of-death data are collected annually in most countries. Information on chronic diseases as causes of disability is increasingly available from health surveys (see

Coefficients and confidence interval

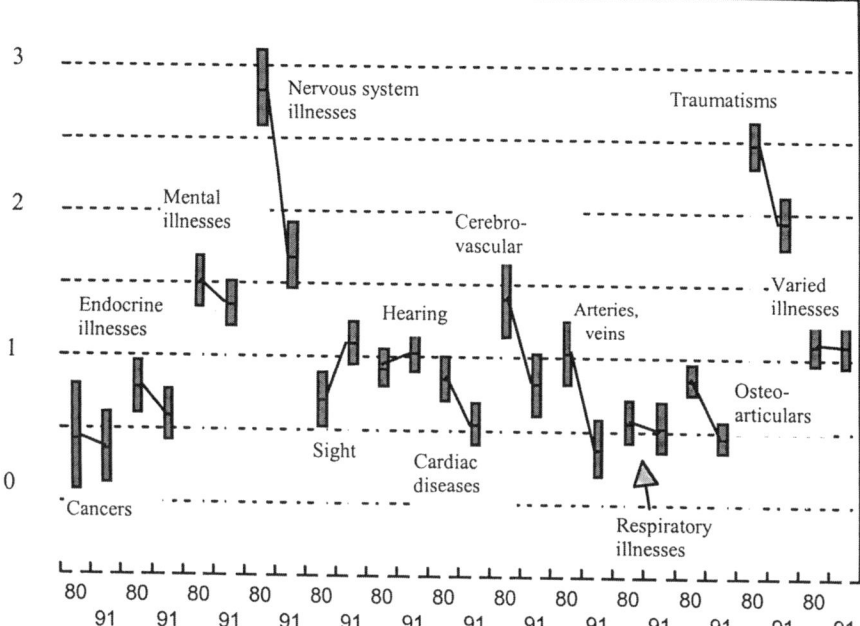

Figure 2.2. Trends in the influence of different disabling diseases on disability, at identical age, from 1980 to 1991 (men). From Robine *et al* (1998). Reprinted by permission of Sage Publications, Inc.

Boult *et al*, 1994; Ettinger *et al*, 1994; Furner *et al*, 1995; Guccione *et al*, 1994). It is obvious that since diseases have an impact both on mortality and on disability, the effect of changes in diseases on health expectancy, and thus on compression of morbidity, is not clear *a priori*. Regarding this effect two factors are important: (1) the relation between these diseases and disability, and (2) the extent to which mortality from these diseases ends disabled and non-disabled life.

Disability

The relation between diseases and disability, and thus between changes in disease prevalence and in the prevalence of disability, is less simple than one might expect. In studying the causes and mechanisms responsible for the *reduction* in disability rates in France between 1981 and 1991 (which caused together with mortality reductions an increase in disability-free life expectancy), Robine and colleagues (Robine *et al*, 1998) found that the prevalence of the main disabling diseases *increased* generally after age 60 or 70 (except for respiratory diseases and traumatisms) rather than decreased. In other words, a reduction in disability prevalence by age was accompanied by an increase in the prevalence of disabling diseases (by age). It was shown that a reduction in the disabling impact of these diseases explained the observed decline in disability rates in 1991 as compared to 1981 (Figure 2.2).

To be more specific, there were lower probabilities of having disabilities in men with a disease of the nervous system, a cardiovascular disease, an osteoarticular disease or a traumatism and higher probabilities in men with an eye disease. For women the results are almost the same, except for the increase in the disabling impact of mental diseases. These outcomes might indicate that the rate of disease progression is slowing down (as suggested by the dynamic equilibrium hypothesis), although it is also possible that the propensity to report diseases, especially the less severe forms, has changed (Robine et al, 1998). Regarding the consequences of changes in diseases for compression of morbidity, two observations arise from this study. First, it is the net effect of changes in the prevalence of chronic diseases and in their disabling impact that counts. Second, an expansion of the period with disabling chronic diseases might co-occur with a compression of the period with disability.

Mortality

The extent to which major causes of death end disabled and non-disabled life was the main subject of a study from Hayward which used an extended multistate life-table model differentiating deaths in the active and inactive state by cause (Hayward et al, 1998). This was the first study to include information on both the health state preceding death (active versus inactive) and the cause of death (heart diseases, cerebral diseases, cancer and other diseases). It was found that functional decline need not necessarily precede death. Most of the deaths (68.5%) in men age 70 occurred in the active state whereas in women at this age deaths are roughly split up between the two health states. At older ages, larger proportions of deaths occurred in the inactive state, but still a sizeable proportion of deaths occurred in persons who were still active. This concentration of active deaths suggests that extending active life could be accomplished partially by lowering mortality rates among persons without functioning problems. A further analysis of the effect of eliminating specific causes of death on active and inactive life expectancy showed that for heart diseases most of the gains in life expectancy at age 70 for men are felt in terms of increased active life. Of the three additional years men can expect to gain when heart disease would be eliminated, almost two years would be added to active life. The results, however, differed by age and sex. With increasing age, a gradual shift was found, such that the elimination of heart diseases at older ages would add more years of inactive life than of active life. In women aged 70 most of the years gained through the elimination of heart diseases would be

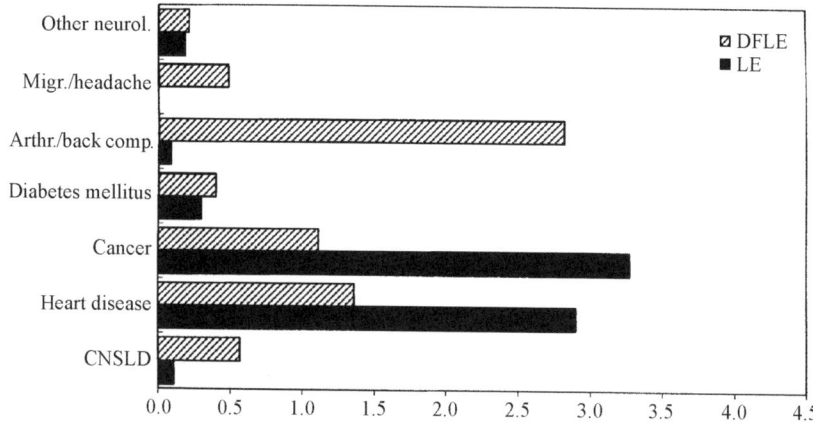

Figure 2.3. Increase in total life expectancy (LE) and disability-free life expectancy (DFLE) with hypothetical elimination of a disease (men, age 15). CNSLD, chronic non-specific lung disease. From Nusselder *et al* (1994). Reproduced with permission

inactive years. The effects of eliminating mortality from cancer and cerebral diseases on the number of active and inactive years would be smaller. Interpretation of the outcomes in terms of compression of morbidity (not included in the original contribution) gives a less optimistic message, as it indicates that reducing mortality from heart disease, cancer and cerebral diseases expands not only the number of active years, but also that of inactive years. That is, elimination of these diseases as a cause of death would cause an expansion of morbidity (in an absolute and in a relative sense).

Mortality and Disability

A study of Nusselder and colleagues (Nusselder *et al*, 1994, 1996b) examined whether a hypothetical elimination of specific chronic diseases, and the consequences in terms of disability and mortality, would lead to a compression of morbidity. They found that eliminating disabling diseases such as arthritis/ back complaints that cause little mortality would lead to an increase in disability-free life expectancy, while total life expectancy would remain more or less constant (Figure 2.3). Consequently, life expectancy with disability would decline and thus a compression of morbidity (both in an absolute and a relative sense) would occur. For cancer, a disease with a high case-fatality, elimination would result not only in a gain in disability-free life expectancy, but also in an – even larger – increase in life expectancy with disability. In the years that people are saved from dying from cancer, they experience disability due to other causes. So people live longer, but most of these years are spent with disability. Elimination of cancer would therefore result in an expansion of morbidity (in absolute and relative sense, according to the adjusted classification). Whether elimination of both disabling and fatal diseases (e.g. heart diseases and chronic non-specific lung disease) would result in compression or expansion of morbidity depends on the extent to which they cause mortality and disability. For example, eliminating heart disease, where the impact on total mortality exceeds the impact on disability, would lead to an expansion of morbidity in both an absolute and a relative sense. As far as chronic non-specific lung disease is concerned, however, elimination would lead to both absolute and relative compression of morbidity.

To summarise, when highly fatal diseases with a low disabling impact are eliminated, or when only the mortal consequences of chronic diseases are eradicated, increased survival will lead to an expansion of the number of years with disability, even if initially the survival of active persons increases. When changes occur earlier in the disease process and disability is prevented as well, a compression of morbidity (in an absolute and a relative sense) occurs, unless prevention of this disease also decreases mortality substantially. In the latter situation, the net effect depends upon the disabling impact of the disease and its case-fatality.

IMPACT OF SPECIFIC RISK FACTORS

Since disability and mortality share common risk factors, the net effect of changes in the risk factor distribution (or in the excess risks associated with exposure to that risk factor) in terms of compression of morbidity is not obvious. Whether reducing the risk-factor exposure would result in a compression of morbidity depends upon the net effect of two opposite effects. First, as a result of the reduction in exposure, lower disability rates produce an increase in life expectancy without disability and a reduction in life expectancy with disability. Second, a reduction in exposure increases survival. As a result, people live longer and will be longer exposed to the (reduced) risk of disability. On balance, life expectancy with disability decreases when the effect of the disability reduction on the number of years with disability exceeds that of increased survival.

Smoking is an important modifiable risk factor which causes substantial mortality (Doll *et al*, 1994; Nam *et al*, 1995; US Department of Health and Human Services, 1990) and disability (Branch, 1985; Guralnik and Kaplan, 1989; Kaplan, 1992; LaCroix *et al*, 1993; Rogers *et al*, 1994). The consequences of a hypothetical elimination of smoking for health expectancy in the Netherlands have been estimated in two studies, which used different data and a different methodology. Based on a multistate life-table model with a non-disabled and a disabled state, Nusselder and colleagues (Nusselder *et al*, 2000) estimated that eliminating smoking would produce a substantially larger gain in disability-free life expectancy (2.5 years in men and 1.9 years in women) than in total life expectancy (1.6 and 0.8 years, respectively). Consequently, smoking elimination would compress life expectancy with disability in an absolute and a relative sense. Thus, despite the fact that life would be extended as a consequence of eliminating smoking, and people would be exposed longer to disability, lower incidence rates of disability and higher recovery rates from disability would produce on balance a reduction in years with disability. Based on a multistate model with different disease states in combination with disability weights (i.e. the DALE approach), Barendregt *et al* (1998) found that smoking elimination would reduce the difference between total life expectancy and disability-adjusted life expectancy (DALE), which means that smoking elimination would produce a compression of morbidity (in an absolute and a relative sense). Recent studies for other countries seem inconclusive as to whether smoking elimination would result in a compression of morbidity (Ferrucci *et al*, 1999; Martel *et al*, 2000; Bronnum-Hansen and Juel, 2001).

CONCLUSION

Ten years of REVES have contributed to the methodological progress necessary for research on compression of morbidity and to the development of a better understanding of the complex interaction between morbidity, mortality and population health in general and of compression of morbidity in particular. Health expectancy proved to be a powerful measure and the life table an important tool in studying compression of morbidity. Besides advocating the use of health expectancy, REVES has been an important platform for discussions on the definition and measurement of compression of morbidity, on different methods to calculate health expectancy, and on the dynamics underlying a compression of morbidity. Nevertheless, much research remains to be done. Research on the ageing and disablement process has stressed the importance of several potential risk factors and effect modifiers in these processes. More research is needed to understand the opposite results from prior studies on the effect of (elimination of) smoking in terms of compression of morbidity and to assess the contribution of risk factors other than smoking. Disease-specific models are needed to assess the effect of changes in different phases of the disease process. The increasing availability of longitudinal studies, which include information on risk factors, chronic diseases, disability and mortality, will offer new challenges for further research on this issue. REVES can keep on playing an important role in exchanging data, discussing methodological problems and interpreting outcomes of these studies, as it did in the last 10 years.

ACKNOWLEDGEMENTS

The writing of this chapter is supported by the Netherlands Organization for Scientific Research (NWO, grant 904-68493).

REFERENCES

Alter, G. and Riley, J.C. (1989) 'Frailty, sickness, and death: models of morbidity and mortality in historical populations', *Population Studies* 43, 25–45.

Barendregt, J.J. and Bonneux, L. (1995) 'Changes in incidence and survival of cardiovascular diseases and their impact on disease prevalence and health expectancy', in Mathers, C., McCallum, J. and Robine, J.-M. (eds) *Advances in Health Expectancies*. Canberra, Australia: Australian Institute of Health and Welfare.

Barendregt, J.J. and Bonneux, L. (1998) *Degenerative Disease in an Aging Population: Models and Conjectures*. Rotterdam, the Netherlands: Erasmus University Rotterdam.

Barendregt, J.J., Bonneux, L. and Van der Maas, P.J. (1994) 'Health expectancy: an indicator for change?', *Journal of Epidemiology and Community Health* 48, 482–487.

Barendregt, J.J., Bonneux, L. and Van der Maas, P.J. (1997) 'How good is Sullivan's method for monitoring changes in population health expectancies' (letter), *Journal of Epidemiology and Community Health* 51, 578.

Barendregt, J.J., Bonneux, L. and Van der Maas, P.J. (1998) 'From a population health indicator to a tool for policy making', *Journal of Aging and Health* 10, 242–258.

Boult, C., Kane, R.L., Louis, T.A., Boult, L. and McCaffrey, D. (1994) 'Chronic conditions that lead to functional limitation in the elderly', *Journal of Gerontology* 49, M28–M36.

Branch, L.G. (1985) 'Health practices and incident disability among the elderly', *American Journal of Public Health* 75, 1436–1439.

Breslow, L. and Breslow, N. (1993) 'Health practices and disability: some evidence from Alameda County', *Preventive Medicine* 22, 86–95.

Bronnum-Hansen, H. and Juel, K. (2001) 'Abstention from smoking extends life and compresses morbidity: a population based study of health expectancy among smokers and never smokers in Denmark', *Tobacco Control* 10, 273–278.

Crimmins, E.M. and Ingegneri, D.G. (1993) 'Trends in health among the American population', in Rappaport, A.M. and Schieber, S.J. (eds) *Demography and Retirement: The Twenty-First Century*. London, UK; Westport, CT: Praeger.

Crimmins, E.M. and Saito, Y. (1993) 'Getting better and getting worse', *Journal of Aging and Health* 5, 3–36.

Crimmins, E.M., Hayward, M.D. and Saito, Y. (1994) 'Changing mortality and morbidity rates and the health status and life expectancy of the older population', *Demography* 31, 159–175.

Deeg, D. (1997) 'Cohort survival history and rates of poor health in older men and women', Paper presented at the tenth International workshop of the International Network on Health Expectancy (REVES-10), October, 1997: Tokyo, Japan.

Doll, R., Peto, R., Wheatley, K., Gray, R. and Sutherland, I. (1994) 'Mortality in relation to smoking: 40 years' observations on male British doctors', *British Medical Journal* 309, 901–911.

Ettinger, W., Jr, Fried, L.P., Harris, T., Shemanski, L., Schulz, R. and Robbins, J. (1994) 'Self-reported causes of physical disability in older people: the Cardiovascular Health Study. CHS Collaborative Research Group', *Journal of the American Geriatric Society* 42, 1035–1044.

Ferucci, L., Izmirlian, G., Leveille, S., Phillips, C.L., Corti, M.C., Brock, D.B. and Guralnik, J.M. (1999) 'Smoking, physical activity, and active life expectancy', *American Journal of Epidemiology* 149: 645–653.

Fried, L.P. and Guralnik, J.M. (1997) 'Disability in older adults: evidence regarding significance, etiology, and risk', *Journal of the American Geriatric Society* 45, 92–100.

Fries, J.F. (1980) 'Aging, natural death, and the compression of morbidity', *New England Journal of Medicine* 303, 130–135.

Fries, J.F. (1983) 'The compression of morbidity', *Milbank Memorial Fund Quarterly/ Health and Society* 61, 397–419.

Fries, J.F. (1984) 'The compression of morbidity: miscellaneous comments about a theme', *The Gerontologist* 24, 354–359.

Fries, J.F. (1989) 'The compression of morbidity: near or far?', *Milbank Quarterly* 67, 208–232.

Fries, J.F. (1993) 'Compression of morbidity: life span, disability, and health care costs', *Facts and Research in Gerontology* 7, 183–190.

Furner, S.E., Rudberg, M.A. and Cassel, C.K. (1995) 'Medical conditions differentially affect the development of IADL disability: implications for medical care and research', *The Gerontologist* 35, 444–450.

Greengross, S., Murphy, E., Quam, L., Rochon, P. and Smith, R. (1997) 'Aging: a subject that must be at the top of the world agendas', *British Medical Journal* 315, 1029–1030.

Gruenberg, E.M. (1977) 'The failures of success', *Milbank Memorial Fund Quarterly/ Health and Society* 55, 3–24.

Guccione, A.A., Felson, D.T., Anderson, J.J., Anthony, J.M., Zhang, Y., Wilson, P. W., Kelly-Hayes, M., Wolf, P.A., Kreger, B.E. and Kannel, W.B. (1994) 'The effects of specific medical conditions on the functional limitations of elders in the Framingham Study', *American Journal of Public Health* 84, 351–358.

Guralnik, J.M. and Kaplan, G.A. (1989) 'Predictors of healthy aging: prospective evidence from the Alameda County study', *American Journal of Public Health* 79, 703–708.

Guralnik, J.M., Land, K.C., Blazer, D., Fillenbaum, G.G. and Branch, L.G. (1993) 'Educational status and active life expectancy among older blacks and whites', *New England Journal of Medicine* 329, 110–116.

Haan, M. (1989) 'Compression of morbidity: the Kaiser Permanente Study of oldest old', in Robine, J-M., Blanchet, M. and Dowd J.E. (eds) *Health Expectancy*. London: HMSO.

Hayward, M.D. and Heron, M. (1999) 'Racial inequality in active life among adult Americans', *Demography* 36, 77–91.

Hayward, M.D., Crimmins, E.M. and Saito, Y. (1998) 'Cause of death and active life expectancy in the older population of the United States', *Journal of Aging and Health* 10, 192–213.

Herrmann, F.R., Michel, J.-P., Bruchez, M., Lalive d'Épinay, C. and Grab, B. (1999) 'Hip fracture and healthy life expectancy', in Egidi, V. (ed.) *Towards an Integrated System of Indicators to Assess the Health Status of the Population*. Rome: ISTAT.

Jagger, C. and Clarke, M. (1988) 'Mortality risks in the elderly: five-year follow-up of a total population', *International Journal of Epidemiology* 17, 111–114.

Kaplan, G. (1992) 'Maintenance of functioning in the elderly', *Annals of Epidemiology* 2, 813–822.

Katz, S., Branch, L.G., Branson, M.H., Papsidero, J.A., Beck, J.C. and Greer, D.S. (1983) 'Active life expectancy', *New England Journal of Medicine* 309, 1218–1224.

Kramer, M. (1980) 'The rising pandemic of mental disorders and associated chronic diseases and disabilities', *Acta Psychiatrica Scandinavica* 62, 382–397.

LaCroix, A.Z., Guralnik, J.M., Berkman, L.F., Wallace, R.B. and Satterfield, S. (1993) 'Maintaining mobility in late life. II. Smoking, alcohol consumption, physical activity, and body mass index', *American Journal of Epidemiology* 137, 858–869.

Manton, K.G. (1982) 'Changing concepts of morbidity and mortality in the elderly population', *Milbank Memorial Fund Quarterly/Health and Society* 60, 183–244.

Manton, K.G. (1988) 'A longitudinal study of functional change and mortality in the United States', *Journal of Gerontology* 43, S153–S161.

Martel, L., Bélanger, A. and Berthelot, J.-M. (2000) 'Smoking and disability-free life expectancy', *Report on the demographic situation in Canada 2000*. Quebec: Statistics Canada.

Mathers, C. (1994) 'Health expectancies in Australia 1993: preliminary results', in Mathers, C., McCallum, J. and Robine, J.-M. (eds) *Advances in Health Expectancies*. Canberra, Australia: Australian Institute of Health and Welfare.

Mathers, C.D. and Robine, J.M. (1997a) 'How good is Sullivan's method for monitoring changes in population health expectancies?' *Journal of Epidemiology and Community Health* 51, 80–86.

Mathers, C.D. and Robine, J.M. (1997b) 'How good is Sullivan's method for monitoring changes in population health expectancies?' (Reply to letter), *Journal of Epidemiology and Community Health* 51, 578–579.

Mathers, C., Robine, J.M. and Wilkins, R., eds (1994) 'Health expectancy indicators: recommendations for terminology', in Mathers, C., McCallum, J. and Robine, J.-M. (eds) *Advances in Health Expectancies*. Canberra, Australia: Australian Institute of Health and Welfare.

McCallum, J. and Shadbolt, B. (1994) 'Ageing and disability in Australia: prevalence and predictors in a longitudinal survey', in Mathers, C., McCallum, J. and Robine, J.-M. (eds) *Advances in Health Expectancies*. Canberra, Australia: Australian Institute of Health and Welfare.

Michel, J. and Robine, J. (1992) 'Example de modélisation du veillissement/Modeling the aging process: an example', Paper presented at the fifth International workshop of the International Network on Health Expectancy (REVES-5), February, 1992: Ottawa, Canada.

Michel, J.P., Arroyo, J., Loew, F., Rizzoli, R. and Robine, J.M. (1993) 'Ageing process: femoral neck fracture', in Robine, J-M., Mathers, C.D., Bone, M. and Romieu, I. (eds) *Calculation of Health Expectancies: Harmonization, Consensus Achieved and Future Perspectives*. Montrouge, France: John Libbey Eurotext.

Mulhorn, K. (1995) 'Disability as a mortality risk factor among the elderly', Paper presented at the tenth International workshop of the International Network on Health Expectancy (REVES-10): REVES paper 296.

Nam, C., Rogers, R. and Hummer, R. (1995) 'Impact of future smoking scenarios on mortality levels of adult population in the U.S. until the year 2050', Paper presented at the eighth International workshop of the International Network on Health Expectancy (REVES-8), October, 1995: Chicago, United States.

Nusselder, W. (1997) *Compression or Expansion of Morbidity: A Life-Table Approach*. Rotterdam, the Netherlands: Erasmus University Rotterdam.

Nusselder, W.J., van der Velden, K., van Sonsbeek, J.L., Lenior, M.E. and van den Bos, G.A. (1994) 'The effect of elimination of selected chronic diseases on the disability-free population: compression or expansion of morbidity?', in Mathers, C., McCallum, J. and Robine, J.-M. (eds) *Advances in Health Expectancies*. Canberra, Australia: Australian Institute of Health and Welfare.

Nusselder, W., Looman, C., Stronks, K. and Mackenbach, J. (1996a) 'Compression of morbidity: an exploration of the conditions', Paper presented at the ninth International workshop of the International Network on Health Expectancy (REVES-9), December, 1996: Rome, Italy.

Nusselder, W.J., van der Velden, K., van Sonsbeek, J.L., Lenior, M.E. and van den Bos, G.A. (1996b) 'The elimination of selected chronic diseases in a population: the compression and expansion of morbidity', *American Journal of Public Health* 86, 187–194.

Nusselder, W.J., Looman, C.W.N., Marang-Van de Mheen, P.J., Van de Mheen, H. and Mackenbach, J.P. (2000) 'Smoking and the compression of morbidity', *Journal of Epidemiology and Community Health* 54, 566–574.

Olshansky, S.J., Rudberg, M.A., Carnes, B.A., Cassel, C.K. and Brody, J.A. (1991) 'Trading off longer life for worsening health', *Journal of Aging and Health* 3, 194–216.

Robine, J.M. and Ritchie, K. (1991) 'Healthy life expectancy: evaluation of global indicator of change in population health', *British Medical Journal* 302, 457–460.

Robine, J.M. and Mathers, C.D. (1993) 'Measuring the compression or expansion of morbidity through changes in health expectancy', in Robine, J-M., Mathers, C.D., Bone, M. and Romieu, I. (eds) *Calculation of Health Expectancies: Harmonization, Consensus Achieved and Future Perspectives*. Montrouge, France: John Libbey Eurotext.

Robine, J., Mormiche, P. and Sermet, C. (1998) 'Examination of the causes and mechanisms of the increase in disability-free life expectancy', *Journal of Aging and Health*, 10, 171–191. Sage Publications Inc.

Rogers, R. (1993) 'Successful aging in the United States', in Robine, J-M., Mathers, C.D., Bone, M. and Romieu, I. (eds) *Calculation of Health Expectancies: Harmonization, Consensus Achieved and Future Perspectives*. Montrouge, France: John Libbey Eurotext.

Rogers, R.G., Nam, C.B. and Hummer, R.A. (1994) 'Activity limitation and cigarette smoking in the United States: implications for health expectancies', in Mathers, C., McCallum, J. and Robine, J.-M. (eds) *Advances in Health Expectancies*. Canberra, Australia: Australian Institute of Health and Welfare.

Rogers, R.R., Rogers, A. and Belanger, A. (1992) 'Disability-free life among the elderly in the United States. Sociodemographic correlates of functional health', *Journal of Aging and Health* 4, 19–42.

Strawbridge, W.J., Camacho, T.C., Cohen, R.D. and Kaplan, G.A. (1993) 'Gender differences in factors associated with change in physical functioning in old age: a 6-year longitudinal study', *The Gerontologist* 33, 603–609.

US Department of Health and Human Services (1990) *The Health Benefits of Smoking cessation: A Report of the Surgeon General*. Rockville, MD: Centre for Chronic Disease Prevention and Health Promotion.

Verbrugge, L.M. (1984) 'Longer life but worsening health? Trends in health and mortality of middle-aged and older persons', *Milbank Memorial Fund Quarterly/ Health and Society* 62, 475–519.

Verbrugge, L.M. and Balaban, D.J. (1989) 'Patterns of change in disability and well-being', *Medical Care* 27, S128–S147.

Verbrugge, L.M. and Jette, A.M. (1994) 'The disablement process', *Social Science and Medicine* 38, 1–14.

Verbrugge, L.M., Reoma, J.M. and Gruber-Baldini, A.L. (1994) 'Short-term dynamics of disability and well-being', *Journal of Health and Social Behaviour* 35, 97–117.

Wilkins, R., Chen, J. and Ng, E. (1994) 'Changes in health expectancy in Canada from 1986 to 1991', in Mathers, C., McCallum, J. and Robine, J.-M. (eds) *Advances in Health Expectancies*. Canberra, Australia: Australian Institute of Health and Welfare.

World Health Organization (1984) *The Uses of Epidemiology in the Study of the Elderly: Report of a WHO Scientific Group on the Epidemiology of Aging*. Geneva: WHO.

3

Patterns of Disability Change Associated with the Epidemiologic Transition

GEORGE C. MYERS*, VICKI L. LAMB[†] and EMILY M. AGREE[‡]

[†]Duke University, Durham, NC, USA and [‡]Johns Hopkins University, Baltimore, MD, USA

INTRODUCTION

Since its inception in 1989, REVES has been not only an international network of researchers, but also a movement with a mission to develop conceptual and methodological tools for examining transitions in health status. In this chapter, we review developments by the REVES network over the past decade related to the interaction of disability trends and overall population health. Three main features of this research are evident: first, improvements in the measurement of disability at the population level; second, attention to changing levels of disability; and third, efforts to create a conceptual framework that describes changes in the extent and distribution of disability that accompany the epidemiologic transition and includes a set of testable propositions about the mechanisms that produce these changes.

In the past decade, there has been an important shift in emphasis from studying the *quantity* of remaining life to examining the *quality* of those years. The primary goal of increasing the active/healthy years of life, along with longevity, has been widely recognized by national health agencies, as well as international organizations such as the World Health Organization (WHO) (Manton, 1999). The changed mandate is clearly congruent with the original aims of REVES, which no doubt accounts in large measure for the continued success and vitality of the network.

*Deceased.

Determining Health Expectancies. Edited by J-M. Robine, C. Jagger, C.D. Mathers, E.M. Crimmins and R.M. Suzman.
© 2003 John Wiley & Sons, Ltd

An emphasis upon quality has broadened perspectives on conceptualizing and measuring health status. The initial term used by many REVES investigators 'disability-free life expectancy' (DFLE) clearly implied that disability was a key concept, but precisely how it should be measured has been widely debated. The WHO International Classification of Impairments, Disabilities and Handicaps (WHO, 1980) and the efforts of the US National Academy of Sciences (Pope and Tarlov, 1991) have offered relatively little help in clarifying the issue. Increasingly, it has been accepted that there is no 'gold standard', but rather that multiple indicators contribute to measuring the quality or, more commonly, the *poor* quality of remaining years (e.g. presence of disease; physical handicaps; subjective evaluations of ability, capacity and performance; actual performance; needs for assistance; mental states). Each approach is meritorious and contributes to capturing the multidimensionality of health, but because of its widespread use in surveys and other collection procedures, the presence and number of self-reported limitations in the activities of daily living (ADL) (Katz *et al*, 1983) has come to be a widely used metric for assessing disability.

A *second* distinctive feature of REVES has been the emphasis on examining changing health conditions over time, which may include both shifts over the individual life course or aggregate changes in population or subgroup levels. This dynamic perspective is widely shared in the fields of public health and has led to repeated periodic data collection efforts. Especially noteworthy in this regard is the growing implementation of longitudinal/panel studies, which permit assessment of age-related shifts on the micro-level for individuals and of aggregate changes on the macro-level. Data from such investigations are crucial in deriving transition probabilities between states of wellness and ill-health, including reversals and recoveries, which are needed for multistate life tables. The importance of transitional analyses and the use of more sophisticated actuarial procedures (e.g. multistate life tables, survival analyses, etc.), which capture the dynamics of the processes, have received considerable attention in REVES.

Third, there has been a long-standing interest within the social sciences and epidemiology in determining the historical sequence and major stages of important socioeconomic and epidemiological transformations and under-standing the corresponding transitions. This has been especially true in the field of demography, in which frameworks to establish the temporal progressions of fertility and mortality were proposed initially in the 1930s by Landry (1934). By the 1940s, the notion of a 'demographic transition' became embedded in the field (Notestein, 1945) to describe fairly universal patterns of declining mortality levels and subsequent declines in fertility, with accompanying characteristic changes in growth rates (both a steady state initially and following the transition) and population structure (from an initial juvenation to an eventual aging of the population). While critics have accepted the main descriptive aspects of this formulation, they have noted the absence of sound explanations for its unfolding. Moreover, there have been repeated questions about the appropriateness of the model to describe conditions in contemporary developing countries. This has led to a series of sub-models differentiated mainly by the pace and timing of the transitions in births and deaths.

The demographic transition provides a generalized model describing changes in vital rates and population composition in human populations that occur in conjunction with social and economic development. The mechanisms behind these changes have been discussed in a series of cognate models that cover the components of population change – transitions in fertility (Douglas *et al*, 1996), mortality (Omran, 1971, 1983), and migration (Zelinsky, 1971; Friedlander, 1983; Rogers, 1989). Moreover, each of these component models has led to sub-component models. In the case of mortality, the epidemiologic transition has given rise to a disability transition model (Myers and Lamb, 1993), a nutritional model (Popkin, 1993), and models that add additional stages to the transition (Barrett *et al*, 1998; Myers and Manton, 1987; Olshansky and Ault, 1986; Rogers and Hackenberg, 1987). In this chapter, we give major attention to the epidemiologic transition formulation and its derivatives.

EPIDEMIOLOGIC TRANSITION

Epidemiologic transition theory focuses upon changes in the complex patterns of disease and mortality associated with the demographic transition (Omran, 1971). The intent of the theory was to direct focus on the shifts in disease patterns and causes of mortality, and the resulting impacts upon life expectation and population growth. Omran (1983) set forth a series of propositions to formulate the theoretical basis of this framework. The major premise of the theory, Proposition 1, assumes mortality to be the fundamental factor in population dynamics.

Omran's propositions form an outline of the stages of the transition, 'whereby pandemics of infection are progressively (but not entirely) displaced by degenerative and man-made diseases as the leading causes of death' (Proposition 2), as well as an overview of causal factors (e.g. rising standards of living and nutritional improvement) for the early Western transitions (Proposition 4). As with the original formulation, Proposition 5 differentiates among four basic models of the epidemiologic transition, depending on the 'distinctive variations in the pattern, the pace, the determinants, and the consequences of population change' (1983, p. 311).

These propositions focus on the epidemiologic transition from a population perspective. Omran also acknowledged differentials in the rates and pace of mortality change within a population (Proposition 3). Mortality improvements are not expected to occur uniformly through a population; but rather, some groups will benefit earlier (e.g. the young and females) while others realize benefits at a slower pace (e.g. the poor and ethnic minorities).

TRENDS IN MORTALITY AND MORBIDITY

The rapid declines in overall mortality in developed countries, especially infant and child mortality, in the immediate post-World War II period gradually gave rise in the 1960s to a fairly stagnant level trend in mortality. Nonetheless, a decade later the declines continued, particularly focused on reductions in mortality rates at older ages. Moreover, the declines were due to reductions in the prevalence of several chronic diseases, contrary to the Omran formulation.

An important question to be considered is whether it is necessary to consider a fourth stage, or new phase, to the epidemiologic or health transition, which in turn, would further impact the incidence and prevalence of disabilities. A number of researchers suggested that the epidemiologic transition framework be extended to include a fourth stage in the Western model (Kan and Kim, 1982; Olshansky and Ault, 1986; Myers and Manton, 1987; Rogers and Hackenberg, 1987). The additional stage was deemed warranted because mortality had continued to decline further than anticipated by Omran in his original framework. In particular, chronic disease mortality had been curtailed (perhaps by delayed age of onset, as suggested by Olshansky and Ault (1986)), though there had been no major medical breakthroughs, and gains continued to be made in life expectation (Myers and Manton, 1987). The depictions of the fourth stage placed emphasis upon the influences of social and cultural factors on population morbidity and mortality rates. Such influences are due to individual lifestyle behaviors (e.g. smoking, exercise, diet), although there is conflict regarding whether the predictions were for greater improvements (Olshansky and Ault, 1986) or self-destruction (Rogers and Hackenberg, 1987).

Interestingly, while some were calling for a new stage due to non-communicable mortality rate declines, others have come to envision a third transition to a new stage in the epidemiologic transition to account for steady gains in infectious diseases (Armstrong et al, 1999; Olshansky et al, 1997). Barrett et al (1998) have provided a thorough review of these developments, which include an unprecedented number of new infectious diseases (e.g. Legionnaire's disease, HIV, Ebola, etc.); re-emerging infections such as malaria and tuberculosis; and re-emerging pathogens that are generating antimicrobial resistant strains. Olshansky et al (1997) also presented an overview of the trend of infectious and parasitic disease emergence and re-emergence; and the demographic, social and environmental factors contributing to the re-emergence of such diseases. Gaylin and Kates (1997) provide special attention to the emergence and spread of the AIDS pandemic. Although some of these developments were anticipated previously (Myers and Manton, 1987), they now have become global issues.

The relationships between mortality and morbidity trends have an important bearing on model formulations, but remain matters largely of conjecture. The naïve initial assumptions have been that they are closely related and therefore follow close trajectories over time. That is, if mortality declines, morbidity also declines. Alter and Riley (1989; Riley and Alter, 1996) have demonstrated, using historical data sources, that morbidity levels tended to rise after mortality declines, rather than the reverse. Moreover, this does not reflect increases in incidence, but rather improvements in case fatality and, at the same time, rising prevalence levels. It is tempting to say that this also includes rising comorbidities, but the evidence for this conclusion is scant historically.

MORBIDITY DETERMINANTS

As countries progress through the later stages of the epidemiologic transition, the traditional indicators of population health, such as mortality, are expected to change very little. Thus, extensions of the model have shifted focus from mortality declines to changing patterns of morbidity (Barrett *et al*, 1998). In his discussion of the determinants of the epidemiologic shifts (Proposition 4), Omran noted three major categories of disease determinants:

> 1. Ecobiologic determinants of mortality indicate the complex balance between disease agents, the level of hostility in the environment, and the resistance of the host...
> 2. Socio-economic, political, and cultural determinants include standards of living health habits, hygiene, and nutrition.
> 3. Medical and public health determinants are specific preventive and curative measures used to combat disease: they include improved public sanitation, immunization and the development of decisive therapies (Omran, 1983, pp. 309–310).

Thus, the incidence and prevalence of morbid conditions, particularly chronic and degenerative diseases, age at onset, and case-fatality rates have become increasingly important concerns in understanding population health. Also important is the consideration of individual behavior and lifestyles, as well as the influence of social conditions and environments and socio-political developments in the form of public health ideologies and movements (Nathanson, 1996).

At the Montpellier REVES meeting, Vallin (1993) addressed the main point of Omran's model, which was the eradication or reduction of mortality due to infectious diseases. This marked the emergence of mortality due to 'degenerative' and 'man-made' diseases and introduced a new phase. He indicated that the new phase was different from earlier ones for two reasons. First, from a pathological point of view, the fight against illness and disease shifted away from the fight against infection to a focus on combating the chronic and degenerative diseases. Second, this change marked a new public health strategy that included the participation of individuals in monitoring their personal behavior and lifestyle. For example, in the US the main rallying cry became 'health promotion and disease prevention'. Such changes have effects on future health trends – both the causes and consequences of morbidities, as well as strategies for prevention or postponement of disease onset.

Diet, sources of nutrition and other environmental factors are found to be instrumental in affecting population health and resistance to disease. Popkin (1993) extended the demographic and epidemiologic transition models to include 'nutrition transition' in which he delineates five broad nutrition patterns associated with diet availability, composition and variety. Fogel and Costa (1997) also emphasize the importance of sustenance on the lives and activities of populations. A key theme of their work is the consideration of the importance of the distribution of nutrition within a population, and the effects of such distributions on the energy available for productive activities. Their work highlights the genetic and physiological linkages to body size and mortality outcomes, as well as the variability of mortality outcomes given the distribution of body stature and weight. More recently, Scott and Duncan (2000) have pointed out the implications of chronic malnutrition for the intergenerational transmission of low birth weight from mothers to daughters and the consequent implications for adult mortality during the transition.

Myers and Manton (1987) suggested that debilitating 'non-life-threatening' (NLT) diseases would assume greater importance in assessments of population health, especially with an aging population. Moreover, research indicates that much of the disability, especially physical limitations, among the elderly is generated by NLT diseases such as arthritis (Manton, 1990; Verbrugge *et al*, 1989, 1991; Verbrugge and Patrick, 1995). Thus, the examination of causal mechanisms associated with population health represents only part of the picture, particularly when there is little change in the vital rates of populations. The consideration of the social effects of individuals' health and morbidity, such as disablement, is of increased importance in the assessment of population health.

DISABILITY TRANSITIONS

The epidemiologic transition framework was extended in a REVES paper to include propositions regarding patterns of disability transitions associated with the transition (Myers and Lamb, 1993). The goal was to bring into focus changes in the causes and levels of disability, and the distribution of disablement within different segments of the population.

The propositions and rationales are as follows:

1. Overall, crude rates of disability incidence are higher in the initial stages of an epidemiologic transition and prevalence levels are lower. As the transition proceeds, a reversal in these levels occurs.

It is necessary to distinguish between the incidence and prevalence of both morbidities and disabilities. Incidence refers to the occurrence of new cases, and is affected by factors such as those associated with susceptibility to contracting certain illnesses (e.g. due to poor health or nutrition), whereas prevalence reflects both current and prior incidence. Prevalence levels are strongly influenced by case-fatality rates and intervention strategies. For example, in the early stages of the transition, high infant and child mortality would tend to eliminate those born with congenital malformations or who were subject to impairments due to severe infectious and parasitic diseases. Such low levels of survival would reduce the prevalence of disabilities in the total population, particularly in the older ages, even while incidence is high. Moreover, changes in the average duration of morbid and disabling conditions will affect prevalence levels. As medical and rehabilitative improvements occur, the likelihood of comorbidities (and codisabilities) for individuals increases, thus leading to greater prevalence levels of disabilities.

2. Underlying causes of disablement shift during the transition from those attributable to communicable diseases to those that result from non-communicable diseases.

In the early stages of the epidemiologic transition, the infectious conditions leading to death are also the major causes of disablement for survivors. A United Nations report on disability indicates that: 'Those developing countries offering the least extensive preventive medicine programmes reported that such diseases as measles, rubella, diphtheria, tetanus, smallpox, meningitis, encephalitis and venereal and endemic diseases such as malaria tended to account for a notable proportion of disability' (United Nations, 1986, p. 11). At later stages of the epidemiologic transition the disease-related disabilities tend to be associated with somatic and metabolic diseases, chronic cardiovascular and degenerative disorders. In the United States arthritis is the major source of disability at older ages, and the major fatal cause of disability is heart disease (Verbrugge and Patrick, 1995).

3. During the transition, disability prevalence levels shift from being higher at younger ages to being higher at older ages.

The incidence, prevalence and distribution by cause of disabilities differ according to age group. Disabilities by age are strongly associated with morbidity trends and, therefore, follow characteristic patterns through the epidemiologic transition. In early stages of the transition, as in many less developed countries where there is a lack of preventive services and primary health care, a larger proportion of the disabled population is young. As the transition proceeds, there is a major reduction in the incidence of infectious and parasitic diseases, and increases in total life expectancy. Thus, more persons survive to old age in reasonably good health and are subject to chronic and degenerative disorders, which are often accompanied by long-term disability.

4. The mean age of overall disability rises during the transition and disability becomes more compressed at older ages.

During the transition, as the age pattern of disability prevalence shifts from younger to older ages, it can be expected that there also will be a shift in disability onset to increasingly high mean ages, as well as a greater concentration of incidence around these means. At the early stages of the transition, infectious and parasitic diseases (the major causes of both death and disablement) affect all ages, and most profoundly the very young and the very old. Therefore the distribution of morbidity and disability incidence is more widely spread across ages, though low levels of life expectancy mean that the peak levels are at the younger ages.

5. During the transition, prevalence levels of disability shift from being higher for males to being higher for females.

The disability transition occurs differentially across age groups, sex, social class and geographic location. At the early stages of the epidemiologic transition young females may have mortality and morbidity levels that are equal to or greater than males, due in part to preferential treatment of boys in allocation of family resources including nutrition and more aggressive responses to illness for male children (DeRose *et al*, 2000; Yount, 1999). Poor nutrition and compromised health can lead to lower resistance of females to infectious diseases and complications associated with childbearing for women of reproductive ages. As the transition progresses, longevity increases and the characteristic survival gap favoring females over males widens, females are at higher risk of becoming disabled at older ages and of living longer with these disabilities.

6. Prevalence levels of disability are greater in lower socioeconomic groups than in higher socioeconomic groups, and the differential becomes stronger through the transition.

It is frequently held that the transmission of communicable diseases is not very selective with regard to the socioeconomic circumstances of persons. In contrast, differences in non-communicable disease incidence and prevalence appear to be strongly related to such indicators. Therefore, as the epidemiologic transition proceeds, and the disease burden shifts to chronic non-lethal causes, socioeconomic status differentials would be expected to assume greater importance. The pace of this change should accelerate during the fourth stage of the transition when factors such as differential access to care, environmental exposure, and lifestyle and behavioral risks are more salient for morbidity and mortality patterns.

7. There is a reversal in the environmental differential in disability prevalence levels so that levels of disability in urban areas become much less than in rural areas during the transition.

There is considerable evidence in industrialized countries that disability levels are lower in urban metropolitan areas than in rural areas. However, there is inconsistent evidence that disability levels are usually higher in rural areas in less developed countries. In early stages of the transition, when infectious and parasitic diseases are most prominent and mortality is high, and public health measures are not widespread (e.g. sewer systems and/or vaccinations), mortality should be higher in urban areas. Consequently, disability should be lower in urban areas. This difference would be especially pronounced in less developed countries (LDCs) in the 20th century because, despite the introduction of medical advances and infrastructural development, problems associated with rapid growth mean that the urban areas of many countries are extremely congested. As the transition proceeds, a number of possible outcomes include: (a) *ceteris paribus* these differentials should narrow because mortality from chronic diseases should – actually – not favor either environment; or (b) migration and residential patterns will increasingly affect the differentials (people with chronic diseases can move, but people with acute life-threatening ailments just die where they are). Thus, the rural/urban differential may reflect other factors, such as differential access to health care.

8. Prevalence levels of disablement increase during the transition due to heightened social awareness of health and disease.

Disability is both a product of physiological impairments and also a social construct that is influenced by factors such as changes in media attention, legislation regarding disabilities, medical assessments of health and disablement, and public expectations regarding age-specific definitions of 'health'. Consequently, reported levels of disability prevalence may be higher at times during the course of the transition, particularly in more developed countries, as individuals become increasingly aware of the symptoms associated with chronic diseases and develop higher expectations of functional health, even at older ages.

9. During the transition, the years of healthy life expectancy (HLE) rise with increasing life expectancy, though the percentage of HLE relative to total remaining life expectancy is expected to decline.

While populations are experiencing increases in life expectation, the issue is whether there also are increases in the number *and* proportion of expected disability-free years. Much of the research by REVES members and others through the early 1990s indicated an increase in the number of years of healthy life, but a decline in the proportion of expected healthy years, which follows the logic of the previous propositions in that the prevalence of disability should increase, particularly at older ages. However, more recent research (e.g. Crimmins *et al*, 1997; Manton *et al*, 1997) has noted a reversal of this trend. Thus, increased population aging may not ultimately result in proportionately larger amounts of disabled life expectancy, particularly at older ages.

TESTING THE PROPOSITIONS

It should be noted that these nine propositions initially were derived from a general understanding of disability trends for developed and developing countries obtained from previous REVES presentations and other sources. They assume that the conditions in developing countries today are reflective of the early phases of the epidemiologic transition, and are similar to the ways in which it unfolded in the past. Additionally, the propositions refer to changes associated primarily with epidemiologic trends. To conduct an adequate assessment of this formulation required a systematic examination of empirical evidence from such sources as historical time series data, as well as from additional cross-national comparative studies.

HISTORICAL RESEARCH

In a series of papers, Elman and Myers (1997, 1999; Myers and Elman, 1996, 2000) use data from the 1880 US census to examine morbidity and disability levels and differentials at the early stages of the modern epidemiologic transition. The census collected information not only about many physical impairments (as did many other 19th century enumerations), but also data about ill-health conditions limiting normal role activities and the specific nature of these conditions. Although there are quality considerations that limit the use of these data, nonetheless they provide national information for individuals in households that has not been available until the past few decades in the US. The data are drawn from the IPUMS (Integrated Public Use Microanalytic Series) automated datasets, which contain US census samples for the periodic censuses since 1850.

The cross-sectional results largely confirm the propositions on disabilities at the early stages of the transition, as presented earlier. The prevalence levels of disabilities (measured in various ways) tend to be low (Proposition 1), and chronic diseases and disabilities rise with age as infectious diseases decline in importance (Propositions 2 and 3), with male morbidity and disability levels greater than for females and of a more serious nature (Proposition 5). Rural prevalence levels of disability were found to be higher than urban in 1880 (Proposition 7). In the United States at the end of the 19th century, morbidity levels, as well as mortality levels, were higher in urban areas due to poorer public health conditions (Condran and Crimmins, 1980). US mortality rates first declined in rural areas (Condran and Crimmins, 1980).

Although these findings are for only one date, they are consistent with what might be expected at this particular time in a transition. Life table calculations also were made and show that life expectancy was generally low, but that proportionate health expectancy was quite high (Myers and Elman, 1996). At age 50, 94.4% of remaining life for males and 95.6% for females could be expected to be lived disability free. Using cohort life table estimates made only small improvements in total life expectancy and health expectancy (Myers and Elman, 2000). These findings are consistent with Proposition 9.

In previous REVES presentations, Alter and Riley (1997; Riley, 1993) have analyzed patterns of sickness incidence and duration, using local friendly society records in Great Britain for the late 18th through early 20th century. The friendly societies were organized to provide partial wage compensation for periods of illness. To join a friendly society, the potential member had to be considered well or fit by society members and the society's medical practitioner. Thus, the records do not represent all adult workers during the periods covered.

The 'sickness' records characterize patterns of limitations in major/work activities, which can be used as a general definition of disability. Their research indicates that from the late 1700s to mid-1800s, the total sickness time for workers was a quite small proportion of the adult life course. During the 19th century the incidence of sickness episodes decreased, whereas the duration of sickness time increased (Riley, 1993). Transition models between wellness, periods of sickness and recovery over time also indicate decreases in sickness incidence and increases in sickness duration for the period 1779–1929 (Alter and Riley, 1997). Both sets of findings lend support to Proposition 1. Although the friendly society data are not representative of all adult workers, the trend of results does follow expected changes in morbidity and disability over the transition with decreases in incidence rates and increases in duration, which leads to higher prevalence rates.

CROSS-NATIONAL COMPARISONS

Since developing the disability transition propositions, Lamb and Myers (1999; Lamb et al, 1994; Lamb, 1996, 1999) have used data from the WHO regional studies of Health and Social Aspects of Aging to compare cross-national patterns of health, disability and healthy life expectancy among older adults.

The WHO regional studies, conducted under the direction of Gary R. Andrews, collected individual-level data from non-institutionalized persons age 60 years and older in the Western Pacific, Eastern Mediterranean and Southeast Asian regions.

In general, the results support a number of the propositions on disability transitions over levels of development. A large proportion of expected life years were to be spent in good health, and countries with higher levels of development (as measured, e.g., by life expectancy at age 65 or the proportion surviving to age 65) had higher prevalences of disability (Lamb *et al*, 1994; Lamb and Myers, 1999; Lamb, 1999). Using a Grade of Membership model of functional and emotional disability profiles, Lamb (1996) found that of nine countries studied, the least developed in terms of health and economic indicators (i.e., Burma (Myanmar) and Indonesia) had the highest probabilities associated with the functionally healthy profiles and lower non-significant probabilities associated with the frail profiles. In a comparative study of successful aging in Indonesia, Sri Lanka and Thailand, Lamb and Myers (1999) indicated that the largest proportion of high successful aging was in Indonesia, the country with the smallest proportion of the population surviving to age 65. Selective survival and high case-fatality rates could work to leave greater proportions of the Indonesian elderly in excellent health. Such findings lend support to Propositions 1 and 3.

Regarding the assessment of socioeconomic differentials, Lamb and Myers have used the self-report of literacy as a measure of economic status. A study of elderly people in Bahrain, Egypt, Jordan and Tunisia indicated that those who were literate had much higher odds for having no problems with six Katz-type activities of daily living (Lamb *et al*, 1994). The largest odds ratio was for Egypt, which had the highest proportion of literate elders.

These results are limited in scope for testing the disability propositions, in that only older adults comprise the samples and there is little information regarding the causal factors associated with functional problems. However, taken together, the trend of these findings warrants further examination of the disability transition propositions with samples of a broader age range in a variety of settings.

THEORETICAL CONSIDERATIONS

Several issues have arisen from consideration of the Omran formulation. The epidemiologic transition has been criticized for its lack of specificity with regard to causes of death in particular. Smith (1994) has questioned whether it needs to fulfill equilibrium considerations (e.g. have feedback that returns the system to a steady state), and whether sequential transition models are appropriate. These are general issues with all theoretical formulations. To take one example, the model is sometimes dismissed as simply a set of 'empirical generalizations'. Don't all valid theories have to conform to empirical testing of their propositions? As long as these propositions are explicitly stated and collectively describe a system, the formulation seems appropriate. In general, there are three issues at stake in these modeling efforts.

One, the patterns of the variables generally form linear and unidirectional sequences over time. It is appropriate to add another stage to the model that reverses course or offers other dimensions, as, for example, in noting a new transition in which infectious diseases increase or non-communicable diseases are reduced.

Two, Omran followed up his original formulation by adding a set of alternative model paths depending mainly on the tempo of change. How suitable is it to create a number of sub-models that describe conditions in various developing and developed regions? There are temporal, social, economic and regional influences on population health. Thus, it would seem appropriate to incorporate such factors in sub-models of disability transitions.

Finally, is not one of the critical elements of a theory, as opposed to a descriptive model, to have sets of explanations? These would include both proximate determinants as well as distal factors, both of which are often lacking from theoretical formulations.

Overall, the transition models and sub-component models of change in population health and morbidity signal the possibility of a transition in the *conceptualization* of population health. When the consequences of illness were death (or recovery), the concern was of population survival. Hence, it was most useful to consider mortality rates as the primary indicator of population health. Comparisons of crude death rates, infant mortality rates or average life expectancy measures are commonly used in such analyses. However, as increasing proportions of populations survive the diseases of infancy and childhood, the emphasis has shifted to a focus on disabilities as a way of representing population health, and particularly adult health. The diseases of later life result in disablement. Thus, the social effects of morbid conditions, especially those that are chronic and degenerative conditions, are the primary concern.

The focus of future research must be on a better understanding of the complex processes that encompass health, disease and disability, particularly among older persons. The examination of such dynamics will aid in an understanding of the determinants of population health. Recent developments in population health and well-being, such as declines in the prevalence of elderly functional disability, the global rise of infectious diseases and the increase in life expectancy at the oldest old ages, signal dynamic changes that continue to occur. At issue is the development of testable propositions and reliable diachronic research to understand change and continuity in population health. For example, we cannot predict solely from theoretical models how comorbidities and disabilities will cluster within a population, especially under conditions of low mortality. It is imperative that future research effectively demonstrates the interplay of interdisciplinary theoretical formulations (from genetics to social networks to social and physical environmental contextual determinants) and diverse research methodologies to model trends of population health and health transitions.

REFERENCES

Alter, G. and Riley, J. (1989) 'Frailty, sickness and death: models of morbidity and mortality in historical populations', *Population Studies* 43, 25–45.

Alter, G. and Riley, J. (1997) 'Sickness, recovery, and sickness redux: transitions into and out of sickness in nineteenth-century Britain', in 10th Work-group meeting REVES, Tokyo, October.

Armstrong, G.L., Conn, L.A. and Pinner, R.W. (1999) 'Trends in infectious disease mortality in the United States during the 20th century', *Journal of the American Medical Association* 281, 61–66.

Barrett, R., Kuzawa, C.W., McDade, T. and Armelagos, G.J. (1998) 'Emerging and re-emerging infectious diseases: the third epidemiological transition', *Annual Review of Anthropology* 27, 247–271.

Condran, G. and Crimmins, E. (1980) 'Mortality differentials between rural and urban areas of states in the northeastern United States 1890–1900', *Journal of Historical Geography* 6, 179–202.

Crimmins, E.M., Saito, Y. and Ingegneri, D. (1997) 'Trends in disability-free life expectancy in the United States, 1970–90', *Population and Development Review* 23, 555–572.

DeRose, L.F., Das, M. and Millman, S.R. (2000) 'Does female disadvantage mean lower access to food?', *Population and Development Review* 26, 517–547.

Douglas, R.M., Jones, G. and D'Souza, R.M. (eds) (1996) 'The shaping of fertility and mortality declines: the contemporary demographic transition', *Health Transition Review* (Suppl.) 6.

Elman, C. and Myers, G. (1997) 'Age and sex-differentials in morbidity at the start of an epidemiological transition: returns from the 1880 US census', *Social Science and Medicine* 45, 943–956.

Elman, C. and Myers, G. (1999) 'Geographic morbidity differentials in the late nineteenth-century United States', *Demography* 36, 429–443.

Fogel, R.W. and Costa, D.L. (1997) 'A theory of technophysio evolution, with some implications for forecasting population, health care costs, and pension costs', *Demography* 34, 49–66.

Friedlander, D. (1983) 'Demographic responses and socio-economic structure: population processes in England and Wales in the nineteenth century', *Demography* 20, 249–272.

Gaylin, D.S. and Kates, J. (1997) 'Refocusing the lens: epidemiologic transition theory, mortality differentials and the AIDS pandemic', *Social Science and Medicine* 44, 609–613.

Kan, S.H. and Kim, Y. (1982) 'Cause-structure of post-transitional mortality decline: the case of Utah', *Social Science Journal* 19, 63–71.

Katz, S., Branch, L.G., Branson, M.H., Papsidero, J.A., Beck, J.C. and Greer, D.S. (1983) 'Active life expectancy', *New England Journal of Medicine* 309, 1218–1224.

Lamb, V.L. (1996) 'A cross-national study of quality of life factors associated with patterns of elderly disablement', *Social Science and Medicine* 42, 363–377.

Lamb, V.L. (1999) *Active life expectancy of the elderly in selected Asian countries*. Tokyo: Nihon University Population Research Institute. (NUPRI Research Paper Series No 69).

Lamb, V.L. and Myers, G.C. (1999) 'A comparative study of successful aging in three Asian countries', *Population Research and Policy Review* 18, 433–449.

Lamb, V.L., Myers, G.C. and Andrews, G.R. (1994) 'Healthy life expectancy of the elderly in Eastern Mediterranean countries', in Mathers, C., McCallum, J. and Robine, J-M. (eds) *Advances in Health Expectancies*. Canberra: Australian Institute of Health and Welfare.

Landry, A. (1934) *La révolution démographique; études et essai sur les problèmes de population*. Paris: Sirey.

Manton, K.G. (1990) 'Mortality and morbidity', in Binstock, R.H. and George, L.K. (eds) *Handbook of Aging and the Social Sciences*. New York: Academic Press.

Manton, K.G. (1999) 'Dynamic paradigms for human mortality and aging', *Journal of Gerontology* 54A, B247–B254.

Manton, K.G., Corder, L. and Stallard, E. (1997) 'Chronic disability trends in the US elderly populations 1982 to 1994', *Proceedings of the National Academy of Sciences* 94, 2593–2598.

Myers, G.C. and Elman, C. (1996) 'Patterns of Health Status in Early America: Results from the 1880 US Census'. Presented at the 9th Meeting of the Network on Health Expectancy (REVES), Rome, Italy.

Myers, G.C. and Elman, C. (2000) 'Morbidity, disability, and mortality in the United States in the late 19th century: differentials and social implications', in 10th Entretiens du Centre Jacques Cartier.

Myers, G.C. and Lamb, V.L. (1993) 'Theoretical perspectives on healthy life expectancy', in Robine, J-M., Mathers, C.D., Bone, M.R. and Romieu, I. (eds) *Calculation of Health Expectancies: Harmonization, Consensus Achieved and Future Perspectives*. Montrouge: John Libbey Eurotext.

Myers, G.C. and Manton, K.G. (1987) 'The rate of population aging: new view of epidemiologic transitions', in Maddox, G.L. and Busse E.W. (eds) *Aging: The Universal Human Experience*. New York: Springer.

Nathanson, C.A. (1996) 'Disease prevention as social change: toward a theory of public health', *Population and Development Review* 22, 609–637.

Notestein, F.W. (1945) 'Demographic studies of selected areas of rapid growth', in *Proceedings of the Round Table on Population Problems, Twenty-second Annual Conference of the Milbank Memorial Fund*. New York: Milbank Memorial Fund.

Olshansky, S.J. and Ault, A.B. (1986) 'The fourth stage of the epidemiologic transition: the age of delayed degenerative diseases', *Milbank Quarterly* 64, 355–391.

Olshansky, S.J., Carnes, B., Rogers, R.G. and Smith, L. (1997) 'Infectious diseases – new and ancient threats to world health', *Population Bulletin* 52(2).

Omram, A.R. (1971) 'The epidemiologic transition: a theory of the epidemiology of population change', *Milbank Memorial Fund Quarterly* 49, 509–538.

Omram, A.R. (1983) 'The epidemiologic transition theory: a preliminary update', *Journal of Tropical Pediatrics* 29, 305–316.

Pope, A.M. and Tarlov, A.R. (eds) (1991) *Disability in America: Toward a National Agenda for Prevention*. Washington, DC: National Academy Press.

Popkin, B.M. (1993) 'Nutritional patterns and transitions', *Population and Development Review* 19, 138–157.

Riley, J.C. (1993) 'Active life expectancy during the long mortality decline: the transition from brief to protracted sickness', in Robine, J-M., Mathers, C.D., Bone, M.R. and Romieu, I. (eds) *Calculation of Health Expectancies: Harmonization, Consensus Achieved and Future Perspectives*. Montrouge: John Libbey Eurotext.

Riley, J.C. and Alter, G. (1996) 'The sick and the well: adult health in Britain during the health transition', *Health Transition Review* 6, 19–44.

Rogers, A. (1989) 'The elderly mobility transition: growth, concentration, and tempo', *Research on Aging* 11, 3–32.

Rogers, R.G. and Hackenberg, R. (1987) 'Extending epidemiologic transition theory: a new stage', *Social Biology* 34, 234–243.

Scott, S. and Duncan, C.J. (2000) 'Interacting effects of nutrition and social class differentials on fertility and infant mortality in a pre-industrial population', *Population Studies* 54, 71–87.

Smith, L.R. (1994) 'Reflections on the next stage of the epidemiological transition', in Mathers, C., McCallum, J. and Robine, J-M. (eds) *Advances in Health Expectancies*. Canberra: Australian Institute of Health and Welfare.

United Nations (1986) *Disability: Situation, Strategies and Policies*. New York: United Nations (ST/ESA/176).

Vallin, J. (1993) 'Life expectancy: past, present and future possibilities', in Robine, J-M., Mathers, C.D., Bone, M.R. and Romieu, I. (eds) *Calculation of Health Expectancies: Harmonization, Consensus Achieved and Future Perspectives*. Montrouge: John Libbey Eurotext.

Verbrugge, L.M. and Patrick, D.L. (1995) 'Seven chronic conditions: their impact on US adults' activity levels and use of medical services', *American Journal of Public Health* 85, 173–182.

Verbrugge, L.M., Lepkowski, J.M. and Imanaka, Y. (1989) 'Comorbidity and its impact on disability', *Milbank Quarterly* 67, 450–484.

Verbrugge, L.M., Lepkowski, J.M. and Konkol, L.L. (1991) 'Levels of disability among US adults with arthritis', *Journal of Gerontology* 46, S71–S83.

World Health Organization (1980) *International Classification of Impairments, Disabilities, and Handicaps*. Geneva: World Health Organization.

Yount, K.M. (1999) 'Persistent inequalities: women's status and the differential treatment of sick boys and girls. A case study of Minia, Egypt', PhD dissertation. Baltimore: Johns Hopkins University.

Zelinsky, W. (1971) 'The hypothesis of the mobility transition', *Geography Review* 61, 219–249.

4

Trends in Health Expectancies

JEAN-MARIE ROBINE, ISABELLE ROMIEU and JEAN-PIERRE MICHEL*

INSERM, Montpellier, France and *Institutions Universitaires de Gériatrie, Geneva, Switzerland

The analysis and interpretation of chronological series of disability-free life expectancy (DFLE) was one of the initial aims of the Network on Health Expectancy and the Disability Process (REVES). The argument was as follows:

> Several countries have now put together chronological series of DFLE using a common procedure: USA (1966–1976), England and Wales (1976, 1981, 1985), Quebec, Canada (1978, 1987). How should observed deviations in DFLE be interpreted? Should the new observed value of DFLE be compared to the preceding one or to an expected value, such as an expected value of DFLE in which mortality alone evolves while disability stagnates? (Introduction to the Network, February 1989)

In the mid-1970s the rapid increase in life expectancy (LE) at birth was assumed to have ended in low mortality countries. The sustained and continuous increase in LE observed over the 1980s was totally unexpected. The drop in the mortality of the oldest old was particularly surprising and led many to wonder whether people only escaped death from heart disease to live in poor health (Fuchs, 1984). This question has fuelled an important debate about the relationship between changes in mortality and morbidity. Historically the increase in LE meant an improvement in the health status of the population. This was no longer necessarily the case, because chronic diseases had replaced, or were progressively replacing, acute diseases such as infectious diseases. The risk of becoming ill was not solely linked to the risk of dying but also to the risk of becoming disabled (Riley, 1990). Thus, with a constant recovery rate, if the risk of dying diminished more than the risk of becoming ill, the risk of being ill increased.

In the absence of pertinent data on changes in morbidity, the relationships between changes in these risks were debated, gradually focusing on three main theories, the expansion of morbidity, dynamic equilibrium and the

Determining Health Expectancies. Edited by J-M. Robine, C. Jagger, C.D. Mathers, E.M. Crimmins and R.M. Suzman.
© 2003 John Wiley & Sons, Ltd

compression of morbidity (Manton, 1982; Robine, 1986; Crimmins, 1990) (see Chapter 2). In the 1980s various observations summarized by Lois Verbrugge in a paper 'Longer life but worsening health' (Verbrugge, 1984)[1] contributed strongly to a pessimistic view about the changes in population health status with declining mortality. The debate has continued until now, continually renewed with the availability of new data on trends in health expectancy and health status (see below).

THE DISABLEMENT PROCESS

The concept of 'health state expectancy' (HSE), a composite measure of morbidity and mortality (DFLE or active life expectancy (ALE)), has been developed in order to monitor the quality of the years of life gained, particularly for older people (Sanders, 1964; Sullivan, 1971). According to Sanders, 'In such an analysis we would not only determine for each age the probability of survival, but also the subsidiary probabilities of those surviving on the basis of their functional effectiveness. This would range from individuals who were completely dependent on others, even for carrying on their daily living activities, to those fully equipped to carry on with no apparent handicap all the functions characteristic of their age and sex' (Sanders, 1964).

Chronic diseases have numerous and varying consequences, ranging from the absence of any discomfort to death, making them the object of an international classification (WHO, 1980, 2001). Adding the risks of disability to the risks of disease permitted a considerable improvement in models of health. The concept of disability allowed rigorous definition of the theories summarized above.

The various theories on changes in the health status of populations could be described in terms of relative changes in LE and various HSE like DFLE (Robine, 1986, 1992). The HSE might be good indicators for estimating change in the health of population while the mortality rate has been falling and the demographic transition has been continuing. For example, the pandemic theory assumes a decrease in the proportion of healthy years in LE (Robine et al, 1991). Precise definitions of the various theories, assumptions and scenarios in terms of relative changes in LE and various HSE were the topics of several studies since the beginning of the REVES network (Robine, 1986, 1991; Robine and Mathers, 1993, Robine et al, 1996a; Nusselder et al, 1996; Nusselder, 1998) (see Chapter 2 dealing with the compression of morbidity). Yet, the application of the general model of health transition (Chapter 2, Figure 2.1) to the 1981 and 1991 French data showed that the increase in LE was accompanied by a parallel increase in

[1] There was obviously a link to the book 'Doing Better but Feeling Worse: Health in the United States' edited by John H. Knowles, in 1975.

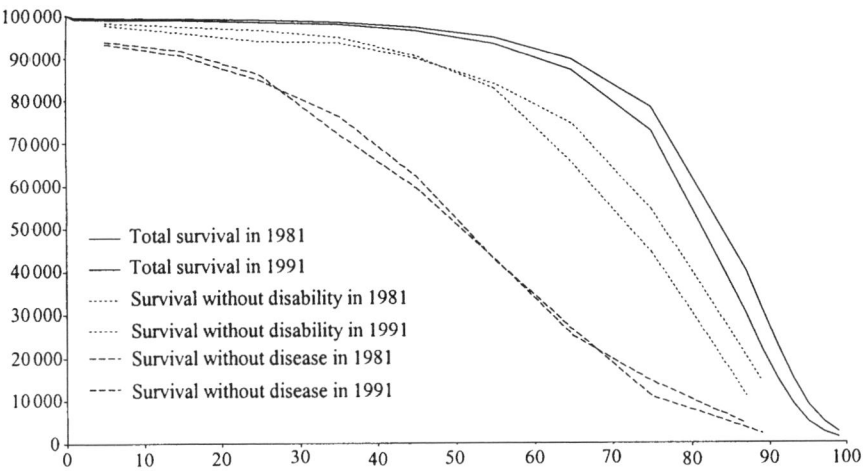

Figure 4.1. Survival without disease and survival without disability (WHO model, 1984) France, 1981 and 1991, females.
Source: Robine, J.M., Mormiche, P. and Cambois, E. (1996) Evolution des courbes de survie totale, sans maladie chronique et sans incapacité en France de 1981 à 1991: application d'un modèle de l'OMS. *Annales de Démographie Historique* 99–115. Reproduced with permission

DFLE, while LE without chronic diseases has remained constant (Robine *et al*, 1996b) (Figure 4.1). This apparent contradiction in the changes in morbidity and disability provides an example of the theory of dynamic equilibrium proposed by Manton in 1982. With the decline in mortality, the prevalence of chronic diseases increased but these diseases were, on average, less severe and less often resulted in disability (Manton, 1982).

In contrast to mortality, notions such as health or morbidity are difficult to define. Health is 'a composite of current state and prognosis (i.e. the probability of moving to other states) that occurs throughout an individual's life' (Fanshel and Bush, 1970). In this way health is not only, 'the ability to function now, but the outlook for future functional ability' (Fanshel, 1972). This life-course definition of health is the justification for the use of health state expectancies as fundamental health indicators for populations, because they measure the lifetime spent in different health states.

CHRONOLOGICAL SERIES

Only provision of time series of both LE and HSE will make it possible to answer the questions raised earlier in this chapter and decide which theoretical approach is supported. This explains why REVES devoted several sessions of its meetings to the presentation and analysis of empirical chronological series on disability or time series on HSE. Since the creation of REVES, several series have been presented:

- Various HSE from Australia, Canada, China, England and Wales, Finland, France, Japan, the Netherlands, Sweden, Taiwan and the United States.[2]
- Mental health series in the Netherlands and in the United States[3] and
- HSE trends by socioeconomic status (SES) in Sweden, Finland, United States and France[4] (see Chapter 5: Social Inequalities).

In addition, several theoretical or methodological papers dealing with the interpretation of chronological series were presented,[5] in particular on changes in disability during the epidemiological transition, in term of incidence, prevalence, severity level, and recovery (see Chapter 3).

TIMES SERIES ON DISABILITY DATA

After the creation of REVES, publications and analysis of time series on disability, without DFLE calculation, continued especially in the United States, focusing on various aspects of functional status. Many authors employed the same data, particularly data from the American National Health Interview Survey (NHIS). Some authors continued to note that an increase in disability is not evident in the old (Verbrugge, 1989). Some authors underlined that changes in the disability prevalence at the older ages were linked to the drop of the mortality rate at these ages (Crimmins, 1990; Riley, 1990).

Pandemic or Disability Decline in North America

In 1991, Crimmins and Ingegneri pointed out that for those aged 45 to 75, activity restriction increased from 1969 to 1975, levelled off from 1975 to 1982 and decreased from 1982 to 1988 (the last year of NHIS observation at that time). Beyond 75 years of age, there was not a clear trend from 1969 to 1988.

---

[2] Australia (Mathers, 1991a, 1994; Mathers and Jain, 1999), Canada (Brunelle, 1991; Wilkins and Adams, 1992; Wilkins et al, 1994; Wilkins and Chen, 1995; Martel and Bélanger, 2000), China (Qiao, 1997), England and Wales (Bone, 1991; Jagger and Clarke, 1991; Bebbington and Wittenberg, 1999; Kelly and Baker, 2000), Finland (Sihvonen et al, 1996), France (Robine, 1994; Cambois and Robine, 1999), Japan (Koizumi, 1994), the Netherlands (Boshuizen, 1991; Perenboom et al, 1993; Deeg et al, 1994, 1996; Perenboom et al, 2000), Sweden (Pettersson, 1995), Taiwan (Tu and Chen, 1992, 1994, 1995; Chen et al, 1996; Tu et al, 1997) and the United States (Colvez, 1992; Corder et al, 1992; Crimmins et al, 1992a, 1992b; Osborn, 1992; Crimmins and Saito, 1997a; McClellan and Yan, 2000).
[3] Perenboom and van de Water, 1997; Sauvaget et al, 1997.
[4] Pettersson, 1995; Sihvonen et al, 1996; Crimmins and Saito, 1993, 2001; Cambois and Robine, 1999; Cambois et al, 2001.
[5] Robine, 1991; van de Water, 1991; Brunelle, 1993; Crystal et al, 1993; Myers and Lamb, 1993; Riley, 1993; Robine and Mathers, 1993; Smith, 1994; Riley and Alter, 1995; Myers and Elman, 1996; Nusselder et al, 1996; Alter and Riley, 1997; Lamb, 1999.

Using comparable data from two other surveys, the 1962 and 1975 Survey of Older Population and the 1984 Supplement on Aging (SOA-NHIS), the same authors showed a slight improvement in health for 65+ people during a 25-year period (Crimmins and Ingegneri, 1991). In 1992 Preston, by analysing the gains in the level of education from one cohort to another, brought out new elements which could explain the improvement in health in older populations in the United States (Preston, 1992).

Manton *et al*, using data from the National Long Term Care Study (NLTCS, 1982, 1984 and 1989), showed that in the 65+ population, the prevalence of IADL (instrumental activities of daily living) disability decreased from 1982 to 1989 whereas the prevalence of ADL disability and the prevalence of institutional placement remained stable (Manton *et al*, 1993a, 1993b). Freedman and Soldo, by combining the NLTCS data (1982–1989) with the NHIS data and the Longitudinal Study of Aging (LSOA, 1984–1990), published a first report on changes in disability in the old in the United States confirming Manton's results (Freedman and Soldo, 1994). Later Manton *et al* extended their conclusions to 1994 (Manton *et al*, 1995, 1997, 1998) and finally to 1999. According to Manton, the main findings are an acceleration of the decline in chronic disability prevalence from 1994 to 1999 compared with 1989 to 1994, the large relative and absolute drop in institutional use and a greater decline for black Americans after 1989 (Manton and Gu, 2001). In addition, the prevalence of severe dementia for the US age 65 and older population appears to decline significantly from 1982 to 1999 when severe dementia is measured by the inability to undergo a cognitive battery such as the Short Portable Mental Status Questionnaire (SPMSQ) or the Mini-Mental State Examination (MMSE) and to answer a questionnaire without the help of a proxy (Corder and Manton, 2001).

In 1995, using once again the NHIS data, Waidmann *et al* reconsidered the existence of a turning point in the 1980s at least in the United States (see above Crimmins and Ingegneri, 1991). Like their predecessors, they re-examined all the available data and did not find a clear trend for the oldest old (70 years and over) from 1969 to 1981. This did not prevent them from taking for granted that the health of the young adult and the elderly deteriorated during the 1970s and then improved during the 1980s. Then, Waidmann *et al*, comparing their results to the 'failure of success' hypothesis (i.e., the pandemic or expansion of morbidity), noted that the improvement in survival was highest among the oldest (over the age of 70), while the apparent deterioration in health was more centred on the youngest from 45 to 69 years of age (Waidmann *et al*, 1995). On the other hand, Crimmins *et al* pointed out that the variations observed with the 1984–1990 LSOA or the 1982–1993 NHIS looked more like fluctuations than clear trends (Crimmins, 1996; Crimmins *et al*, 1997b).[6] However, in the

---

[6] See also Crimmins and Ingegneri 1993; Crimmins, 1997; Crimmins and Saito, 1997b.

age range from 30 to 69 years disability increased for the later born cohorts (Reynolds *et al*, 1998) and the ability to work improved significantly for those in their 60s (Crimmins *et al*, 1999).

But, while there was a growing body of evidence for a decline in disability rates among the elderly, estimates of the extent of the fall of these disability rates were imprecise. A few studies showed smaller declines or no sustained increase in disability. Others, which in the past had shown either increasing disability or no change over time, now showed statistically significant declines in elderly disability rates (Waidman and Manton, 1998). Documenting her argument with data from the Union Army pensions, indicating a long-term decline in chronic diseases for older men in the United States (50 to 74 years) between 1900–1910 and more recent periods, Costa showed that the shift from manual to white-collar jobs was the main determinant of this transition (Costa, 2000). In the Framingham Heart Study covering the second part of the 20th century, at the same age between 55 and 70 years, there was substantially less disability in the offspring cohort than in the original cohort. The secular decline in disability was strongly evident among individuals with chronic diseases. In addition, fewer offspring perceived their health as fair or poor and fewer had chronic diseases (Allaire *et al*, 1999). For the last years of the 20th century, using the 1992–1996 Medicare Current Beneficiary Surveys (MCBS), Waidmann and Liu found at age 65 years and over a consistent decline in the rate of IADL disability.[7] Trends toward a more educated elderly cohort, already indicated by Preston (see above), could only partially explain the disability decline (Waidmann and Liu, 2000; Crimmins *et al*, 1999).

Analysis carried out by Freedman and Martin, using data from the Survey of Income and Program Participation (SIPP), shown that between 1984 and 1993 four functional abilities – vision of printed characters, lifting and carrying a sack of roughly 10 lb, climbing stairs and walking a quarter of a mile (about three city blocks) – increased significantly (Freedman and Martin, 1998). Setting aside the question of vision, which depends partly on the wearing of glasses, these results clearly suggested an improvement in physical vigour. Among the four considered explanatory variables, education was the most important in accounting for this trend. This analysis suggested that future changes in education would continue to contribute to improvements in functioning (Freedman and Martin, 1999). In addition, using the 1993 Asset and Health Dynamics of the Oldest Old study (AHEAD) and the Health and Retirement Survey (HRS), Freedman *et al* showed that the percentage of the non-institutionalized population aged 70 years and older with severe cognitive impairment declined from 6.1% in 1993 to 3.6% in 1998. According to the authors, this cognitive functioning improvement

---

[7] The decline in ADL disability was largely concentrated in the last year, in 1996.

might account for much of the observed improvement in IADL function (Freedman *et al*, 2001).

Again analysing the NHIS data from 1982 to 1996 for persons aged 70 and over, Schoeni *et al* have recently shown that most of the decline in disability took place between 1982 and 1986 with little change after 1986. Most of the decline involves routine activity needs, not personal care needs. The only group to experience improvements were elderly persons with more than a high school degree (Schoeni *et al*, 2001). Thus the most recent results from the NHIS (Schoeni *et al*, 2001), the NLTCS (Manton *et al*, 1997; Manton and Gu, 2001) and the MCBS (Waidmann and Liu, 2000) brought contradictory conclusions for the United States, raising again concerns about the disability trend among old people.

For Canada as a whole, despite similar methodology, large increases in disability were observed in the results of the Health and Activity Limitations Survey (HALS) between 1986 and 1991. However, the differences were not significant beyond the age of 55 (LaRoche and Morin, 1994). On the other hand, researchers concluded from a Manitoba study that there was a deterioration in the functional health in the elderly population, but the ADL questions were markedly changed between the two surveys (Roos *et al*, 1993). In Quebec, where the 1998 Health and Activity Limitations Survey is comparable to the 1986 and 1991 surveys, an increase in disability prevalence has been observed for all age groups, resulting from a large increase in mild disability combined with a decrease in moderate and severe disability (Saucier and Lafontaine, 2001).

Disability Changes in Europe and Japan

Outside of North America, during the same period of time, different studies have shown an improvement in functional health for the elderly in terms of ADL in Sweden (Svanborg, 1988) and in the United Kingdom (Jagger *et al*, 1991; Spiers *et al*, 1996). In this last country, the decrease in the inability to carry out ADL was particularly clear over the period from 1976 to 1994 (Grundy, 1997). In France, an improvement in the health of the elderly living at home was observed between 1980 and 1991, as well as the near stability in health of those residing in institutions. Despite an increase in the survival of older people in France, the health of the elderly population, wherever their place of residence, improved between 1980 and 1991 (Robine *et al*, 1998). These results were similar to those already found in the Paris area for the 1965–1980 period (Mizrahi and Mizrahi, 1989, 1993, 1994).

In Finland, contradictory results were published. On the one hand, an increase in the proportion of people reporting long-standing illness from 1964 to 1996, especially among the elderly, was reported. On the other hand, a decrease in the proportion of people with ADL disabilities was noted from 1986 to 1994.[8] A third Finnish study attested a decrease in the proportion of people reporting poor or rather poor health in the age group 55 to 64 years from 1979 to 1998 (Aromaa *et al*, 1999). In Switzerland, in the French cantons, from 1979 to 1994 there was a clear increase in ADL performances and in mobility. Hearing abilities improved over the age of 80 and perceived health improved for all the older population (Lalive d'Epinay *et al*, 2000).

According to Grundy *et al* the prevalence of disability reported in the 1996/7 UK disability survey was much higher than in the earlier 1985 survey of disabled adults in private households. The authors underlined that this last result was not in accordance with trends from the United States (Grundy *et al*, 1999). It was more in line with the Labour Force Survey in Great Britain which showed an important increase, year after year, in the disability rate at working age for the period 1984–1996 (Cousins *et al*, 1998). However, the detailed data revealed a decrease in the prevalence of the most severe levels of disability and an increase in the prevalence of the least severe levels, especially above the age of 75 years. The decrease in the prevalence of the most severe levels of disability was in line with the decrease in the inability to carry out ADL for the period 1976–1994, noted above (Grundy, 1997).

In Japan, the data from the 1992, 1995 and 1998 Comprehensive Survey of Living Conditions of the People on Health and Welfare suggest a trend to worsening health when looking at the ability/inability of people aged 65 and over (the most severe disability level) to perform at least one ADL even if the need for help with ADL in general declined (Saito, 2001).

A Paradoxical Situation

Finally, the situation in the United States and in Europe was quite paradoxical. On the one hand, most of the studies on disability found a general rise in disability. On the other hand, close examination of all these studies, particularly those studying the United States, showed the following: (1) the differences recorded in children (learning difficulties, etc.) were strongly linked to the development of different educational programmes; (2) the inability to work in adults was strongly linked to the development of social programmes (development and promotion of disability pensions) and to the condition of the labour market; (3) ADL disabilities did not increase in the elderly, and these measures were the least susceptible to changes in the social environment; (4) and finally, whatever the age studied, the most severe forms of disability were not increasing (Robine, 2000). To summarize the whole body of data collected since the end of the 1960s, it appeared that not a single study in the United

---

[8] However, two cohort studies have shown the opposite, at a local level, for an earlier period (Anttila, 1991; Winblad, 1993).

States clearly identified deterioration in functional health in the elderly. During the 1980s, other countries began to collect data. Most series indicated an improvement in functional health, namely for ADL in England and Wales (1976–1994), Finland (1986–1994), Switzerland (1979–1994) or for discomfort in daily life in France (1980–1991). In the 1990s, American studies using new data (1984 and 1993 SIPP; 1992 and 1996 MCBS; 1993 AHEAD and 1998 HRS) suggested that global functional health (including cognitive functioning) and/or IADL disability of the elderly had improved significantly over the last few years. But other series showed contradictory results: the American NHIS data indicated no precise disability trend, while two UK disability surveys showed a global increase in disability. What could be the explanations for such differences? This was all a bit chaotic.

Extreme caution must be exercised before drawing general conclusions. But globally the results suggested that the functional status of the elderly population has improved over the last thirty years. The drop in mortality at older ages has continued to increase the proportion of over-65 survivors. This change should have or could have led to an increase in disability rates at the top of the scale, but this was not the case. However, the different components of morbidity – e.g. disease, functional status and perceived health – did not necessarily evolve in unison (Crimmins, 1996; Spiers et al, 1996). The concept of 'functional health' itself consisted in functional limitations, difficulties in performing tasks, activity restriction, and dependence. The improvement over time in ADL and IADL performances was not necessarily linked with the improvement in physical and sensory abilities such as mobility, agility, vision or hearing (Manton et al, 1993b; Freedman and Martin, 1998) or in cognitive abilities (Freedman et al, 2001).

Two hypotheses can be raised. Firstly, the fall in mortality was accompanied by a redistribution of the levels of disability with, on the one hand, a decrease in the prevalence of the most severe levels and, on the other hand, an increase in the prevalence of the least severe levels. Changes in the total prevalence of disability would depend on these opposing changes. This hypothesis, initially raised in France (Tartarin and Bouget, 1994), can be empirically verified in England and Wales (Figure 4.2). It is also observed in Quebec between 1986 and 1998 (Saucier and Lafontaine, 2001). This redistribution would explain the result of Waidmaan and Liu showing an increase over time in the proportion of physical limitations but not of disability (Waidmann and Liu, 2000). Secondly, the disability attributed to disease or old age would be in fact the consequence of the low educational and training level of the earliest cohorts. Better educated and better trained, most recent cohorts had better cognitive performances and therefore better performances for activities requiring mental skills. Cognitive abilities and IADL measures would be affected by changes in level of education. These hypotheses provide further justification for distinguishing between various concepts of health, chronic morbidity, perceived health, and

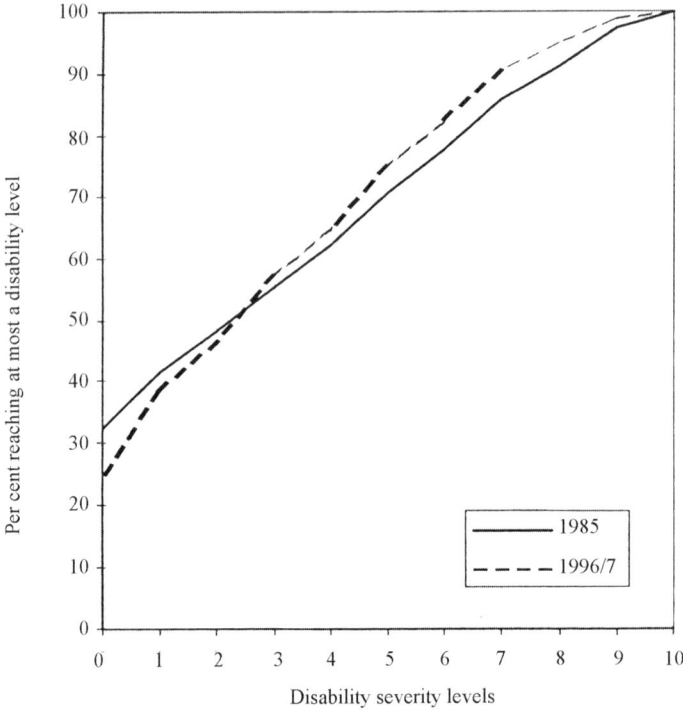

Figure 4.2. Cumulated distribution of disability severity levels, Great Britain, 1985 and 1996/7, both sexes at age 80 and over.
Source: Grundy, E., Ahlburg, D., Ali, M., *et al* (1999) *Disability in Great Britain.* HMSO, Department of Social Security (Research Report 94). Reproduced with permission

functional health. It is this multifaceted point of view which allows the calculation of health state expectancy.

CHRONOLOGICAL SERIES ON HEALTH EXPECTANCIES

In 1991, a first synthesis of time series on HSE for three countries – Australia, England and Wales and the US – concluded that overall the studies supported the theory of the 'pandemic of disabilities' (Robine *et al*, 1991). However, this work based on various DFLE calculations showed that the series of LE without severe disability supported the 'theory of equilibrium'. Following this first synthesis, most authors differentiated severe and non-severe disability in the analysis and the presentation of new series. The most recent synthesis integrated calculations from almost 50 countries including 15 time series performed in low mortality countries: Western Europe, Nordic countries, North America, Australia, Japan and New Zealand (Robine and Romieu,

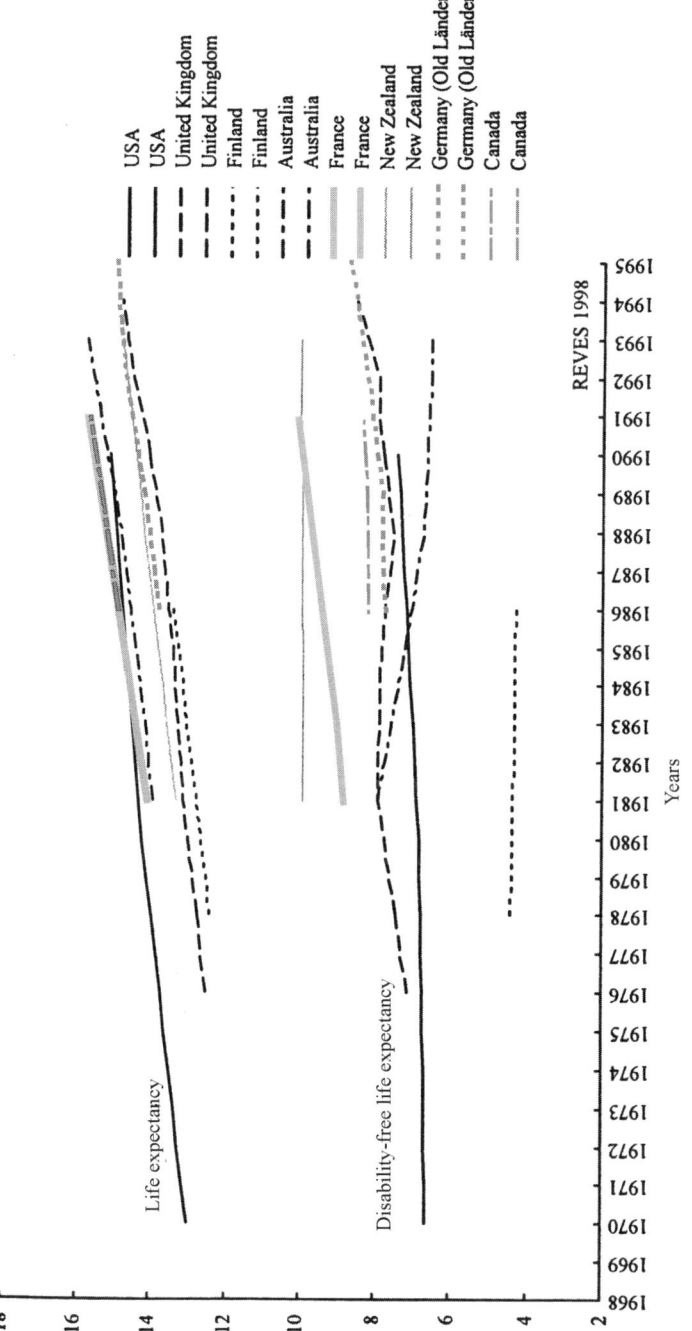

Figure 4.3. Changes in life expectancy and disability-free life expectancy – *all levels of disability combined* – at 65 years of age, in different countries, men.

Sources: Crimmins *et al*, 1989, 1997a; Bebbington and Darton, 1996; Sihvonen, 1994; Mathers, 1991b, 1996; Robine and Mormiche, 1994; Davis and Graham, 1997; Brückner, 1997; Wilkins *et al*, 1994

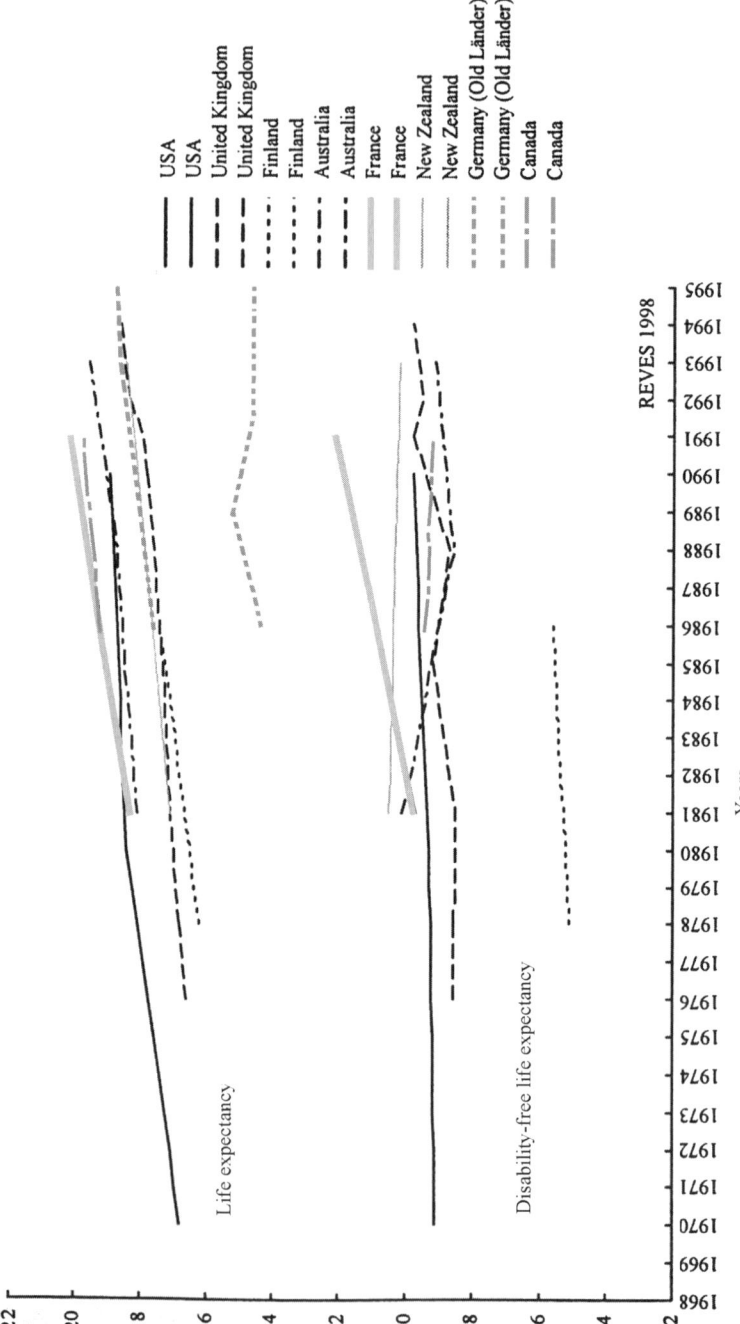

Figure 4.4. Changes in life expectancy and in disability-free life expectancy – *all levels of disability combined* – at 65 years of age, in different countries, women.
Sources: Crimmins *et al*, 1989, 1997a; Bebbington and Darton, 1996; Sihvonen, 1994; Mathers, 1991b, 1996; Robine and Mormiche, 1994; Davis and Graham, 1997; Brückner, 1997; Wilkins *et al*, 1994

1998; Robine *et al*, 1999). The data gathered cover a 25-year period, from 1970 to 1995, and could be used to compare changes in LE and DFLE (all levels of disability combined), with changes in severe DLFE.

Figures 4.3 and 4.4 show that although the increase in LE at age 65 appeared universal and regular in the low mortality countries, the same is not true for the DFLE – all disability levels combined – which appeared to have stagnated. The gains in LE might be years with disability.

Figure 4.3 presents series ranging from 1970 to 1995 of total LE and DFLE – all disability levels combined – at age 65 in men in eight different countries: Australia, Canada, Finland, France, Germany, New Zealand, the United States and the United Kingdom. The analysis of the earliest series demonstrated that DFLE – all levels combined – was stagnating. However, the relationship over time differed across countries. For instance, the Canadian and Finnish series still suggested that DFLE was levelling off, whereas the American, British, German, and French series showed that DFLE was increasing (the increase was particularly strong in France). In contrast, the Australian series showed a decrease in DFLE. Hence, no general conclusion can be firmly drawn even if the general feeling, when looking at Figure 4.4, was that while LE was increasing for the various countries, DFLE – all severity levels combined – was apparently stagnating.

Figures 4.5 and 4.6 show that severe DFLE evolved in parallel with LE in all the countries in which data were available, namely, Australia, Canada, France, Japan, the United States and the United Kingdom. This means that if the years gained in LE were years of life with disability, they were not with severe disability. A more careful look at the figures and a thorough knowledge of the data used allows one to distinguish between

- 'very' severe DFLE (institutionalization and/or bed confinement), which had been evolving at the same rate as LE since 1970 (American, French and Japanese series), and
- severe DFLE (or ALE), which had been evolving at the same rate as LE since the end of the 1980s for females (Australian and UK series, see Figure 4.6).

All these figures give the impression that (1) 'very' severe DFLE has been increasing along with LE since data has been available, (2) severe DFLE has been clearly increasing only for the last 10 years, and (3) DFLE – all levels of disability combined – has basically stagnated over the same period of time, even if most of the data show a tendency toward a slight increase at the end of this period.

Therefore, it clearly appears that DFLE has evolved very differently depending on the severity level of disability: a decrease for the most severe levels of disability (institutionalization and/or bed confinement), and an increase for the less severe levels of disability (no ADL dependency). Changes in DFLE – all levels of disability combined – are nothing else than the result of these opposite changes.

In Great Britain, for instance, between 1981 and 1995, LE at 65 years of age increased continuously from 13.0 to 14.7 years for males and from 16.9 to 18.3 years for females. But LE free of long-standing illness increased only slightly from 7.6 to 8.3 years for males and from 8.5 to 9.5 years for females (Kelly and Baker, 2000). This suggests that applying the general model of health transition (WHO, 1984) to the available data in England and Wales (Bone et al, 1995; Grundy, 1997; Grundy et al, 1999; Kelly and Baker, 2000) would bring similar conclusions to those of its previous application to French data (Robine et al, 1996b). An increase in LE in England and Wales between 1981 and 1995 was accompanied by a parallel increase in severe DFLE (or ALE). During the same period of time, LE free of limiting long-standing illness remained constant or increased slightly and DFLE – all levels combined – stagnated.

DFLE calculations and analysis suggest that a vital key to the interpretation of time series is the level of severity of disability. The more severe the levels, the more similar the changes. The less severe the levels, the more the change varies from one country to another. The analysis of time series of DFLE by severity level in comparison to trends in total LE and LE without disabling chronic disease or LE without long-standing illness supports the 'theory of dynamic equilibrium', which partly explains the increase in LE by a slowing down in the rate of progression of chronic diseases (Manton, 1982). In the low mortality countries, the decline in mortality among the oldest old during the 1980s and the 1990s is accompanied by an increase in the prevalence of chronic diseases, and maybe by an increase in the total prevalence of disability, but these diseases are on the average less severe and lead less often to severe levels of disability. The results indicate that at worst the increase in LE is accompanied by a pandemic of light and moderate, but not of severe disabilities.

One of the most recent studies, distinguishing functional limitations (seeing, hearing, walking difficulties) which can be seen as a pre-disability level from activity restrictions, provides another example illustrating a possible redistribution of disability severity levels. In Quebec, between 1986 and 1998, LE increased by two years whereas life expectancy without functional limitation (seeing, hearing) decreased by one year. But during the same period, LE without activity restriction (all levels combined) stagnated whereas LE without moderate and severe activity restriction increased in parallel with LE (Pampalon et al, 2001). Another recent study using microcensus data for the years 1978, 1983, 1991 and 1998 suggests that both LE in good perceived health and the ratio of healthy years to LE increased between 1978 and 1998 in Austria, leading to the conclusion that elderly people in the 21st century may not only live longer but also live longer in good health (Doblhammer and Kytir, 2001).

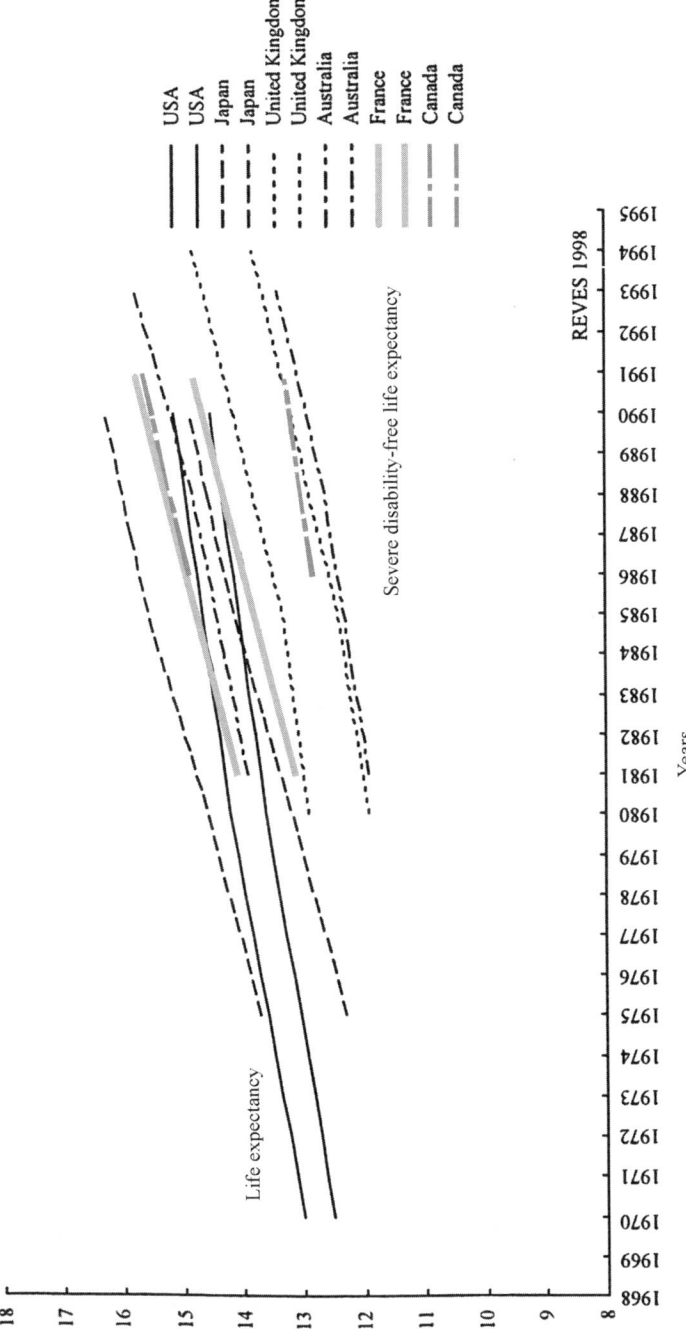

Figure 4.5. Changes in life expectancy and in *severe* disability-free life expectancy at 65 years of age, in different countries, men. *Sources:* Crimmins *et al*, 1989, 1997a; Crimmins and Saito, 1993; Inoue *et al*, 1997; Bebbington and Darton, 1996; Mathers, 1991b, 1996; Robine and Mormiche, 1994; Wilkins *et al*, 1994

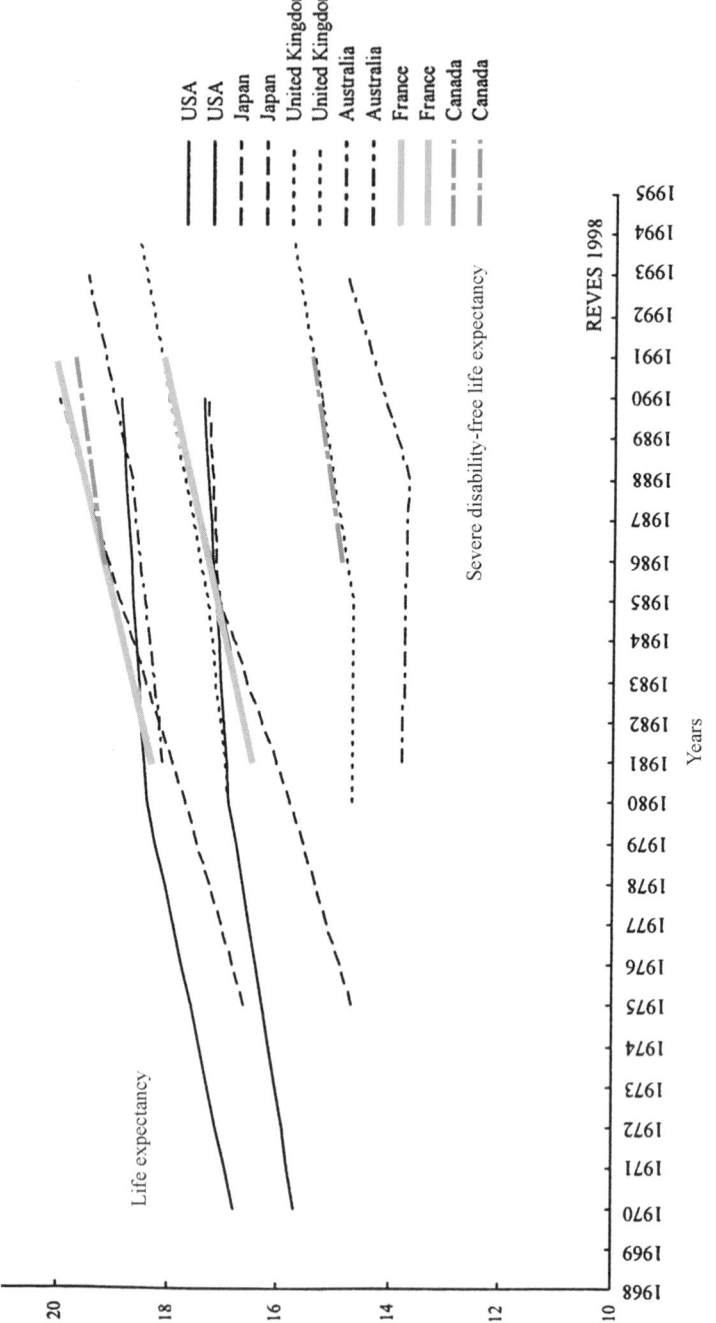

Figure 4.6. Changes in life expectancy and *severe* disability-free life expectancy at 65 years of age, in different countries, women. *Sources*: Crimmins *et al*, 1989, 1997a; Crimmins and Saito, 1993; Inoue *et al*, 1997; Bebbington and Darton, 1996; Mathers, 1991b, 1996; Robine and Mormiche, 1994; Wilkins *et al*, 1994

CAUSES AND MECHANISMS

To go further in the analysis several authors studied specific changes in the statistical relationships linking chronic morbidity to disability. Using the data from the French National Health Surveys, the presence of chronic disabling diseases led significantly less often to disability in 1991 than in 1981, suggesting that the reported morbidity was less severe in 1991 (Robine *et al*, 1998). American studies confirmed the French study with the data of the Supplement on Aging (SOA) to the 1984 and 1994 NHIS (Crimmins and Saito, 2000; Freedman and Martin, 2000). Although chronic conditions increased, the percentage of older Americans with upper body limitations (reaching up over one's head; reaching out; and using one's finger to grasp or handle) declined from 5.1% to 4.3% between 1984 and 1994. Those with lower body limitations (walking for a quarter mile; walking up 10 steps without resting; standing for about two hours; stooping, crouching or kneeling; and lifting or carrying a 25 lb object) declined from 34.2% in 1984 to 28.5% in 1995 (Freedman and Martin, 2000). When the gender differentials were examined there were no functioning and disability changes for old men with disease and an improvement in Nagi functions (Nagi, 1976) and IADLs for women with disease. On the other hand, there was no improvement in ADL disability for either sex (Crimmins and Saito, 2000). The Framingham Heart Study essentially confirmed these results (Allaire *et al*, 1999).

CONCLUSION

The time series on health expectancies have contributed significantly to our current knowledge on changes in the health of populations experiencing declining mortality in the oldest old. The hypothesis of a rectangularization of the survival curves at extreme ages is largely questioned today. The shape of the survival curve, the mortality trajectories at the extreme ages and the limits of human life span need to be reassessed (Nusselder and Mackenbach, 1995; Mesrine, 1997; Barbi *et al*, 1999; Olshansky and Carnes, 1995, 2000).

Health expectancy and HSE time series enabled comparisons of changes in the three fundamental dimensions of a population's health, namely mortality, chronic morbidity and disability. In particular, the series offered a unified framework to support international comparisons and synthesis analyses whereas accumulation of empirical studies of prevalence of disability series led essentially to contradictory results. But behind these general conclusions, heterogeneity has been noted between comparable countries and needs to be understood. For example, not all the developed countries have the same fall in mortality among the oldest old (Nusselder and Mackenbach, 2000). The decrease in ADL disability, noted in several European countries, is not verified in North America although such a decrease could be expected given the hypothesis of redistribution of disability by severity levels. France has experienced a large decrease in its disability rates – all disability levels combined – whereas a stagnation or even an increase has been observed in England and Wales.

However, limitations in the times series are real and need to be avoided in the future. Presently, most series are too short. Current protocols from the surveys used to constitute the statistical series have to be preserved as long as possible to allow the continuation of the series. Disability severity levels are still poorly defined and standardized, complicating analyses as well as communication with policy makers. Standardization of disability as well as general health measures should become a priority.

Health state expectancies series could be improved, but they are still relevant and provide meaningful series for policy making. They do not aim to replace life expectancies but, on the contrary, they enable the assessment of whether the increase in life expectancy is accompanied by a compression or expansion of morbidity or disability. Recent studies show that people with lower risks (defined on the basis of smoking, body mass index, and exercise patterns) not only live longer, but experience fewer years of disability before death (Vita et al, 1998; Ferrucci et al, 1999; Nusselder et al, 1999, 2000). None of these studies suggests that there is a trade-off between quantity and quality of life, but rather, at least for two of them, that there is a possible compression of disability, with quantity and quality of life going hand in hand. Thus, if future increases in life expectancy are due to better behaviours, they could also be accompanied with larger increases in disability-free life expectancy leading to a compression of disability. In fact, in the United States some forecasts of disability in elderly populations are very optimistic (Manton et al, 1997; Manton and Gu, 2001). Improvement in the level of education of successive cohorts impacts directly on the cognitive performance of older people and therefore indirectly on the decrease in IADL restrictions. A recent study in the United States showed through calculation of DFLE from 1970 to 1990 that compression of morbidity has begun among those of higher educational status, whereas those of lower status are still experiencing expansion of morbidity, and underlined again the possible role of education (Crimmins and Saito, 2001). In France, when comparing DFLE and LE for males, compression of disability between 1980 and 1991 is verified for all occupational groups (Cambois et al, 2001). Moreover, several recent studies have shown an improvement in perceived health of older people (Aromaa et al, 1999; Lalive d'Epinay et al, 2000), with life expectancy increasing together with life expectancy in good perceived health in Austria from 1978 to 1998 (Doblhammer and Kytir, 2001).

We conjecture that a positive synergy between improving levels of education, improving nutritional status, better working conditions and better health behaviours (including better management of early impairments) should improve the functional abilities and performance of essential activities for daily life of future cohorts. We hypothesize there will be a redistribution of the levels of severity of disability. To prove our hypothesis we need to continue the HSE time series as well as distinguishing between and standardizing disability severity levels.

REFERENCES

Allaire, S.H., LaValley, M.P., Evans, S.R., *et al* (1999) 'Evidence for decline in disability and improved health among persons aged 55 to 70 years: the Framingham Heart Study', *American Journal of Public Health* 89(11), 1678–1683.

Alter, G. and Riley, J.C. (1997) 'Sickness, recovery, and Redux: Transitions into and out of sickness in the nineteenth-century Britain', in 10th Work-group meeting REVES, Tokyo, REVES paper 294.

Anttila, S. (1991) 'Functional capacity in two elderly populations aged 75 or over: comparisons at 10 years' interval', *Journal of Clinical Epidemiology* 44, 1181–1186.

Aromaa, A., Koskinen, S. and Huttunen, J. (1999) *Health in Finland*. Helsinki: National Public Health Institute.

Barbi, E., Caselli, G. and Vallin, J. (1999) 'Trajectories of extreme survival in heterogeneous populations', in 11th Work-group meeting REVES, London, REVES paper 326.

Bebbington, A.C. and Darton, R.A. (1996) *Healthy Life Expectancy in England and Wales: Recent Evidence*. London: PSSRU.

Bebbington, A. and Wittenberg, R. (1999) 'The implications for long term care finance of trends in healthy life expectancy', in 11th Work-group meeting REVES, London, REVES paper 332.

Bone, M. (1991) 'Changing disability rates over time in Great Britain', in 4th Work-group meeting REVES, Leiden, REVES paper 55.

Bone, M.R. (1992) 'International efforts to measure health expectancy', *Journal of Epidemiology and Community Health* 46, 555–558.

Bone, M.R., Bebbington, A.C., Jagger, C., Morgan, K. and Nicolaas, G. (1995) *Health Expectancy and its Uses*. London: HMSO.

Boshuizen, H. (1991) 'Trends in health expectancy in the Netherlands in the period 1980–1990; some preliminary results', in 4th Work-group meeting REVES, Leiden, REVES paper 58.

Brückner, G. (1997) 'Health expectancy in Germany: what do we learn from the reunification process?', in 10th Work-group meeting REVES, Tokyo, REVES paper 290 (NUPRI Research paper series no. 72, February 2001).

Brunelle, Y. (1991) 'The evolution of recognized disability/L'évolution de l'incapacité reconnue', in 4th Work-group meeting REVES, Leiden, REVES paper 56.

Brunelle, Y. (1993) 'Understanding changes in the health status', in Robine, J-M., Mathers, C.D., Bone, M.R. and Romieu, I. (eds) *Calculation of Health Expectancies; Harmonization, Consensus Achieved and Future Perspectives* (*Calcul des espérances de vie en santé: harmonisation, acquis et perspectives*). Paris: John Libbey Eurotext.

Cambois, E. and Robine, J-M. (1999) 'Differentials in health expectancy for three socio-professional groups in the French male population, 1980–1991', in 11th Work-group meeting REVES, London, REVES paper 357.

Cambois, E., Robine, J-M. and Hayward, M.D. (2001) 'Social inequalities in disability-free life expectancy in the French male population, 1980–1991', *Demography* 38(4), 513–524.

Chen, K., Tu, J., Chang, M. and Yang, C. (1996) 'Morbidity and chronic disability in an elderly population: Taiwan, 1989–1993', in 9th Work-group meeting REVES, Rome, REVES paper 278.

Colvez, A. (1992) 'Changes in disability-free life expectancy in the USA between 1966 and 1976', in Robine, J-M., Blanchet, M. and Dowd, J.E. (eds) *Health Expectancy*. London: HMSO.

Corder, E.H. and Manton, K.G. (2001) 'Change in prevalence of severe dementia among older Americans: 1982 to 1999', XXIV IUSSP General Population Conference. IUSSP, Salvador.

Corder, L., Manton, K.G. and Stallard, E. (1992) 'Change in the functional level of the United States population in the 1980s', in 5th Work-group meeting REVES, Ottawa, REVES paper 92.

Costa, D.L. (2000) 'Understanding the twentieth-century decline in chronic conditions among older men', *Demography* 37(1), 53–72.

Cousins, C., Jenkins, J. and Laux, R. (1998) 'Disability data from the LFS: comparing 1997–98 with the past', *Labour Market Trends* June, 321–335.

Crimmins, E.M. (1990) 'Are Americans healthier as well as longer-lived?', *Journal of Insurance Medicine* 22(2), 89–92.

Crimmins, E.M. (1996) 'Mixed trends in population health among older adults', *Journal of Gerontology: Social Sciences* 51B(5), S223–S225.

Crimmins, E.M. (1997) 'Trends in mortality, morbidity, and disability: what should we expect for the future of our ageing population', in IUSSP/UIESP (eds) *International Population Conference (Congrès International de la Population)*. Beijing, October 11–17, 1997. Liège: IUSSP/UIESP.

Crimmins, E.M. and Ingegneri, D.G. (1991) 'Trends in health among the American population' Paper prepared for the Pension Research Council Symposium.

Crimmins, E.M. and Ingegneri, D.G. (1993) 'Trends in health among the American population', in Rappaport, A. and Schieber, S.J. (eds) *Demography and Retirement: the 21st Century*. Westport, CT; London: Praeger.

Crimmins, E.M. and Saito, Y. (1993) 'Trends in disability-free life expectancy in the United States, 1970–1990: Gender, racial and socioeconomic differences', Paper prepared for the 1993 IUSSP General Convention in Montreal.

Crimmins, E.M. and Saito, Y. (1997a) 'Trends in disability-free life expectancy in the United States, 1970–1990: gender, racial, and socio-economic differences', in 10th Work-group meeting REVES, Tokyo, REVES paper 292.

Crimmins, E.M. and Saito, Y. (1997b) 'Getting better and getting worse: transitions in functional status among older Americans', *Journal of Aging and Health* 5, 3–36.

Crimmins, E.M. and Saito, Y. (2000) 'Changes in the prevalence of diseases among older Americans: 1984–1994', *Demographic Research* 3; article 9.

Crimmins, E.M. and Saito, Y. (2001) 'Trends in healthy life expectancy in the United States 1970–1990: gender, racial, and educational differences', *Social Science and Medicine* 52, 1629–1641.

Crimmins, E.M., Saito, Y. and Ingegneri, D. (1989) 'Changes in life expectancy and disability-free life expectancy in the United States', *Population and Development Review* 15, 235–267.

Crimmins, E.M., Saito, Y. and Ingegneri, D. (1992a) 'Changes in life expectancy and disability-free life expectancy in the United States', in: Robine, J-M., Blanchet, M. and Dowd, J.E. (eds) *Health Expectancy*. London: HMSO.

Crimmins, E.M., Hayward, M.D. and Saito, Y. (1992b) 'The relationship between changing mortality rates, changing morbidity rates and the health status of the population', in 5th Work-group meeting REVES, Ottawa, REVES paper 91.

Crimmins, E.M., Saito, Y. and Ingegneri, D. (1997a) 'Trends in disability-free life expectancy in the United States, 1970–90', *Population and Development Review* 23, 555–572.

Crimmins, E.M., Saito, Y. and Reynolds, S.L. (1997b) 'Further evidence on recent trends in prevalence and incidence of disability among older Americans from two sources: the LSOA and the NHIS', *Journal of Gerontology: Social Sciences* 52B(2), S59–S271.

Crimmins, E.M., Reynolds, S.L. and Saito, Y. (1999) 'Trends in health and ability to work among the older working-age population', *Journal of Gerontology: Social Sciences* 54B(1), S31–S40.

Crystal, S., Sambamoorthi, U. and Merzel, C. (1993) 'Compression versus expansion of morbidity: modeling the impact of antiviral therapy in HIV disease', in Robine, J-M., Mathers, C.D., Bone, M.R. and Romieu, I. (eds) *Calculation of Health Expectancies; Harmonization, Consensus Achieved and Future Perspectives* (*Calcul des espérances de vie en santé: harmonisation, acquis et perspectives*). Paris: John Libbey Eurotext.

Davis, P. and Graham, P. (1997) 'Personal communication to REVES'.

Deeg, D.J.H., Kriegsman, D.M.W. and van Zonneveld, R.J. (1994) 'Trends in fatal chronic diseases and disability in the Netherlands 1956–1993 and projections 1993–1998', in Mathers, C.D., McCallum, J. and Robine J-M. (eds) *Advances in Health Expectancies*. Canberra: Australian Institute of Health and Welfare, AGPS.

Deeg, D.J.H., Smit, J.H., Kriegsman, D.M.W. and Van Zonneveld, R.J. (1996) 'Transition in health limitations in the Netherlands: comparison across four decades', in 9th Work-group meeting REVES, Rome, REVES paper 270.

Doblhammer, G. and Kytir, J. (2001) 'Compression or expansion of morbidity? Trends in healthy-life expectancy in the elderly Austrian population between 1978 and 1998', *Social Science and Medicine* 52, 385–391.

Fanshel, S. (1972) 'A meaningful measure of health for epidemiology', *International Journal of Epidemiology* 1(4), 319–337.

Fanshel, S. and Bush, J.W. (1970) 'A health-status index and its application to health-services outcomes', *Operations Research* 18, 1021–1066.

Ferrucci, L., Izmirlian, G., Leveille, S.G., Phillips, C.L., Corti, M.C., Brock, D.B. and Guralnick, J.M. (1999) 'Smoking, physical activity and active life expectancy', *American Journal of Epidemiology* 149(7), 645–653.

Freedman, V.A. and Martin, L.G. (1998) 'Understanding trends in functional limitations among older Americans', *American Journal of Public Health* 88(10), 1457–1462.

Freedman, V.A. and Martin, L.G. (1999) 'The role of education in explaining and forecasting trends in functional limitations among older Americans', *Demography* 36(4), 461–473.

Freedman, V.A. and Martin, L.G. (2000) 'Contribution of chronic conditions to aggregate changes in old-age functioning', *American Journal of Public Health* 90(11), 1755–1760.

Freedman, V.A. and Soldo, J.S. (1994) *Trends in Disability at Older Ages*. Washington, DC: National Academy Press.

Freedman, V.A., Aykan, H. and Martin, L.G. (2001) 'Aggregate changes in severe cognitive impairment among older Americans: 1993 and 1998', *Journal of Gerontology: Social Sciences* 56B(5), S100–S111.

Fuchs, V.R. (1984) 'Through much is taken: reflections on aging, health and medical care', *Milbank Memorial Fund Quarterly/Health and Society* 62, 143–165.

Grundy, E. (1997) 'The health and health care of older adults in England and Wales, 1841–1994', in Charlton, J. and Murphy, M. (eds) *The Health of Adult Britain 1841–1994*. London: The Stationery Office (vols 1 and 2).

Grundy, E., Ahlburg, D., Ali, M., *et al* (1999) *Disability in Great Britain*. London: HMSO, Department of Social Security (Research Report 94).

Inoue, T., Shigematsu, T. and Nanjo, Z. (1997) 'Health life tables in Japan, 1990: a quality of the longest life expectancy in the world', *Minzoku Eisei* 63(4), 226–240.

Jagger, C. and Clarke, M. (1991) 'The changing disability profile of the elderly', in 4th Work-group meeting REVES, Leiden, REVES paper 57.

Jagger, C., Clarke, M. and Clarke, S.J. (1991) 'Getting older – feeling younger: the changing health profile of the elderly', *International Journal of Epidemiology* 20, 234–238.

Kelly, S. and Baker, A. (2000) 'Healthy life expectancy in Great Britain, 1980–96, and its use as an indicator in UK Government strategies', in 12th Work-group meeting REVES, Los Angeles, REVES paper 406.

Koizumi, A. (1994) 'Life expectancy and quality of life in Japan', in Mathers, C.D., McCallum, J. and Robine J-M. (eds) *Advances in Health Expectancies*. Canberra: Australian Institute of Health and Welfare, AGPS.

Lalive d'Epinay, C., Bickel, J.F., Maystre, C., *et al* (2000) *Vieillesses au fil du temps 1979–1994,* Lausanne: Editions Réalités sociales.

Lamb, V.L. (1999) 'The effects of population development on elderly health and disablement', in 11th Work-group meeting REVES, London, REVES paper 346.

LaRoche, S. and Morin, J.P. (1994) *Etude des variations entre les taux d'incapacité de l'ESLA de 1986 et de 1991*. Ottawa, Canada: Statistique Canada, Division des méthodes d'enquêtes sociales.

Manton, K.G. (1982) 'Changing concepts of morbidity and mortality in the elderly population', *Milbank Memorial Fund Quarterly/Health and Society* 60, 183–244.

Manton, K.G. and Gu, X. (2001) 'Changes in the prevalence of chronic disability in the United States black and nonblack population above age 65 from 1982 to 1999', *Proceedings of the National Academy of Sciences USA* 98, 6354–6359.

Manton, K.G., Corder; L.S. and Stallard, E. (1993a) 'Estimates of change in chronic disability and institutional incidence and prevalence rates in the US elderly population from the 1982, 1984, and 1989 National Long Term Care Survey', *Journal of Gerontology: Social Sciences* 48(4), S153–S166.

Manton, K.G., Corder, L.S. and Stallard, E. (1993b) 'Changes in the use of personal assistance and special equipment from 1982 to 1989: results from the 1982 and 1989 NLTCS', *The Gerontologist* 33(2), 168–176.

Manton, K.G., Stallard, E. and Corder, L.S. (1995) 'Changes in morbidity and chronic disability in the US elderly population: Evidence from the 1982, 1984 and 1989 National Long Term Care Survey', *Journal of Gerontology: Social Sciences* 50B(4), S194–S204.

Manton, K.G., Corder, L.S. and Stallard, E. (1997) 'Chronic disability trends in elderly United States populations: 1982–1994', *Proceedings of the National Academy of Sciences USA* 94, 2593–2598.

Manton, K.G., Stallard, E. and Corder, L.S. (1998) 'Dynamics of dimensions of age-related disability 1982 to 1994 in the US elderly population', *Journal of Gerontology: Biological Sciences* 53A(1), B59–B70.

Martel, L. and Bélanger, A. (2000) 'Report on the demographic situation in Canada 1998–1999. An analysis of the change in dependence-free life expectancy in Canada between 1986 and 1996', in 12th Work-group meeting REVES, Los Angeles, REVES paper 407.

Mathers, C.D. (1991a) 'Australian trends in disability-free and handicap-free life expectancy 1981–1988', in 4th Work-group meeting REVES, Leiden, REVES paper 52.

Mathers, C.D. (1991b) *Health Expectancies in Australia, 1981 and 1988*. Canberra, ACT: Australian Institute of Health Publications.

Mathers, C.D. (1994) 'Health expectancies in Australia 1993: preliminary results', in Mathers, C.D., McCallum, J. and Robine, J-M. (eds) *Advances in Health Expectancies*. Canberra: Australian Institute of Health and Welfare, AGPS.

Mathers, C.D. (1996) 'Trends in health expectancies in Australia 1981–1993', *Journal of the Australian Population Association* 13, 1–15.

Mathers, C.D. and Jains, S. (1999) 'Trends in health expectancies in Australia 1981–1998 and preliminary results from the Australian burden of disease study', in 11th Work-group meeting, London, REVES paper 339.

McClellan, M. and Yan, L. (2000) 'Understanding disability trends in the US elderly population: The role of disease management and disease prevention', in 12th Work-group meeting REVES, Los Angeles, REVES paper 404.

Mesrine, A. (1997) 'Form of the mortality curve at the end of life?', in 10th Work-group meeting REVES, Tokyo, REVES paper 300.

Mizrahi, A. and Mizrahi, A. (1989) *Evolution de l'état de santé. Risque vital et invalidité*. Paris: CREDES, no. 814.

Mizrahi, A. and Mizrahi, A. (1993) *Evolution des déficiences et des soins aux personnes âgées en institution, France 1977–1988*. Paris: CREDES, no. 966.

Mizrahi, A. and Mizrahi, A. (1994) *L'évolution paradoxale de l'état de santé des personnes âgées en France: amélioration du pronostic vital, diminution de l'incapacité et augmentation du nombre de maladies. Conference 'Economics of Aging'*. Paris: CREDES, no. 1027.

Myers, G.C. and Elman, C. (1996) 'Patterns of health status in early America: Results from the 1880 US Census', in 9th Work-group meeting REVES, Rome, REVES paper 269.

Myers, G.C. and Lamb, V.L. (1993) 'Theoretical perspectives on healthy life expectancy', in Robine, J-M., Mathers, C.D., Bone, M.R. and Romieu, I. (eds) *Calculation of Health Expectancies; Harmonization, Consensus Achieved and Future Perspectives (Calcul des espérances de vie en santé: harmonisation, acquis et perspectives)*. Paris: John Libbey Eurotext.

Nagi, S.Z. (1976) 'An epidemiology of disability among adults in the United States', *Milbank Memorial Fund Quarterly/Health and Society* 54(4), 439–467.

Nusselder, W. (1998) *Compression or Expansion of Morbidity: a Life-table Approach*. Amsterdam, the Netherlands: Erasmus University Rotterdam.

Nusselder, W.J. and Mackenbach, J.P. (1995) 'Rectangularization of the survival curve in the Netherlands in the 1980s: an analysis of underlying causes-of-death: preliminary results', in 8th Work-group meeting REVES, Chicago, REVES paper 237.

Nusselder, W.J. and Mackenbach, J.P. (2000) 'Lack of improvement of life expectancy at advanced ages in the Netherlands', *International Journal of Epidemiology* 29, 140–148.

Nusselder, W.J., Looman, C.W.N., Stronks, K. and Mackenbach, J.P. (1996) 'Compression of morbidity: an exploration of the conditions', in 9th Work-group meeting REVES, Rome, REVES paper 268.

Nusselder, W.J., Looman, C.W.N., Marang van de Mheen, P.J. and Mackenbach, J.P. (1999) 'Smoking and the compression of morbidity', in 11th Work-group meeting REVES, London, REVES paper 347.

Nusselder, W.J., Looman, C.W.N., Marang van de Mheen, P.J., van de Mheen, H. and Mackenbach, J.P. (2000) 'Smoking elimination produces compression of morbidity', *Journal of Epidemiology and Community Health* 54, 566–574.

Olshansky, S.J. and Carnes, B.A. (1995) 'Living on manufactured time: health implications of exceeding the biological limit to life', in 8th Work-group meeting REVES, Chicago, REVES paper 235.

Olshansky, S.J. and Carnes, B.A. (2000) 'Anatomical oddities and design flaws of the human body', in 12th Work-group meeting REVES, Los Angeles, REVES paper 382.

Olshansky, S.J., Rudberg, M.A., Carnes, B.A., Cassel, C.K. and Brody, J.A. (1991) 'Trading off longer life for worsening health: the expansion of morbidity hypothesis', *Journal of Aging and Health* 3, 194–216.

Osborn, R. (1992) 'Cohort changes in chronic disease and activity limitation', in 5th Work-group meeting REVES, Ottawa, REVES paper 110.

Pampalon, R., Choinière, R. and Rochon, M. (2001) 'L'espérance de santé au Québec', in *Enquête québécoise sur les limitations d'activité 1998*. Ste-Foy: Les Publications du Québec.

Perenboom, R.J.M. and van de Water, H.P.A. (1997) 'Mental health expectancy in the Netherlands, 1989–1995', in 10th Work-group meeting REVES, Tokyo, REVES paper 312.

Perenboom, R.J.M., Boshuizen, H.C. and van de Water, H.P.A. (1993) 'Trends in health expectancies in the Netherlands, 1981–1990', in Robine, J-M., Mathers, C.D., Bone, M.R. and Romieu, I. (eds) *Calculation of Health Expectancies; Harmonization, Consensus Achieved and Future Perspectives* (*Calcul des espérances de vie en santé: harmonisation, acquis et perspectives*). Paris: John Libbey Eurotext.

Perenboom, R.J.M., Van Herten, L.M. and Mulder, Y.M. (2000) 'Trends in DFLE in the Netherlands: Dynamic Equilibrium', in 12th Work-group meeting REVES, Los Angeles, REVES paper 405.

Pettersson, H. (1995) 'Trends in health expectancy for socio-economic groups in Sweden', in 8th Work-group meeting REVES, Chicago, REVES paper 214.

Preston, S.H. (1992) 'Cohort succession and the future of the oldest old', in Suzman, R.M., Willis, D.P. and Manton, K.G. (eds) *The Oldest Old*. New York, Oxford: Oxford University Press.

Qiao, X. (1997) 'Health expectancy of China', in 10th Work-group meeting REVES, Tokyo, REVES paper 305.

Reynolds, S.L., Crimmins, E.M. and Saito, Y. (1998) 'Cohort differences in disability and disease presence', *The Gerontologist* 38(5), 578–590.

Riley, J.C. (1990) 'The risk of being sick: morbidity trends in four countries', *Population and Development Review* 16(3), 403–432.

Riley, J.C. (1993) 'Active life expectancy during the long mortality decline: the transition from brief to protracted sickness', in Robine, J-M., Mathers, C.D., Bone, M.R. and Romieu, I. (eds) *Calculation of Health Expectancies; Harmonization, Consensus Achieved and Future Perspectives* (*Calcul des espérances de vie en santé: harmonisation, acquis et perspectives*). Paris: John Libbey Eurotext.

Riley, J.C. and Alter, G. (1995) 'How long does wellness or sickness predict future health?', in 8th Work-group meeting REVES, Chicago, REVES paper 239.

Robine, J-M. (1986) *Disability-free life expectancy (DFLE) indicators: General indicators of the health of population*. Québec: Conseil des Affaires Sociales et de la Famille (Scientific Report).

Robine, J-M. (1991) 'Changes in health conditions over time', in 4th Work-group meeting REVES, Leiden, REVES paper 60.

Robine, J-M. (1992) 'Disability-free life expectancy', in Robine, J-M., Blanchet, M. and Dowd, J.E. (eds) *Health Expectancy*. London: HMSO.

Robine, J-M. (1994) 'Disability-free life expectancy trends in France 1981–1991, international comparison', in Mathers, C.D., McCallum, J. and Robine J-M. (eds) *Advances in Health Expectancies*. Canberra: Australian Institute of Health and Welfare, AGPS.

Robine, J-M. (2000) 'Can an we expect to live both a longer and a healthier life?', in Jàvor, A., van Eimeren, W. and Duru, G. (eds) *System Science in Health Care*. Budapest: ISSSHC.

Robine, J-M. and Mathers, C.D. (1993) 'Measuring the compression or expansion of morbidity through changes in health expectancy', in Robine, J-M., Mathers, C.D., Bone, M.R. and Romieu, I. (eds) *Calculation of Health Expectancies; Harmonization, Consensus Achieved and Future Perspectives (Calcul des espérances de vie en santé: harmonisation, acquis et perspectives)*. Paris: John Libbey Eurotext.

Robine, J-M. and Mormiche, P. (1994) 'Estimation de la valeur de l'espérance de vie sans incapacité en France en 1991', *Solidarité Santé* (1), 17–36.

Robine, J-M. and Romieu, I. (1998) *Healthy Active Ageing: health expectancies at age 65 in the different parts of the world*. Montpellier: REVES/INSERM, REVES paper 318.

Robine, J-M., Bucquet, D. and Ritchie, K. (1991) 'L'espérance de vie sans incapacité, un indicateur de l'évolution des conditions de santé au cours du temps; vingt ans de recul', *Cahiers Québécois Démographie* 20, 205–235.

Robine, J-M., Mathers, C. and Brouard, N. (1996a) 'Trends and differentials in disability-free life expectancy: concepts, methods and findings', in Caselli, G. and Lopez, A. (eds) *Health and Mortality among the Elderly Populations*. Oxford: Clarendon Press.

Robine, J-M., Mormiche, P. and Cambois, E. (1996b) 'Evolution des courbes de survie totale, sans maladie chronique et sans incapacité en France de 1981 à 1991: application d'un modèle de l'OMS', *Annales de Démographie Historique*, 99–115.

Robine, J-M., Mormiche, P. and Sermet, C. (1998) 'Examination of the causes and mechanisms of the increase in disability-free life expectancy', *Journal of Aging and Health* 10(2), 171–191.

Robine, J-M., Romieu, I. and Cambois, E. (1999) 'Health expectancy indicators', *Bulletin of the World Health Organization* 77, 181–185.

Roos, N.P., Havens, B. and Black, C. (1993) 'Living longer but doing worse: assessing health status in elderly persons at two points in time in Manitoba, Canada', *Social Science and Medicine* 36, 273–282.

Saito, Y. (2001) 'The changes in the level of disability in Japan: 1992–1998', in XXIV IUSSP General Population Conference. IUSSP, Salvador, August 2001.

Sanders, B.S. (1964) 'Measuring community health levels', *American Journal of Public Health* 54(7), 1063–1070.

Saucier, A. and Lafontaine, P. (2001) 'Prévalence et gravité de l'incapacité dans la population québécoise', in *Enquête québecoise sur les limitations d'activité 1998*. Ste-Foy: Les Publications du Québec.

Sauvaget, C., Tsuji, I., Haan, M.N. and Hisamichi, S. (1997) 'Trends in dementia-free life expectancy among the elderly in the United States of America', in 10th Work-group meeting REVES, Tokyo, REVES paper 311.

Schoeni, R.F., Freedman, V.A. and Wallace, R.B. (2001) 'Persistent, consistent, widespread, and robust? Another look at recent trends in old-age disability', *Journal of Gerontology: Social Sciences* 56B(4), S206–S218.

Sihvonen, A.P. (1994) *Suomalaisten toimintakykyiset elinvuodet. Metodinen tarkastelu ja mittaaminen (Health expectancy in Finland. Methodological considerations and measurement)*. Helsinki: STAKES (Report no. 148).

Sihvonen, A.P., Lahelma, E. and Valkonen, T. (1996) 'Changes in the educational pattern in health expectancy from 1986 to 1994 in Finland', in 9th Work-group meeting REVES, Rome, REVES paper 264.

Smith, L. (1994) 'Reflections on the next stage of the epidemiological transition', in Mathers, C.D., McCallum, J. and Robine, J-M. (eds) *Advances in Health Expectancies*. Canberra: Australian Institute of Health and Welfare, AGPS.

Spiers, N., Jagger, C. and Clarke, M. (1996) 'Physical function and perceived health: Cohort differences and interrelationships in older people', *Journal of Gerontology: Social Sciences* 51B(5), S226–S233.

Sullivan, D.F. (1971) 'A single index of mortality and morbidity', *HSMHA Health Reports* 86, 347–354.

Svanborg, A. (1988) 'Cohort differences in the Göteborg studies of Swedish 70-year olds', in Brody, J.A. and Maddox, G.L. (eds) *Epidemiology and Aging*. Berlin: Springer.

Tartarin, R. and Bouget, D. (1994) 'Une allocation dépendance: simulation et projections', *Retraite et Société* No. Spécial.

Tu, E.J.C. and Chen, K. (1992) 'Changes in active life expectancy in Taiwan: compression or expansion?', in 5th Work-group meeting REVES, Ottawa, REVES paper 104.

Tu, E.J.C. and Chen, K. (1994) 'Recent changes in active life expectancy in Taiwan', in Mathers, C.D., McCallum, J. and Robine, J-M. (eds) *Advances in Health Expectancies*. Canberra: Australian Institute of Health and Welfare, AGPS.

Tu, E.J.C. and Chen, K. (1995) 'Recent changes in healthy life expectancy and their implications for medical costs in Taiwan', in 8th Work-group meeting REVES, Chicago, REVES paper 201.

Tu, E.J.C., Chen, K. and Chang, M.C. (1997) 'Changes in morbidity and chronic disability in an elderly population: Taiwan, 1989–1993', in 10th Work-group meeting REVES, Tokyo, REVES paper 307.

van de Water, H.P.A. (1991) 'Health expectancy and change over time: Compression or Pandemia', in 4th Work-group meeting REVES, Leiden, REVES paper 54.

Verbrugge, L.M. (1984) 'Longer life but worsening health? Trends in health and mortality of middle-aged and older persons', *Milbank Memorial Fund Quarterly/ Health and Society* 62(3), 475–519.

Verbrugge, L.M. (1989) 'Recent, present, and future health of American adults', *Annual Reviews in Public Health* 10, 333–361.

Vita, A.J., Terry, R.B., Hubert, H.B. and Fries, J.F. (1998) 'Aging, health risks, and cumulative disability', *New England Journal of Medicine* 338, 1035–1041.

Waidmann, T.A. and Liu, K. (2000) 'Disability trends among elderly persons and implications for the future', *Journal of Gerontology: Social Sciences* 55B(5), S298–S307.

Waidmann, T. and Manton, K.G. (1998) *International Evidence on Disability Trends among the Elderly*, Washington, DC: US Dept of Health and Human Services, Office of Disability, Aging, and Long-Term Care Policy.

Waidmann, T., Bound, J. and Schoenbaum, M. (1995) 'The illusion of failure: trends in self-reported health of the US elderly', *The Milbank Quarterly* 73(2), 253–287.

Wilkins, R. and Adams, O.B. (1992) 'Health expectancy trends in Canada, 1951–1986', in Robine, J-M., Blanchet, M. and Dowd, J.E. (eds) *Health Expectancy*. London: HMSO.

Wilkins, R. and Chen, J. (1995) 'Measures of health expectancy based on physical independence handicap: demographic, regional and social dimensions for Canada in 1986 and 1991', in 8th Work-group meeting REVES, Chicago, REVES paper 209.

Wilkins, R., Chen, J. and Ng, E. (1994) 'Changes in health expectancy in Canada from 1986 to 1991', in Mathers, C.D., McCallum, J. and Robine, J-M. (eds) *Advances in Health Expectancies*. Canberra: Australian Institute of Health and Welfare, AGPS.

Winblad, I. (1993) 'Comparison of the prevalence of disability in two birth cohorts at the age of 75 years and older', *Journal of Clinical Epidemiology* 46(3), 303–308.

World Health Organization (1980) *International Classification of Impairments, Disabilities, and Handicaps: A manual of classification relating to the consequences of disease*. Geneva: WHO.

World Health Organization (1984) *The Uses of Epidemiology in the Study of the Elderly: Report of a WHO scientific group on the epidemiology of aging*. Geneva: WHO (Technical Report Series 706).

World Health Organization (2001) *ICIDH-2: International Classification of Functioning, Disability and Health: Full version*. Geneva: WHO.

PART II

The Relevance of Health Expectancies

Introduction

EILEEN M. CRIMMINS

University of Southern California, Los Angeles, CA, USA

The central policy problem facing modern society is the potential conflict between living longer and improving the quality of life (van de Water, 1993). Health expectancy measures provide information to help us to design policy to address this conflict. Additional areas of policy to which health expectancy measures speak include: monitoring health trends, examining equity between subgroups of populations, providing a basis for health care planning, and linking interventions to potential outcomes (Bone *et al*, 1995, 1998). The chapters in this section provide numerous examples of research done over the past 10 years relevant to a variety of policy choices. Policy relevance of the health expectancy approach is also directly addressed in a number of papers in the literature (Barendregt *et al*, 1998; Bone *et al*, 1994, 1998; van de Water, 1993).

MONITORING OF HEALTH TRENDS AND EVIDENCE ON THE COMPRESSION OF MORBIDITY

The issue of compression or expansion of morbidity has only recently arisen with the rapid decline in mortality at older ages from chronic conditions. When the concept was introduced, it was appealing but empirical evidence of the compression or expansion of morbidity was totally lacking. The development of indicators summarizing mortality and morbidity has provided an important tool for understanding how health status and length of life change in actual populations and whether there has been an expansion or contraction of healthy life. This indicator provides a yardstick for measuring the achieved balance between increasing the length of life and increasing the quality of life. Simulation studies based on the healthy life model have been extremely important in clarifying the links between mortality change and morbidity

Determining Health Expectancies. Edited by J-M. Robine, C. Jagger, C.D. Mathers, E.M. Crimmins and R.M. Suzman.

change. These have played a key role in alerting governments to the potential for increases in years lived with disability and disease unless there are reductions in the rate of morbidity onset or increases in the age at onset. The importance for population health of preventing disease and delaying its progression when mortality is declining has been made clear through the use of the health expectancy model.

Many governments have adopted measures of healthy life expectancy to clarify past trends in the length of healthy life and to provide future projections of the length of life of a given quality. These include among others Canada, Britain (Bone *et al*, 1995, 1998), the Netherlands, Belgium and the United States. Examples of these are provided in the chapters in Part IV of this volume. Most governments have relied on available data to produce estimates of the trend in healthy life for their own countries. Some countries such as the United States have set targets for future achievement in terms of healthy life expectancy.

Empirical evidence of the change in health expectancy for many countries has been important in identifying international similarities in the type and direction of change. Reliability of results across countries has been reinforcing in terms of assessing the validity of change in any one country and in clarifying that the compression of morbidity is an aim that has yet to be fully realized in any one country. The similarity across countries of trends in healthy life for the 1970s alerted governments to the potential for differential trends in the prevalence of disability and mortality. The similarity of more recent findings of some compression of morbidity has also been an indicator of reliability.

A number of governments also have been active in supporting research to determine the policy uses of a variety of potential measures of health expectancy. For instance, the Department of Health in Britain commissioned British researchers to perform a set of pilot studies in order to evaluate the policy uses of the health expectancy approach (Bone *et al*, 1995, 1998). Statistics Canada as well as a number of Canadian provincial governments have supported substantial research on and monitoring of healthy life expectancy (Wilkins, 2001). The governments of France, the Netherlands and the United States have supported significant research on methods of estimating health expectancy. In addition, international agencies such as WHO and the European Union have implemented or are in the process of implementing the collection of data to monitor international trends in health expectancy and to further develop methods of monitoring changes in health quality.

EQUITY BETWEEN SUBGROUPS OF THE POPULATION

Health policy in most countries aims both to improve population health and to reduce differentials in health. The papers in this section on Social Inequalities

(Chapter 5 – Crimmins and Cambois) and Sub-national Variations (Chapter 6 – Bebbington and Bajekal) document the significant focus on differentials in the work on health expectancies. Many governments have found health expectancies to be a useful tool for summarizing health differentials within subgroups of their populations. The conclusions of this work are inescapable: health expectancies generally clarify the compounding effect of differences in mortality and morbidity between the advantaged and the disadvantaged. The summary effect of social differences can be illustrated with the health expectancy approach. While these chapters point out the differences in results that have been observed across numerous studies, the similarities of major conclusions across countries are most impressive.

In many countries health policy is made or administered at a sub-national geographic level. Geographically based indicators provide a basis for distributing resources at these levels (Bone *et al*, 1994). The use of health indicators to distribute resources geographically might seem relatively straightforward: those with shorter healthy life should be provided with greater resources. Bebbington and Bajekal (Chapter 6) clarify that other factors must be considered: migration effects may cause differences that will not respond to resources, incentives to 'game' the system should not be provided, and there should be a link between the indicator of poor health and the resources provided.

HEALTH CARE PLANNING AND LINKING INTERVENTIONS TO OUTCOMES

Barendregt and coauthors (1998) note that the role of health policy is to maintain and improve public health within the constraints of limited resources. Policy makers are forced to choose between a dazzling array of potential interventions that affect both the causes and consequences of health problems. Healthy life expectancy can provide a common metric with which to evaluate the potential benefits of a wide variety of interventions as well as to project the implications of changes in population and technology. Barendregt *et al* (1998) also clarify the importance of being able to understand the whole process of health change from risk factors, through disease onset to its resulting problems of disability and death. They provide examples of the potential uses of the health expectancy approach for summarizing the effects of changes in risk factors such as smoking and for technological changes that affect a specific disease such as cardiovascular conditions.

Most health policy in most countries is organized about disease-based interventions. For many policy applications, it is desirable to link diseases to the outcomes such as disability and death to clarify the relative effect of potential interventions. Mathers (Chapter 7) outlines the various approaches that have been taken to attribute loss of healthy life to specific causes and conditions. The health expectancy approach provides a common metric for use with any number of health conditions. The length of healthy life lost to various diseases lays the basis for policy making that takes into account the relative burden of different conditions. Although coupling these estimates with the potential cost and possible techniques for eliminating and reducing disease is necessary before advocating any specific policy.

One of the diseases or conditions identified as having a major role in reducing healthy life is mental illness. Ritchie and Polge (Chapter 8) clarify the value of the health expectancy approach in the area of mental health. They detail the diagnostic tools that have been developed for identifying the prevalence of mental health problems with emphasis on dementia. Their compilation of estimates for life with and without dementia at the older ages for many countries is impressive because of the similarity in the burden of this problem across societies. Ritchie and Polge have also used the life table technique to clarify the age structure of the demented population. While many researchers applying the healthy life expectancy approach have limited their analyses to the expectation of life values from the life table, additional life table values indicating the population health status can be very useful for policy makers. The healthy life expectancy approach is well suited to evaluating the potential impact of treatments currently proposed for cognitive loss. If early dementia were treated regularly with drugs to delay its progression, it is quite likely that the length of life with dementia will be increased.

Mathers (Chapter 7) outlines approaches to incorporating risk factors and medical interventions into models of healthy life. While these approaches have yet to become widespread, their value as a tool for health planning is clear. Again, one of the more interesting outcomes from this work is the demonstration that medical intervention can actually result in a less healthy population. The potential for increasing the prevalence of heart disease in the Netherlands by reducing death from cardiovascular conditions and even delaying incidence at the younger ages has been demonstrated.

CONCLUSION

The use of a health expectancy approach has resulted in almost world-wide recognition of the need to focus not only on the length of life but on the length of life of a given quality. This approach is being widely used by governments to monitor trends in population health and the compression of morbidity as well as socioeconomic and geographic differences. The policy value of the healthy life expectancy approach arises from its integrative and comparative features. There is significant potential to develop both methods and data to clarify the value of health interventions in terms of ability to change healthy life. Many different approaches to healthy life are valuable; which one is used depends on the type of policy being considered and the type of intervention or forecast needed.

REFERENCES

Barendregt, J., Bonneux, L. and van der Maas, P. (1998) 'Health expectancy: From a population health indicator to a tool for policy making', *Journal of Aging and Health* 10, 242–258.

Bone, M., Bebbington, A. and Nicolaas, G. (1994) 'Policy relevance and comparability problems of health expectancy indicators', in Mathers, C.D., McCallum, J. and Robine, J.M. (eds) *Advances in Health Expectancies*. Canberra: Australian Institute of Health and Welfare, AGPS.

Bone, M., Bebbington, A., Jagger, C., Morgan, K. and Nicolaas, G. (1995) *Health Expectancy and Its Uses*. London: HMSO.

Bone, M., Bebbington A. and Nicolaas, G. (1998) 'Policy applications of health expectancy', *Journal of Aging and Health* 10, 136–153.

van de Water, H. (1993) 'Policy relevance and the further development of the health expectancy indicator', in Robine, J.M., Mathers, C.D., Bone, M.R. and Romieu, I. (eds) *Calculation of Health Expectancies: Harmonization, Consensus Achieved*. Paris: John Libbey Eurotext.

Wilkins, R. (2001) 'Healthy life expectancy in low mortality countries: The Canadian experience', Paper presented at meetings of the Longevity and Health Committee, IUSSP, Beijing.

5

Social Inequalities in Health Expectancy

EILEEN M. CRIMMINS and EMMANUELLE CAMBOIS*

University of Southern California, Los Angeles, CA, USA and *INSERM, Montpellier, France

INTRODUCTION

The average length of life and the healthiness of that life are related to socioeconomic status in all societies. Differences in mortality and morbidity by social class have been the focus of public health concern for over a century and reductions in these differentials are currently a major concern of both international agencies and individual governments (Bone *et al*, 1995; WHO, 1998).

Measures of health expectancy summarize the combined effects of mortality and morbidity on the length of healthy and unhealthy life. Differences by social class in the length of expected healthy life provide a summary of the effects of both mortality and morbidity in causing inequality in healthy life. Because health expectancy indicators are comparable across groups with different age structures, they are of particular use for comparing socioeconomic differences at one point in time or changing differentials over time.

Many studies representing a number of countries have focused on socioeconomic inequality in expected total and healthy life (see Table 5.1). While the details of these studies will be discussed below, most studies find that higher social class is linked to longer life and longer healthy life and that differences by social class in expected healthy life are larger than differences in total life expectancy.

Determining Health Expectancies. Edited by J-M. Robine, C. Jagger, C.D. Mathers, E.M. Crimmins and R.M. Suzman.
© 2003 John Wiley & Sons, Ltd

BACKGROUND

The differences in both mortality and morbidity by social status that result in differences in health expectancy have long been recognized. Recent increases in mortality differentials observed in some countries have been cause for growing concern about differential population health (Townsend and David, 1982; Marmot *et al*, 1987; Preston and Elo, 1995). In addition, there is evidence for the United States of recent increases in the size of morbidity differentials (Crimmins and Saito, 2001).

The earliest studies of healthy life expectancy highlighted differences between social groups. In his 1971 paper, Sullivan documented differences in healthy life for racial groups in the United States (Sullivan, 1971). Differences between poor and non-poor and by social class were also a focus of studies in the early 1980s (Katz *et al*, 1983; Wilkins and Adams, 1983a, 1983b). Since that time, a large number of studies have addressed socioeconomic inequality in healthy life in many individual countries.

Before detailing the general findings of these studies, we will discuss some of the issues that must be considered in looking at differences by social status in estimates of healthy life. First, we explain why it is difficult to compare the numerical estimates of healthy life by socioeconomic status across the large number of studies listed. We clarify how definitions of health and social status as well as the methodological approach affect the comparability of results. Secondly, while we do not directly compare the numerical estimates of expected healthy life, we discuss the remarkably consistent general conclusions that can be drawn from existing studies addressing social inequality in healthy life.

DEFINITIONS OF SOCIAL STATUS

There are many indicators that can be used to distribute the population along a continuum from low to high socioeconomic status. Those most frequently employed are education, income and occupation. The use of these measures builds on a long tradition in the field of social stratification and applications in the field of public health.

In order to develop estimates of healthy life expectancy for socioeconomic subgroups of the population, it is necessary to have age-specific mortality rates or life tables for the appropriate groups. Life tables for social groups must be constructed by linking data on social status for large numbers of individuals to subsequent death records. The scarcity of such information is one factor that limits the ability to produce estimates of healthy life by social group. In countries with population registers, the linking of the characteristics of living persons and deaths can be accomplished more easily. In other countries, the necessary socioeconomic information may not be available for decedents without a specialized study. Because life tables sometimes can be more readily constructed by characteristics related to, but not direct indicators of social status, such as race/ethnicity and geographic location, these social groups are sometimes used in examinations of inequality in healthy life (Bebbington, 1993; Crimmins *et al*, 1989; Hayward and Heron, 1996). In countries where race and/or ethnicity are used as a proxy for socioeconomic position, it is because they are strongly related to the more direct measures like education and income.

The size of the socioeconomic differences in health expectancy observed depends on the indicator of status employed. For instance, both Guralnik *et al* (1993) and Crimmins *et al* (1996) find that educational differences in healthy life expectancy are greater than racial differences. Nault *et al* (1996) find that income differences in life expectancies and in health expectancy are larger than educational differences for males. For females, while income and educational differences in life expectancy are similar, educational differences in health expectancy are larger than income differences.

Education is the most commonly used indicator of social status in studies of social inequality in health for a number of reasons. After adulthood is reached, education remains relatively constant across the life span. It is not subject to the same temporal variability as income or occupation, both of which may experience both ups and downs, some of which are transient. At some parts of the age range, e.g. old age when pension programs are the major source of income, income may not be an appropriate indicator of lifetime social status because the dispersion of income is often reduced by pension programs. In old age, family income may become a close proxy for marital status or living arrangements where income is related to the number of household members. For both of these reasons income in old age may not be an appropriate indicator of lifetime social status.

Studies of social inequality in health assume that causation runs from social status to health. Significant work, particularly by economists, is directed at determining the direction of causation between levels of various measures of socioeconomic status and health. Education is not as likely to be affected by health as other measures of social status such as income or occupation. Those who are unable to work because of health reasons may have a reduced income or a changed occupation. One must be alert to the fact that health can affect socioeconomic status, especially after middle age.

An additional asset of education as an indicator of socioeconomic status is that every adult can be categorized by individual educational level, whereas many adults in a society may not have an occupation or an income at any given time. This lack of data on members of the population results in the omission of groups of people from the research population; for instance, women and those out of the labor force may be omitted from studies based on occupation.

Another approach is to assign family characteristics to those for whom data are not available, e.g. family income may be assigned to those without income. This raises the additional issue of whether per capita or household income is the more appropriate measure by which to characterize individuals.

Issues in devising indicators of social status for examination of temporal change in health inequality are greater. Even studies which use the same indicator of socioeconomic status for multiple time points in the same country face problems because of changes in measures and the meaning of social status indicators over time. For instance, in later time periods, or for more recent cohorts, educational and income levels have increased and occupational distributions have shifted from manual or blue collar to professional or white collar. As a result, the meaning of any specific level of socioeconomic status in terms of relative status, e.g. 12 years of schooling, may change from one decade to the next.

Two approaches to examining change over time have been employed. The first is to keep the definition of social status constant and examine change within groups that reflect different absolute positions in the social hierarchy (Crimmins and Saito, 2001); the second is to try to keep the relative positions in the social hierarchy constant and to let the absolute definition of social status change over time (Sihvonen et al, 1998). These approaches will, of course, answer different questions about change over time. The absolute approach indicates whether there has been change in the length of healthy life for people with a fixed status; the relative approach indicates whether the length of healthy life for people representing a set proportion of the social distribution has changed. Both approaches are complicated by the fact that persons in the population represent cohorts who have lived in different social environments.

Comparisons across countries in expected years of healthy life are also difficult. For instance, years of schooling completed has a different meaning from country to country because of administrative differences in the years of schooling considered primary, secondary, and higher education. International comparisons are also hampered by differences in income levels and definitions of poverty as well as differences in occupational distributions. For these comparisons an absolute or relative approach could also be employed.

DEFINITION OF HEALTHY LIFE

As with any study of healthy life, the definition of healthy life employed will affect the results. Studies of inequality in healthy life have employed indicators of a number of dimensions of health: self-reported health, disability, functioning deficits, and the presence of long-standing illness or of specific physical and mental conditions. Social inequality is greater in some outcomes than in others. For this reason, the size of socioeconomic differentials in healthy life differs by definition of health, and change across socioeconomic groups will vary with the type of health outcome investigated (Pettersson, 1995a; Crimmins *et al*, 1996; van de Water *et al*, 1996; Valkonen *et al*, 1997; Doblhammer and Kytir, 1999).

METHODS OF LIFE TABLE ESTIMATION

Most studies of social inequality in healthy life expectancy are based on the cross-sectional or Sullivan approach. Because of data availability, the longitudinal approach is limited to studies based on surveys of the older US population (Crimmins *et al*, 1996; Guralnik *et al*, 1993; Manton *et al*, 1997). The method used – cross-sectional or longitudinal – affects the estimated length of healthy life, the size of differentials observed and changes in these differentials over time. Because cross-sectional methods are based on prevalence estimates of ill-health, unhealthy life is affected by life-time health experiences. Differential health over the entire length of the life course will influence results. Longitudinal methods are based only on recent health events, so current age-specific differentials will be the basis of the estimates of healthy life. If there have been differential recent changes in mortality or health processes for socioeconomic groups, estimates of healthy life based on longitudinal methods may produce different health differentials from those based on cross-sectional methods.

RESULTS FROM STUDIES OF INEQUALITY IN HEALTH EXPECTANCY

Table 5.1 lists studies which focus on socioeconomic differences in healthy life expectancy. It includes studies which use a variety of definitions of health, a number of different indicators of socioeconomic status, both cross-sectional and longitudinal methods, and which compute life expectancy and healthy life expectancy at many different ages. While results are not comparable for all studies, we attempt a sample of comparisons to clarify the generalizations we draw.

Differentials in health expectancy are larger than differentials in life expectancy; inequality in mortality and morbidity combine to make larger social differences in years of expected healthy life than in total years of life. Those with lower social status have the shortest life expectancy, the shortest health expectancy, and usually the longest period of unhealthy life. Figure 5.1 shows the differential between high and low educational groups from five countries in both total life expectancy and health expectancy. In these studies health expectancy is based on perceived health and estimated for adult males. The scale of the x axis representing life expectancy is only half that of the y axis representing health expectancy. The difference between social groups in

Table 5.1. Studies examining socioeconomic differences in healthy life expectancy

Country	Authors	Health measures	SES indicators	Population	Method	Findings
Austria	Doblhammer and Kytir (1999)	Functional disability, perceived health	Education	Austria, age 30–75	Sullivan	Lower SES groups live fewer healthy and unhealthy years; differences between SES groups are greater in functional disability than in self-perceived health
Belgium	Bossuyt, van Oyen and Page (2000)	Composite of self-perceived health and disability	Education	Belgium, over age 25	Sullivan	Differences in health expectancy larger than in life expectancy; low education results in lower life expectancy and health expectancy, more years of ill-health
Canada	Nault, Roberge and Berthelot (1996)	Disability Education	Income	Canada, over age 30	Sullivan	Differences in healthy life expectancy larger than in total life expectancy. Larger gaps for men than women
Canada	Wilkins and Adams (1983a, 1983b) (2 studies)	Disability	Income quintile	Canada	Sullivan	Those in the upper quintile of the income distribution have longer life and higher proportion of life free of disability
Finland	Valkonen, Sihvonen and Lahelma (1994, 1997) (2 studies)	Limiting long-standing illness, functional disability, self-perceived health	Education	Finland, over age 25	Sullivan	Higher education is linked to higher life expectancy and disability-free life expectancy. Differences in disability-free life expectancy are larger than in life expectancy

Country	Authors	Health measure	SES measure	Population	Method	Findings
Finland	Kaprio, Sarna, Fogelholm and Koskenvuo (1996)	Receipt of disability pension	Occupation	Finland, men in good health age 20 to age 65	Sullivan	Those in higher status occupations have longer life expectancy and larger proportion of life free of occupationally incapacitating disability
France	Cambois, Robine and Hayward (2001)	Disability	Occupation	Males > 35, currently working or with past activity	Sullivan, two time points	Differences in healthy life larger than differences in life expectancy. Manual workers have the shortest total and longest life expectancy with disability. Change over time has been similar for all groups – inequality has not changed – all have had a compression of morbidity
Great Britain	Bebbington (1993)	Limiting long-standing illness	Occupational social class	Males over age 20	Sullivan	Differences in mortality and morbidity combine to make larger socioeconomic differences in health expectancy than in life expectancy
Netherlands	Boshuizen, van de Water and Perenboom (1994)	Self-reported health	Education	Males, all ages	Sullivan	Larger SES differences in health expectancy than in life expectancy
Netherlands	van den Bos and van der Maas (1993)	Presence of chronic conditions, disability	Index of income, education, and occupation	Persons 55–79, Amsterdam	Sullivan	Lower SES groups have lower life and health expectancy. The years spent with disability are greater for low status men. For women the differences vary by age. Years spent with chronic conditions are higher for women of lower status. For men there is variability by age

(continued)

Table 5.1. (*continued*)

Country	Authors	Health measures	SES indicators	Population	Method	Findings
Norway and Finland	Sihvonen, Kunst, Lahelma, Valkonen and Mackenbach (1998)	Limiting long-standing illness, functional disability, self-perceived health	Education	Persons 25–74	Sullivan	Socioeconomic differences are greatest in healthy life expectancy. More healthy years and fewer unhealthy years for those of higher status
Sweden	Pettersson (1995a)	Health Measure: Composite of limiting long-standing illness and self-perceived health	Occupation	Sweden, 16–84	Sullivan, Trends	Higher SES group lives longer healthy and fewer unhealthy years. Widening gap due to less favorable development of lowest status group
United States	Crimmins, Saito and Ingegneri (1989)	Disability	Race	US	Sullivan, Trends	Greater racial differences in health expectancy than life expectancy. Change between 1970 and 1980 in same direction for race groups
United States	Hayward, Heron	Disability	Race/ethnicity	Persons over age 20	Sullivan	Pattern more complex than observed in most other studies. Some groups have longer lives and fewer years of disability – Asians; others have longer lives and longer disability – Native Americans. Blacks have shorter lives with a higher proportion disabled than whites or Hispanics. Longer life does not always mean better health

Country	Author	Measure	Determinant	Population	Method	Findings
United States	Guralnik, Land, Blazer, Fillenbaum and Branch (1993)	Disability – ADL impairment	Education – race	North Carolina Counties	Increment/ decrement life tables	Education is more strongly related to life expectancy and active life than is race. Generally, the differences between groups are larger in total life than active life. No differences by education in proportion of life active. Differences between blacks and whites depend on age
United States	Crimmins, Hayward and Saito (1996)	ADL and IADL impairment	Education	US population 70 and over	Multistate	Socioeconomic differences in active life expectancy exceed those in total life expectancy. At oldest ages – differences in life expectancy by race are not found but blacks live fewer active years and more inactive years. Those with lower education live more years inactive and fewer active. Even at age 70, there are differences by education in total life expectancy
United States	Crimmins and Saito (2001)	Disability	Education and race	US population over 30	Sullivan	Differences in healthy life are greater than differences in total life expectancy. Differences in healthy life expectancy by education have been widening over time

(continued)

Table 5.1. *(continued)*

Country	Authors	Health measures	SES indicators	Population	Method	Findings
United States	Katz, Branch, Branson, Papsidero, Beck and Greer (1983)	ADL impairment	Poor versus non-poor. Poor indicated by receipt of income or medical care from means-tested pro-grams	Non-institutionalized population of the state of Massachusetts, 1974	Double decre-ment	Active life is shorter for the poor
United States	Manton, Stallard and Corder (1997)	Functioning	Education	US population 65 +		Dynamic assessment of change, stochastic process life tables Findings: Higher education results in longer life expectancy; a longer life expectancy without disability; shorter life with disability and a lower proportion of life with disability

ADL, activities of daily living; IADL, instrumental activities of daily living; SES, socioeconomic status.

expected years of healthy life always is considerably above the diagonal in the figure, meaning that the ratio is above 2:1. The largest socioeconomic difference in life expectancy was about 6 years; the largest difference in the length of expected healthy life was about 18 years or three times as long. In general, larger socioeconomic differences in total life expectancy are linked to larger socioeconomic differences in healthy life expectancy. The excess length of unhealthy life among the low status men in these five countries (not shown in the figure) ranges from 2 years to 12 years. This means that persons of low status have longer unhealthy lives as well as shorter healthy lives.

As mentioned above, the size of inequality in the length of healthy life depends on the indicator of health used. In Table 5.2 the differential between the highest and lowest status groups in length of healthy life is shown for a set of studies that include measures of healthy life based on both perceived health and disability. For men, socioeconomic differences in the length of healthy life are always greater using the perceived health measure although the differences between that and the disability measure are small in most cases. The size of social differentials is not consistently greater using either measure among women in the examples shown in Table 5.2. In two of the examples, however, the social differences for women are much larger using the perceived health measure. This may be because perceived health is based on a composite of health dimensions all of which may differ by socioeconomic status in these countries. It is also possible that people of different social status in different countries and of different genders are more or less willing to report ill-health of different types (Laditka and Jenkins, 1999).

It is difficult to draw a conclusion about gender differences in social inequality. Comparing the figures for men and women from the same study in Table 5.2 indicates that the socioeconomic differential in length of disability-free life is fairly similar for men and women – although the differences are slightly greater for men. Given the generally shorter life expectancies of men, this would mean that the proportional differences would be somewhat greater. The differences by gender in the size of the social difference in length of healthy life defined by perceived health are larger but they are inconsistent in direction by gender.

Inequality in healthy life persists into old age. Studies of health differentials in the oldest years find substantial relationships between indicators of socioeconomic status and mortality and morbidity. One issue in examining age differences in socioeconomic differences in health expectancy is that the composition of the surviving cohort is affected by the very process under examination. Those less likely to survive – those of lower status – will not be in the older years when the measures are taken. This feature has resulted in the supplementation of measures of health expectancy – years of healthy life lived – with measures of health gaps – which includes years not lived – in some analyses of social differences in length of healthy life (Crimmins and

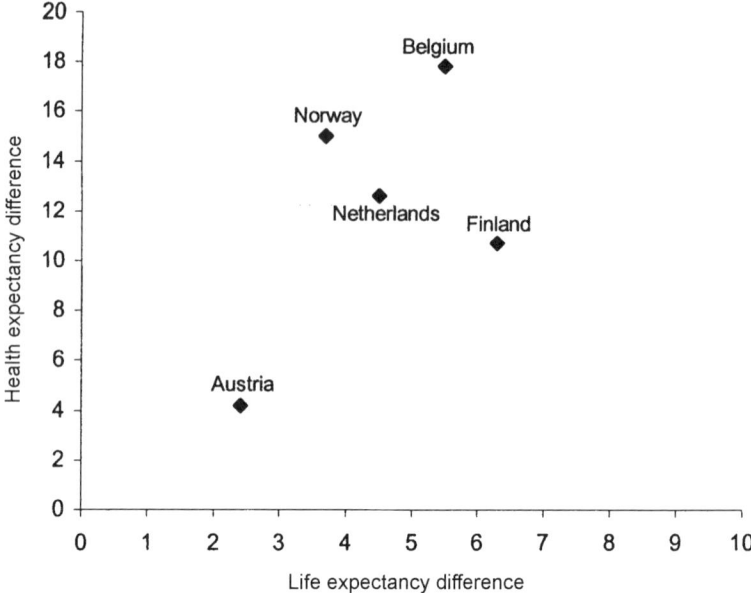

Figure 5.1. Differences between high status and low status groups in health expectancy (perceived health) and life expectancy (adult males in five countries)
Sources: Boshuizen *et al* (1994); Bossuyt *et al* (2000); Doblhammer and Kytir (1999); Valkonen *et al* (1994, 1997)

Table 5.2. Difference between high status and low status groups in length of healthy life by two definitions, perceived health and disability: men and women in five countries

| | Difference in healthy life | | |
	Perceived health	Disability	Age
Men			
Belgium	17.8	17.2	25
Finland	10.7	9.9	25
Austria	4.2	3.8	30–75
Norway	15	9.1	25–74
US whites		10.8	30
Women			
Belgium	24.5	17.3	25
Finland	6.4	7.8	25
Austria	2.2	2.3	30–75
Norway	14.8	8.4	25–74
US whites		9.5	30

Sources: Bossuyt *et al* (2000); Crimmins and Saito (2001); Doblhammer and Kytir (1999); Valkohen *et al* (1994, 1997).

Saito, 2001; Sihvonen *et al*, 1998). This allows examination of three components of social class differences in the length of life: years not lived, years lived in good health, and years lived in poor health.

CHANGE OVER TIME IN INEQUALITY

Only a few studies have addressed change over time in inequality in healthy life. Studies of French occupational groups during the 1980s indicated no change in inequality in healthy life but rather similar improvement across occupational groups (Cambois *et al*, 2001). On the other hand, three other studies point to a recent widening of differentials. A study of occupational differences in Sweden indicated an increase in the difference in length of healthy life for manual and non-manual workers between 1975–1980 and 1986–1990 (Pettersson, 1995a). Examination of change in occupational differentials from 1980–1981 and 1992–1993 led to the same conclusion (Davis *et al*, 1999). In the United States from 1970 to 1990 there was an increase in educational differences in healthy life expectancy due to a widening of differentials in both mortality and morbidity (Crimmins and Saito, 2001).

CONCLUSION

Inequality in health outcomes is one of the major problems faced by policy makers at the beginning of the 21st century. Measures of health expectancy provide useful summaries of the effect of social inequality on mortality and morbidity. While it is difficult to make comparisons across countries, the numerical estimates provide useful guides to the relative size of social differences within countries. Attention to consistency of surveys and to the incorporation of measures which are not influenced by attitudes related to social status is important for monitoring national health differentials. Particular attention needs to be paid to the development of objective indicators for the examination of change over time

REFERENCES

Bebbington, A. (1993) 'Regional and social variations in disability-free life expectancy in Great Britain', in Robine, J-M., Mathers, C., Bone, M. and Romieu, I. (eds) *Calculation of Health Expectancy: Harmonization, Consensus Achieved and Future Perspectives*. Montrouge: John Libbey Eurotext.

Bone, M.R., Bebbington, A.C., Jagger, C., Morgan, K. and Nicolaas, G. (1995) *Health Expectancy and Its Uses*. London: HMSO.

Boshuizen, H., van de Water, H. and Perenboom, R. (1994) 'Socioeconomic differences in health expectancy in the Netherlands', in Mathers, C., McCallum, J. and Robine, J-M. (eds) *Advances in Health Expectancies*. Canberra: Australian Institute of Health and Welfare.

Bossuyt, N., van Oyen, H. and Page, H. (2000) 'Healthy life expectancy and disability-free life expectancy by educational attainment in Belgium', Paper presented at the 12th meeting of REVES.

Bronnum-Hansen, H. (1999) 'Socio-economic differentials in health expectancy in Denmark', Communication at the 11th REVES meeting, London 1999.

Cambois, E., Robine, J.M. and Hayward, M. (2001) 'Social Inequalities in disability-free life expectancy in the French male population, 1980–1991', *Demography* 38(4), 513–524.

Crimmins, E. and Saito, Y. (2001) 'Trends in disability-free life expectancy in the United States, 1970–1990: Gender, racial, and educational differences', *Social Science and Medicine* 52(11), 1629–1641.

Crimmins, E., Saito, Y. and Ingegneri, D. (1989) 'Changes in life expectancy and disability-free life expectancy in the United States', *Population and Development Review* 15, 235–267.

Crimmins, E., Hayward, M. and Saito, Y. (1996) 'Differentials in active life expectancy in the older population of the United States', *Journal of Gerontology: Social Sciences* 51B(3), S111–S120.

Crimmins, E., Saito, Y. and Ingegneri, D. (1997) 'Trends in disability-free life expectancy in the United States, 1970–90', *Population and Development Review* 23, 555–572.

Davis, P., Graham, P. and Pearce, N. (1999) 'Health expectancy in New Zealand 1981–1991: Social variation and trends in a period of social and economic change', *Journal of Epidemiology and Community Health* 53, 519–527.

Doblhammer, G. and Kytir, J. (1999) 'Social inequalities in mortality and morbidity: Consequences for DFLE', in Egidi, V. (ed.) *Towards an integrated system of indicators to assess the health status of the population*. Rome: ISTAT, 1999 [Essays no. 4].

Guralnik, J., Land, K., Blazer, D., Fillenbaum, G. and Branch, L. (1993) 'Educational status and active life expectancy among older blacks and whites', *New England Journal of Medicine* 329, 110–116.

Hayward, M. and Heron, M. (1996) 'Racial inequality in active life among adult Americans', *Demography* 36, 77–91.

Kaprio, J., Sarna, S., Fogelholm, M. and Koskenvuo, M. (1996) 'Total and occupationally active life expectancies in relation to social class and marital status in men classified as healthy at 20 in Finland', *Journal of Epidemiology and Community Health* 50, 653–660.

Katz, S., Branch, L., Branson, M., Papsidero, J., Beck, J. and Greer, D. (1983) 'Active life expectancy', *New England Journal of Medicine* 309, 1218–1224.

Laditka, S.B. and Jenkins, C.L. (1999) 'Effects of disability measurement scales on active life expectancy estimates'. Presented at Network on Health Expectancy REVES 11 Conference, London, 15–17 April.

Manton, K.G., Stallard, E. and Corder, L. (1997) 'Education-specific estimates of life expectancy and age-specific disability in the US elderly population, 1982 to 1991'. *Journal of Aging and Health* 9, 419–450.

Marmot, M.G., Kogevinas, M. and Elston, M.A. (1987) 'Social/economic status and disease', *Annual Review of Public Health* 8, 111–135.

Nault, F., Roberge, R. and Berthelot, J. (1996) 'Espérance de vie et espérance de vie en santé selon le sexe, l'état matrimonial et le statut socio-économique au Canada', *Cahier Quebecois de Demographie* 2, 241–259.

Pettersson, H. (1995a) 'Trends in health expectancy for socio-economic groups in Sweden', in 8th Work-group meeting REVES, International Research Network for Interpretation of Observed Values of Healthy Life expectancy, Chicago.

Pettersson, H. (1995b) 'Längre och friskare liv för tjänstemän', *VälfärdsBulletinen* 1, 10–13.

Preston, S.H. and Elo, I.T. (1995) 'Are educational differentials in adult mortality increasing in the United States?' *Journal of Aging and Health* 7, 476–496.

Sihvonen, A., Kunst, A., Lahelma, E., Valkonen, T. and Mackenbach, J. (1998) 'Socioeconomic inequalities in health expectancy in Finland and Norway in the late 1980s', *Social Science and Medicine* 47, 303–315.

Sullivan, D. (1971) 'A single index of mortality and morbidity', *HSMHA Health Reports* 86, 347–354.

Townsend, P. and David, N. (eds) (1982) *Inequalities in Health: The Black Report.* London: Penguin Books.

Valkonen, T., Sihvonen, A. and Lahelma, E. (1994) 'Disability-free life expectancy by level of education in Finland', in Mathers, C., McCallum, J. and Robine, J-M. (eds) *Advances in Health Expectancies.* Canberra: Australian Institute of Health and Welfare.

Valkonen, T., Sihvonen, A. and Lahelma, E. (1997) 'Disability-free life expectancy by level of education in Finland', *Social Science and Medicine* 44, 801–808.

van den Bos, G. and van der Maas, P.J. (1993) 'Social inequalities in the basic components of health expectancy: chronic morbidity, disability, and mortality', in Robine, J-M., Mathers, C., Bone, M. and. Romieu, I. (eds) *Calculation of Health Expectancy: Harmonization, Consensus Achieved and Future Perspectives.* Montrouge: John Libbey Eurotext.

van de Water, H., Boshuizen, H. and Perenboom, R. (1996) 'Health expectancy in the Netherlands: 1983–1990', *European Journal of Public Health*, 6, 21–28.

Wilkins, R. and Adams, O. (1983a) 'Health expectancy in Canada, late 1970s: demographic, regional, and social dimensions', *American Journal of Public Health* 73, 1073–1080.

Wilkins, R. and Adams, O. (1983b) *Healthfulness of Life: A Unified View of Mortality, Institutionalization and Non-institutionalized Disability in Canada, 1978.* Montreal: The Institute for Research on Public Policy.

World Health Organization – Regional Office for Europe (1998) *Health 21: The Health for All Policy for the WHO European Region: 21 Targets for the 21st Century.* Regional Committee for Europe, 48th Session, Copenhagen, 14–18 September.

6

Sub-national Variations in Health Expectancy

ANDREW BEBBINGTON and MADHAVI BAJEKAL*
University of Kent, Canterbury, Kent, UK and *National Centre for Social Research, London, UK

INTRODUCTION

Regional and local variations within countries are, along with social class, education, gender and ethnicity variations, an important aspect of equity which health expectancy[1] measures have been used to examine. While location variations are perhaps less immediate to an individual's personal circumstances than the other socio-demographic factors, there are three reasons why they are important. First, health services delivery is essentially geographically determined, and must be administered locally. In countries where the management of health care is centralised, identifying health variations as a basis for regional and local resource allocation is a major policy issue. Second, the collection of evidence about health, such as mortality statistics, is invariably organised locally, so figures for local variations are often more readily available, more reliable, and more detailed, than those based on, for example, social class. Third, some social characteristics which are relevant to equity issues are themselves closely linked to locality: such as comparisons between urban and rural dwellers, the needs of deprived neighbourhoods.

This chapter reviews a number of studies that have been concerned with the sub-national dimension in health expectancy variations. Two types of enquiry can be distinguished:

---

[1] Health expectancy here includes all related measures that combine life expectancy with states of health, such as active life expectancy, disease-free life expectancy, years free of long-term health care use, quality-adjusted life years, and other health measures which are based on years of life lived at particular health states, to which relative valuations may be applied. Note that unless stated otherwise, results in this chapter generally relate to health expectancy at birth.

Determining Health Expectancies. Edited by J-M. Robine, C. Jagger, C.D. Mathers, E.M. Crimmins and R.M. Suzman.

- *Comparative.* Studies that are intended to measure and describe health expectancy variations between regions and localities generally, sometimes through time. Such studies may be designed to influence national policies for health planning and resource allocation.
- *Analytic.* Studies that are intended to describe health expectancy differences between *particular types* of areas. Many of these studies are concerned with urban–rural comparisons. Another type of study investigates local variations not for their own sake, but in order to identify whether deprivation or other socio-demographic factors measured at local level can be associated with local variations in health expectancy.

Some of the papers we cite include both types of enquiry.

This chapter also reviews two methodological problems that are specific to regional/local measures:

- The sample sizes needed for making comparisons.
- The effect of internal migration for Sullivan's method.

Finally, we discuss two issues of particular relevance to these studies:

- The role of health expectancy as a tool for regional or local resource allocation.
- The relationship between local life expectancy and the proportion of life in good health.

COMPARATIVE STUDIES

Without exception, comparative studies have used Sullivan's method. This combines local mortality registration statistics with measures of health derived from a large-scale survey (adjusted to allow for the institutional population), or in some cases health data from a census. The countries which have been most active in producing comparative sub-national estimates for health expectancy are Canada, England and Wales, France and Spain. The following paragraphs summarise what is available from these and some other countries.[2]

CANADA

The first regional comparisons for any country were made by Wilkins and Adams (1983). They used the 1978–1979 Canada Health Survey, based on self-reported disability. Results are presented by province, with smaller provinces being grouped together, into five regions in total. The authors also combined

---

[2] Published health expectancy regional/local estimates are not reproduced in this chapter. These figures will be made available from the REVES website at http://www.prw.le.ac.uk/reves/.

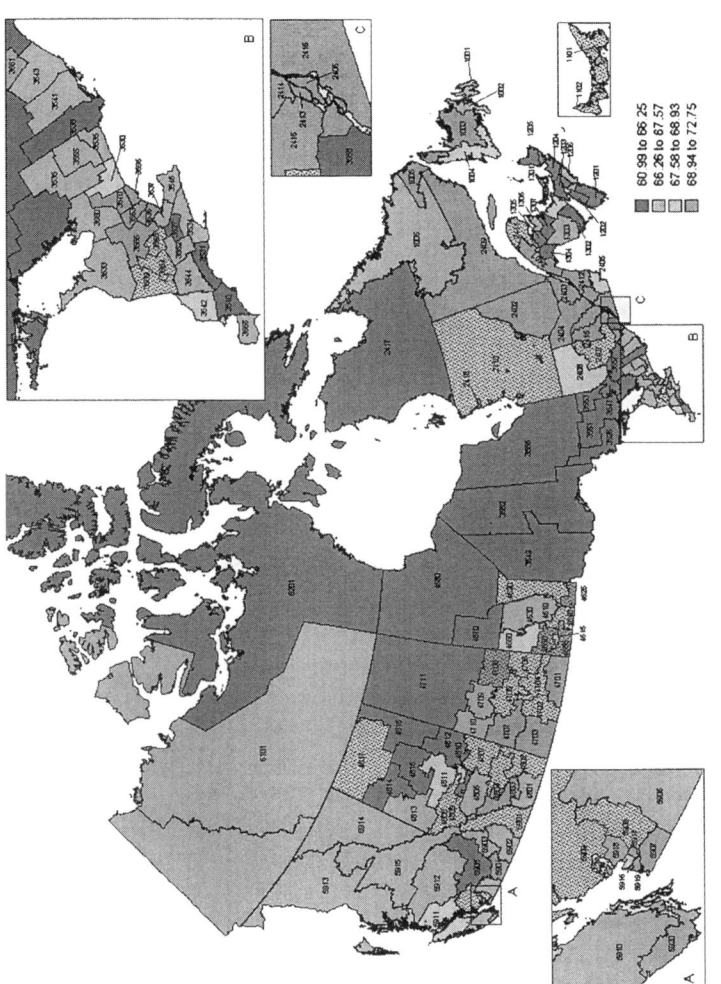

Figure 6.1. Disability-free life expectancy by quartile in Canada, both sexes, 1996.
Source: Mayer *et al* (2001). Reproduced by permission of Statistics Canada. Statistics Canada information is used with the permission of the Minister of Industry, as Minister responsible for Statistics Canada. Information on the availability of the wide range of data from Statistics Canada can be obtained from Statistics Canada's Regional Offices, its World Wide Web site at http://www.statcan.ca, and its toll-free access number 1-800-263-1136.

various levels of disability into what they termed a quality-adjusted life expectancy: one of the few times that such estimates of any kind have been presented by geographical area.

Subsequent Canadian studies were more localised. Wilkins (1986) gave estimates for localities in Montreal based on similar data. Lafontaine *et al* (1991) provide estimates for 18 districts of Quebec province. Manuel *et al* (2000) provide estimates for the 42 health districts of Ontario, using the Health Utilities Index based on the 1990 Ontario Health Survey. They found wide variation in health expectancy, with rural and northern areas lowest, but admitted that the sample size was not sufficient to establish local differences with sufficient precision.

The most comprehensive Canadian study to date, Mayer *et al* (2001), used the question on long-term limiting disablement in the 1996 census to estimate disability-free life expectancy (DFLE) for 138 health regions across Canada (Figure 6.1). Apart from two small outliers, average life expectancy (males and females combined) ranged by 8 years from 73.5 to 81.2, while DFLE ranged by 11.5 years from 61.3 to 72.8. High DFLE is generally observed in health regions in large urban centres, with services availability, high affluence and high immigration – 'Canada main street'. Like Manuel *et al* (2000), Mayer *et al* found that the lowest DFLE is generally in rural or northern regions.

Wilkins *et al* (2001) have prepared health expectancies by neighbourhood for all urban areas based on the 1996 census question on activity limitations, but at the time of writing these figures are unpublished.

ENGLAND AND WALES

Three studies in England and Wales have examined geographical variations in health expectancies. Bebbington (1993) used the 1985–1988 National Disability Survey, with its elaborate 10-factor definition of disability based on an initial sample of around 100 000 households, to prepare estimates across the 10 Standard Regions, for men and women separately (Figure 6.2).[3] Bone *et al* (1995) made use of the limiting longstanding illness question in the 1991 census to prepare estimates for the 10 Standard Regions, the 15 Health Regions, and the 115 Local Administration Areas of England and Wales. Bajekal (2001b) has presented estimates for the 100 or so health authorities of England using the Health Survey for England 1994–1998 (combined sample size 90 000), with the standard 5-point self-rating of health as the basis for health expectancy. All three of these studies, though separated through time and using different measures, identified a very similar pattern in the distribution of health expectancies, with the south-east of England having the highest expectancies

---

[3] Figures 6.2, 6.3 and 6.5 are for males only, to save space. Corresponding figures for females are provided in the sources, and in each case show broadly similar patterns to those for males.

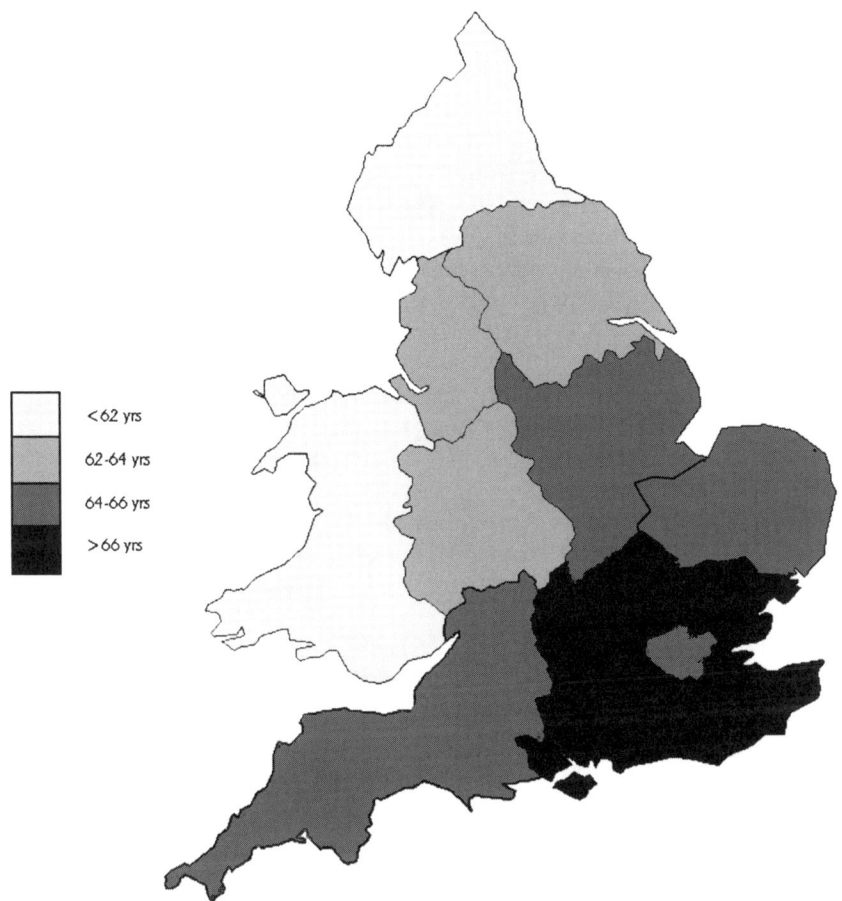

Figure 6.2. Disability-free life expectancy in England and Wales, men, 1985. *Source:* Bebbington (1993, from Table 6)

and the north-west having the lowest. With a comparatively small sample size per area, Bajekal's estimates did have quite wide confidence intervals, typically of around ± 2 years per area. Bissett *et al* (2001) examined the stability of these results by comparing them with ones prepared from the General Household Survey, aggregated over the years 1992–1998. The two measures correlate ($\rho = 0.84$) across health authorities.

FRANCE

Early papers by Colvez *et al* (1983) and Robine *et al* (1986) raised many of the issues associated with regional variations in chronic ill-health and the potential role of health expectancy. But the best source of information is by Robine *et al* (1998) who produced statistics for nine regions of France, for men and women separately. This study is particularly interesting because of its focus on changes through time. It was based on data from the Enquiry on Health and Medical Needs of 1980–1981 and 1991–1992, applied to life tables centred on 1982 and 1990. This used confinement within the home as a measure of disability. Although the general pattern of life expectancy was similar between the two dates, with a distinct north–south gradient, there were some striking changes in the age pattern of disability between the two dates. Four distinct change patterns were observed, applying to different regions though similar between men and women:

1. Strong decline in the disability rate among older people, above 60 (e.g. Nord-Pas-de-Calais).
2. Strong decline in the disability rate in the late middle-aged, 50–69, (e.g. Lorraine/Alsace).
3. Little change (e.g. Rhone-Alps/Auvergne).
4. Rise in the disability rate among younger people, below 50 (e.g. Ile-de-France).

The consequence is that the pattern of healthy life expectancy is remarkably different between the two estimates (Figure 6.3). In particular, the Ile-de-France region around Paris switched from being one of the best to one of the worst areas. The standard errors of regional estimates are at most one year, and so these changes are statistically significant.

SPAIN

Regional comparisons through time are also available for Spain. Gispert and Gutiérrez-Fisac (1995) summarise a programme of work on variations in health expectancy measures, for the 17 autonomous regions of Spain (Figure 6.4). Disability-free life expectancy was determined from a national survey of Disabilities, Impairments and Handicaps in 1986, while Regidor *et al* (1995) used the same source to show variations in functional limitation-free expectancy. More recently, Gutiérrez-Fisac *et al* (2000) have reanalysed the disability-free estimates for the 50 provinces into which Spain is now divided, with an analysis of the causes of these variations. Gispert and Gutiérrez-Fisac (1995) also report healthy life expectancy (HLE) (self-reported health) from the National Health Interview Surveys of 1986 and 1991. As with France, the pattern of change through time is confused, with some regions (Murcia, Navarra) gaining up to 4 years of HLE while another (Asturias) loses almost as much.

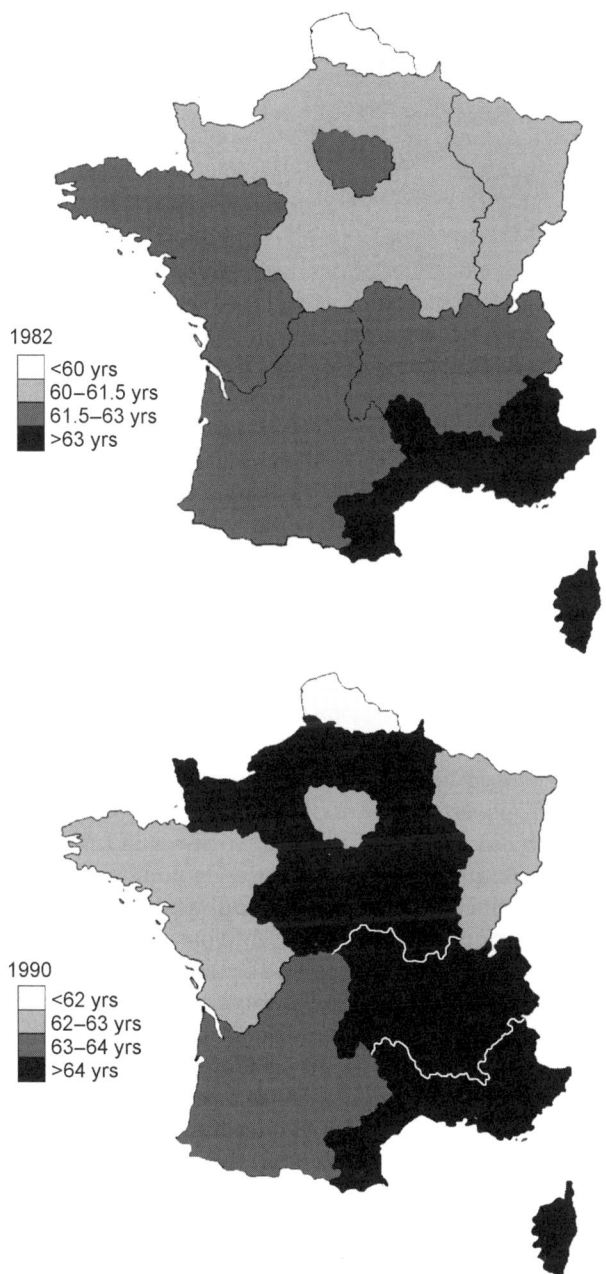

Figure 6.3. Life expectancy without disability in France, men, 1982 and 1990.
Source: Robine *et al* (1998, from Table 3)

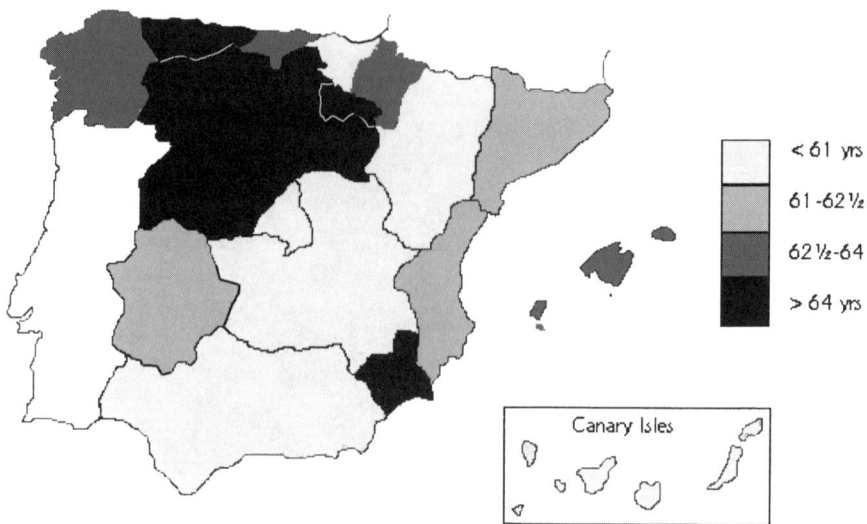

Figure 6.4. Disability-free life expectancy in Spain, both sexes, 1986.
Source: Gispert and Gutiérrez-Fisac (1995, from Figure 1). Reproduced with permission

OTHER COUNTRIES

Mathers (1991) reported up to eight years' difference in disability-free life expectancy across the eight states of *Australia*. Disability-adjusted life years for 1996 in the 78 local government areas of Victoria State have recently been published by Victoria Department of Human Services (2001) based on the Victoria Burden of Disease Study. Buratta and Crialesi (1993, cited by Robine and Romieu, 1998) contrast three regions of *Italy*. Compared with other studies the regional variations are remarkably small, with the Centrale region having both the highest life expectancy and healthy life expectancy, for both men and women. Van Oyen *et al* (1996) compared the Flemish and Walloon regions of *Belgium* using self-perceived health in a survey of about 2600. Walloons have not only a shorter life but a shorter healthy life. Nayar (1994) has presented life expectancies and rates of self-reported morbidity by state in *India*, based on a 1973–1974 health survey; though healthy life expectancies as such do not appear to have been calculated. Kerala, with the highest life expectancy, has by far the worst rates of self-reported morbidity. In view of the very large number of studies examining socio-demographic variations, there is surprisingly little published on state variations in the *United States*. For example, in presenting state variations in reported healthy days per month, CDC (1998) suggested that health expectancies had not been used as they would have been less sensitive to local variations in population health. Whether this is true may be questioned. But many of the 'variations' studies in the US now use longitudinal data, which is unsuitable for detailed inter-state variations because of the sample sizes required.

STUDIES OF SPECIFIC HEALTH CONDITIONS AND SERVICE USE

There are a few studies that have examined local variations in health expectancy for specific conditions. Richie *et al* (1994) compared dementia-free life expectancy in Aquitaine with *France* as a whole, arguing that France in future would be like Aquitaine and the proportion of dementia-free life might therefore be expected to fall slightly. A related type of study focuses on health care use. Bérod and Santos-Eggimann (1999) estimated life expectancy at 65 free of formal care use, for five areas of *Switzerland*. They found that although the expected number of years with care was constant across areas, the balance between home care and nursing home care varied considerably. Bebbington (2001) examined regional differences in *England* in healthy life expectancy of people admitted to care homes. The considerable differences were attributed to admissions policies. Both these last two studies argued for more uniformity in health care provision.

ANALYTIC STUDIES

Analytic studies exist at different levels of complexity. The simpler ones are designed to examine variations between types of area, generally based on a social survey where individuals are classified according to area type. A more complex type of study uses variations between local areas as the basis of an ecological analysis of the factors which affect, or perhaps determine, health expectancies.

URBAN AND RURAL AREAS

For developing countries such comparisons serve not just to demonstrate that differences exist, but to identify emerging health care issues, particularly where rapid urbanisation is taking place, or where governments are becoming concerned to extend health services systematically to rural areas, taking into account both the access problems and lifestyle differences. Brown (1993) compared life, active life and impaired health expectancies in *Ethiopia*, as between Addis Ababa, urban, and rural areas of Arsi Province, based on a survey in 1984. Life expectancy was highest among the urban Arsi, while for males both the active life expectancy and the unimpaired health expectancy is highest in rural Arsi. The implication drawn was that reductions in mortality would result in increased levels of impairment. Qiao *et al* (1993) examined

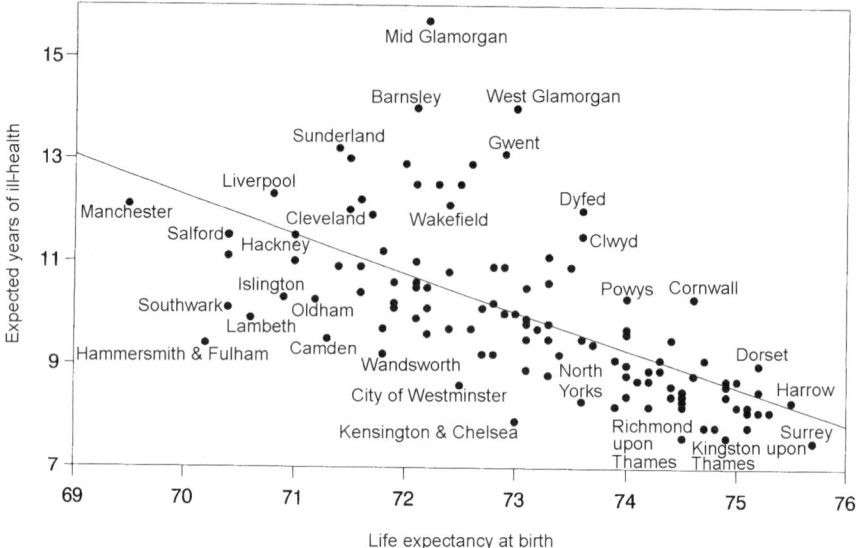

Figure 6.5. Life expectancy and expected years of ill-health, local authorities in England and Wales, 1991, men.
Source: Bone *et al* (1995). Reproduced with permission

urban–rural differences in Xichang, a prefecture of about 170 000 people in *China*, based on a 1989 survey which measured ADL (activities of daily living) and IADL (instrumental activities daily living) disability. Life expectancy at age 15 was about 3 years higher in urban areas compared with rural areas, and health expectancy free from all problems about 5 years higher. Nearly all the extra years of disability were, however, at the lesser end of need, difficulties rather than inability, IADL rather than ADL. Urban–rural differences were far more noticeable than in an identically designed *Canadian* survey. By contrast, in the *US*, Geronimus *et al* (2001) report that rural dwellers outlive urban residents, though their extra years of life are primarily inactive. Charlton (1996) concludes that in *England and Wales*, the health advantage of rural areas increased between 1981 and 1991.

AFFLUENT AND DEPRIVED NEIGHBOURHOODS

Bajekal (2001a) examined healthy life expectancy variations according to the deprivation of the locality (electoral ward) in *England*, between 1994 and 1999. Wards were divided into 10 groups according to affluence and then individuals in the Health Survey for England were classified according to the ward where they lived. Differences in both life expectancy and healthy life expectancy proved considerable across affluence deciles. This inequality is higher for self-reported general health than for self-reported functional disability. Two similar analyses have been undertaken in *Canada*. Pampalon *et al* (2001) used the 1998 Quebec Health and Social Survey, with deprivation measured at enumeration district, by two factors derived from a number of deprivation measures. They report considerable differences in disability and handicap-free life expectancies according to the neighbourhood deprivation scores. Interestingly, the relationship between healthy life expectancy and the two forms of deprivation appears to be stronger in metropolitan Montreal than elsewhere in Quebec, and the authors cite other work (e.g. Haynes and Gale, 2000) which has shown that the relationship between deprivation and poor health is stronger in urban areas. Wilkins *et al* (2001) categorised neighbourhoods across Canada by income quintiles. They found that poorer neighbourhoods have lower life expectancy with more years of activity limitations. The gradient is clearer for women.

ECOLOGICAL CORRELATION STUDIES

Some studies have attempted to identify the socio-demographic correlates of healthy life expectancy by area analysis. This method is attractive where longitudinal data is unavailable and mortality statistics cannot be reanalysed in relation to individual social characteristics. Bone *et al* (1995) used multiple regression analysis with a range of factors for 115 local government areas in *England and Wales* to show that low healthy life expectancy (based on the 1991 census) is linked to areas of low social class, high unemployment, low population density; while it was higher than average (other factors being allowed for) in retirement areas and areas of ethnic diversity (Figure 6.5). Gutiérrez-Fisac *et al* (2000) took a similar approach in their analysis of the disability-free life expectancies in 50 provinces of *Spain*. Multiple regression analysis on 12 area indicators showed that low DFLE is associated with the illiteracy rate, unemployment rate and percentage of smokers in the population, in that order of significance.

SYNTHETIC AND MULTI-LEVEL MODELLING

Where epidemiologists are not able to study the correlates of mortality directly, they often infer relationships from the type of area where mortality is high. A well-known example is how international variations in heart disease have been linked to differences in diet. The next step is to quantify this relationship: by attributing local variations to the factor, using a form of synthetic estimation. Bone *et al* (1995, Chapter 7) used this approach to estimate mortality rates for different ethnic groups as part of the estimation of healthy life expectancy. While the results were plausible, like all synthetic estimations the approach is very prone to yield biased answers if factors other than that which is of primary interest contribute to local variations. Further insight on this is provided by Pampalon *et al* (1999), who used multi-level modelling to consider whether there are distinct compositional (individual characteristics) and contextual (local area) effects on health perception. While not itself a study of health expectancy, the results are of direct relevance to all ecological measures of health. They showed the existence of local variations in health perception even after allowing for individual characteristics such as gender, lifestyle, socio-economic circumstances, etc.

METHODOLOGICAL ISSUES IN STUDIES OF SUB-NATIONAL VARIATIONS

Local comparisons are easier than international comparisons in that the problems of ensuring a uniform methodology are generally less, and with a common system of health care provision it seems reasonable to suppose that people will share assumptions which will cause them to answer questions about health in a comparable manner. But the results of Nayar (1994) and Pampalon *et al* (1999), for India and Canada respectively, and research in the UK showing that people in higher social classes are more likely to declare less serious conditions (Blaxter, 1990), do indicate that caution is needed.

In addition there are other methodological problems specific to local comparisons of health expectancies which should be borne in mind.

DETECTING SIGNIFICANT DIFFERENCES

Where the estimation of health expectancy depends on a national survey to provide the age-specific rates of ill-health, a common problem is providing sufficiently large sample size to enable statistically significant subgroup comparisons to be made. This is particularly true for local variations where, as the examples in the 'Comparative studies' section above show, researchers wish to subdivide their country into anything from 10 to 100 or more small areas. Robine *et al* (1998) were sensitive to this in their study of changes in regional variations in France, and as we have noted Manuel *et al* (2000) were concerned that their sample sizes were not large enough for the types of comparison they wished to make. But often it is not appreciated how large the sample size needs to be to make subgroup comparisons.

Mathers (1991) gave a method for estimating standard errors of healthy life expectancy estimates from Sullivan's method which has become standard, reproduced for example by Jagger (1996). The standard error generally depends mostly on the sampling errors associated with the estimates of ill-health prevalence, and since many health surveys use locally clustered sampling designs, it is particularly important to make allowance for the design effect.

Table 6.1. Size of the sample and significant differences

Sample size	SE	95% CI ($\pm$ years of HLE)
1000	1.26	2.5
2000	0.89	1.7
4000	0.63	1.2

Source: Bajekal (2001b).

Once standard errors (SE) are estimated, since the locality estimates are independent, a test for detecting significant differences between healthy life expectancy (HLE) in two areas A and B involves the Z score:

$$Z = (\text{HLE}_A - \text{HLE}_B)/(\text{SE}_A + \text{SE}_B).$$

Z values greater than 1.96 are significant at the 95% level. The same test can be used for comparing one area with the national average, the latter assumed to be independent if the number of localities is large.

With several localities, the concern may be to test collectively whether they are different. If it can be assumed that the standard errors of all areas are the same (subject to sampling error), then they can be averaged and a standard one-way analysis of variance test is appropriate.

While we cannot provide guidance in every case, an example will provide an indication of the sort of sample size that is likely to be required (Table 6.1). This example is based on the data used by Bajekal (2001b).[4]

In this example, we have assumed that other than the size of the sample, no other parameter changes, that is identical rates of mortality, illness ratios and design effects. The design effect (deft) has been estimated as 1.2 in this survey.

The example shows that with a sample size of 1000, our estimate of HLE is only accurate to within 2½ years: our local estimate would need to be at least this much different from the national average for us to conclude it was significantly higher or lower (with 95% certainty). And if we wished to compare this locality with another for which a sample size of 1000 was available, the difference between them would need to be 5 years for us to draw conclusions. With a sample of 4000 in each area, these differences need only be half as much for significance. But with say 10 areas to compare, this implies a minimum sample size of 40 000. This example highlights the need for large sample sizes for regional comparisons.

---

[4] Based on one health authority (Cambridge and Huntingdon) in England with a population of about 500 000 (an average sized health authority). HLE at birth was calculated to be 63.3, against an England average of 60.2, for the period 1994–1998. These figures are based on HLE estimates derived from the Health Survey for England, and the pooled sample size for the area was 1000, out of a national total of 90 603.

EFFECT OF MIGRATION ON LOCAL HEALTH ESTIMATES

Almost all local estimates are constructed by Sullivan's method. This method combines the prevalence of ill-health in each age range into an overall life expectancy, to create a summary measure of the healthfulness of the locality. However, one of the attractions of health expectancy as a measure is that it provides estimates in a way that has a meaningful interpretation for individuals. Indeed, it has been shown that in a static population where health and mortality rates are unchanging, Sullivan's measure will provide a realistic estimate for a newborn child.

This assumption will break down if people living in an area aged say, 20, cannot expect to have the same morbidity rates as those aged 60 now, when they reach that age. Migration is one important reason why this may not be so. At national level, immigration rates are often sufficiently small that national health expectancies are unlikely to be affected. In small localities, though, the majority of people born in an area will probably move away at some point. In England, for example, 15% of the population had changed county (communities averaging 1 million people) between 1981 and 1991. Rural areas in England experience significant out-migration of young adults in search of work, to be replaced by people closer to retirement who have been successful in professional careers and who prefer to live away from the conurbations where they worked. They may not be at all like the people that have left. Such a locality could have period based life and healthy life expectancies far higher than the true expectation of a newborn child in the area.

Brimblecombe et al (2000) found from the British Household Panel Survey that the health of people moving from high to low mortality districts could be explained by lifetime advantage, and indeed that male migration accounts for nearly all the differences in mortality rates among districts in Britain. Bebbington et al (1996) examined limiting longstanding illness of migrants between 1981 and 1991 in England from the National Longitudinal Survey and found that London exports many ill people, while the more affluent retirement areas tend to import the relatively healthy.

Migration might therefore create a false impression about the relative healthfulness of areas, particularly where the areas are small and movement rates are high. For example, the improving health of rural as opposed to urban areas in Britain is not necessarily due to the favourable environment or the better formal and informal care that is available, but simply the result of recent migration preferences. Healthy life expectancy calculated by Sullivan's method may give a misleading impression of the static position – it might even discourage policy makers from identifying real preventative health care needs among the young, if older people in the area have a good level of health.

DISCUSSION

HEALTH EXPECTANCIES AND RESOURCE ALLOCATION

Countries like England and Wales, Canada and Spain are interested in local variations in health expectancy estimates because of their potential for guiding resource allocation decisions. While the intention is to provide resources on the basis of individual need, health care services and in general administrative arrangements must be geographically based. So equity objectives – such as equal opportunity of access for equal health need – have prompted publicly funded health care systems to develop methods for encouraging the fair geographic distribution of health care resources.

Conceptually, a summary population health indicator that combines morbidity and mortality rates is an attractive measure – certainly a better health needs adjustment factor than mortality rates which have been used in the UK, as it takes into account both the length and health-related quality of life. In the past, researchers have used self-assessed health status on its own or as part of a composite health expectancy indicator as the 'gold standard' to inform resource allocation decisions by validating the choice of alternative, more accessible, health needs measures that correlate highly with it (Birch *et al*, 1996; Mays *et al*, 1992). Recently, however, a number of commentators have advocated the use of health expectancy as a direct measure of health needs for local resource allocation (Wilkins, 1986; Bone *et al*, 1995) or in modified form (Ferland *et al*, 1996). This shift in emphasis is partly the result of the growth in the body of scientific research on health expectancy and partly a reflection of the shift in policy focus to valuing people's judgements about their health. To date, health expectancy has not, as far as we know, been used for the actual distribution of resources between areas either locally or for regional allocations.

For an indicator to be considered suitable for use in resource allocation, it should ideally have the following attributes:

- The measure should be evidence-based and use widely accepted methodologies.
- The measure should be reasonably robust, stable, and not contain systematic biases in recording or reporting.
- The required data should be routinely available on a consistent basis of adequate quality for all geographical units of allocation.
- The indicator should be acceptable to stakeholders and not liable to create perverse incentives to 'game' the system.
- The link between the indicator and resource needs should be self-evident.

What then are the advantages and concerns about health expectancies? Usually they are based on self-reported health status information generally collected through surveys, leading to concerns about the reliability of subjective self-rated assessments compared with objective (medical) assessment of health. An international review by Idler and Benyamini (1997) shows that simple measures of self-rated global health status consistently predict subsequent morbidity and mortality after controlling for risk factors, diagnosed conditions and current health state. These studies appear to confirm the epidemiological validity of self-reported health as an objective measure of individuals' health status.

However, as was mentioned in the previous section on methodological issues, self-reported health status is also known to vary systematically between population subgroups and over time by differences in expectations and cultural norms for health (Ryan, 1992). This issue of a systematic reporting bias and its potential impact on the magnitude of local variations in health expectancy remains a barrier to the widespread acceptability of the indicator for equity-based resource allocation.

A second set of issues relate to the frequency and reliability of the data available. Often, the morbidity data for calculating local level indicators are derived from national or regional health surveys. Over the past decade, the recording – in terms of survey design and instruments used – and the method of calculation have been developed through the agency of the REVES network. However, the size of the sample for a local area in any one year is rarely large enough to calculate reliable rates. Data over several years often need to be aggregated to get a measure that is precise enough to discriminate between areas. In England, where temporal trends in HLE are smooth and fairly stable over the medium term, pooling together data collected in an identical way over several years remains an acceptable solution to the problem of small numbers. But this condition may not apply uniformly over time or space. As already noted, in France (Robine *et al*, 1998), and Spain (Gutiérrez-Fisac *et al*, 2000), regional health expectancy measures do not seem particularly stable through time.

Where a health/disability measure is included in the census, the measure meets the criteria of reliability and population coverage. In the UK, a question on limiting longstanding health was included in the decennial census in 1991 and both this and another question on self-perceived health have been asked in the recent 2001 census. The inclusion of these questions means that HLE estimates can be calculated for small areas and for different population subgroups (by class, ethnicity etc.) provided that mortality data are also available by identical categories. However, the accuracy afforded by census-based measures needs to be balanced against the fact that data are not therefore *routinely* available and quickly become out of date, particularly at the small area level.

Finally, there is the uncertainty as to how to translate inequalities in health expectancies as a metric for resource needs. It is difficult to devise any outcome-related reimbursement system that avoids perverse incentives. Increasing the resources to areas with poor outcomes may well create a disincentive to improve. It is of interest to compare the potential in this respect of two families of summary measures: health expectancies and health gaps (burden of disease measures, e.g. disability-adjusted life years (DALYs)/years of life lost (YLL)) (Murray *et al*, 2000). Both families of indicators are potentially competing candidate measures for inclusion in formula-based resource allocation. Health expectancy measures offer a number of advantages. They do not depend upon the particular age structure of a population (whereas health gaps do, but can be age-standardised). Because of its similarity with life expectancy, the concept of health expectancy is easier to understand. A further advantage is that expectancies calculated using prevalence measures of ill-health directly incorporate changes in mortality and morbidity rates over time. The main drawback of health expectancies compared with health gaps is that the latter provide an overall summary measure that can be partitioned into cause-specific components. This property of additive decomposition has obvious advantages for the purpose of prioritising action to reduce health inequalities resulting from causes of ill-health and premature mortality that are amenable to health care intervention.

LIFE EXPECTANCY AND THE PROPORTION OF ILL-HEALTH

Studies of inequalities in health expectancies frequently comment on the relationship between life expectancy and the expectation of ill-health. For example, it is now firmly established that almost everywhere women have a higher life expectancy than men but that a greater proportion of this is likely to be in ill-health (Robine and Romieu, 1998). Is there any such simple rule for geographical variations?

Bone *et al* (1995) drew attention to a very striking negative correlation between life expectancy and years of ill-health across 115 administrative areas in England and Wales (see Figure 6.5). Results from Mayer *et al* (2001), for 138 health regions across Canada confirm the same.[5] And Wilkins (1986) also found this relationship in Montreal.

But when the analysis is based on larger regions, this result is far less clear. Bebbington (1993) found the same pattern held at regional level in England, as did Van Oyen *et al* (1996) in Belgium. But an attempt by Robine *et al* (1998) to see if a similar relationship held across nine regions of France produced mixed results. In 1982, years of life with disability are significantly negatively correlated with life expectancy, as in England. However, by 1990, the

---

[5] This may be inferred from their diagram plotting life expectancy against DFLE, since, ignoring two small outliers, the slope of the regression line is greater than 1 and so the slope of the regression line between life expectancy and life expectancy in disability must be negative.

correlation is positive, as a result of considerable changes in the rank order of regions. For Spain, the evidence at regional level from both Regidor *et al* (1995) and Gispert and Gutiérrez-Fisac (1995) is of a strong *positive* correlation between life expectancy and years of ill-health. The same is true for Buratta and Crialesi's (1993) regional analysis of Italy. Wilkins and Adams (1983) found little relationship in their pioneering study of regional variation in Canada.

If there is a negative correlation at local level between life expectancy and years of ill-health, then it would appear that where people live longest, they have the least amount of ill-health. It is tempting to attribute this to some form of 'compression of morbidity'. This postulates that as an upper limit to life expectancy is reached, further health improvements can only serve to compress ill-health into the last few years of life. While this is essentially an argument about change through time, it might also be applied across space, if areas of high life expectancy can be regarded as more 'advanced' in health terms. An alternative explanation is that there are sharp social and wealth variations between local areas in both England and Canada, and so the results we cited above are actually a consequence of these social differences. It seems to be generally true – and certainly so in England – that people in low social classes, poorer, and with lower educational attainment have lower life expectancy and can expect a greater proportion of their life in ill-health. A third possibility is that the internal migration of 'healthy' people to particular areas in a country, particularly at retirement, has the dual consequence of both enhancing period life expectancy estimates and reducing the age-specific rates of ill-health. Areas of out-migration will correspondingly apparently suffer.

CONCLUSION

Sub-national variations in health expectancy provide a useful summarisation of the health distribution in countries, and help us understand how urban–rural and social deprivation variations affect health. It must not be forgotten that the observed pattern may be affected by internal migration, and so may not entirely reflect the inherent healthfulness of areas. Health expectancy measures appear to offer potential as a criterion for regional and local resource allocation, but there remain conceptual and methodological barriers to their use in this role.

REFERENCES

Bajekal, M. (2001a) 'Inequalities in healthy life expectancy at small area level: magnitude and trends in England, 1994–1998', Conference presentation REVES 13, Vancouver.

Bajekal, M. (2001b) 'Healthy life expectancy at Health Authority level – preliminary estimates based on the Health Survey for England, 1994–98', NHS Executive Resource Allocation Technical Advisory Group 2001/06.

Bebbington, A.C. (1993) 'Regional and social variations in disability-free life expectancy in Great Britain', in Robine, J-M., Mathers, C.D., Bone, M. and Romieu, I. (eds) *Calculation of Health Expectancies: Harmonization, Consensus Achieved and Future Perspectives*. Montrouge, France: John Libbey Eurotext.

Bebbington, A.C. (2001) 'Healthy life expectancy and inequalities in survival among older people following long-term admission to care homes in England', Conference presentation REVES 13, Vancouver.

Bebbington, A.C., Darton, R.A. and Nicolaas, G. (1996) 'Healthy Life Expectancy in England and Wales: Recent Evidence', Canterbury, UK: University of Kent DP1205 (available via http://www.ukc.ac.uk/pssru/, publications index).

Bérod, A.C. and Santos-Eggimann, B. (1999) 'Long-term formal-care free life-expectancy in Switzerland', Conference presentation REVES 11, London.

Birch, S., Eyles, J. and Newbold, B. (1996) 'Proxies for healthcare need among populations: validation of alternatives – a study in Quebec', *Journal of Epidemiology and Community Health* 50, 564–569.

Bissett, B., Bajekal, M., Purdon, S. and Kelly, S. (2001) 'Healthy life expectancy in England at sub-national level: a comparison of two survey instruments', Conference presentation REVES 13, Vancouver.

Blaxter, M. (1990) *Health and Lifestyles*. London: Tavistock/Routledge.

Bone, M., Bebbington, A.C., Jagger, C., Morgan, K. and Nicolaas, G. (1995) *Health Expectancy and its Uses*. London: HMSO.

Brimblecombe, N., Dorling, D. and Shaw, M. (2000) 'Migration and geographical inequalities in health in Britain', *Social Science and Medicine* 50, 861–878.

Brown, S.C. (1993) 'Health expectancy values in developing countries: Ethiopia as a case study', in Robine, J-M., Mathers, C.D., Bone, M. and Romieu, I. (eds) *Calculation of Health Expectancies: Harmonization, Consensus Achieved and Future Perspectives*. Montrouge, France: John Libbey Eurotext.

Buratta, V. and Crialesi, R. (1993) 'Salute e speranza di vita', in *Studi di Popolazione. Nuovi approcci per la descrizione e l'interpretazione. Convegno dei Giovani studiosi dei problemi di Popolazione.* Rome: Università La Sapienza, dipartimento di Scienze Demografiche.

Centers for Disease Control (1998) 'State differences in reported healthy days among adults, United States, 1993–6', *Mortality and Morbidity Weekly Reports* 47, 239–243.

Charlton, J. (1996) 'Which areas are healthiest?' *Population Trends* 83,17–24.

Colvez, A. and Blanchet, M. (1983) 'Potential gains in life expectancy free of disability: a tool for health planning?', *International Journal of Epidemiology* 12, 86–91.

Ferland, P., Pampalon, R. and Sauve, J. (1996) 'Un indicateur de besoins pour l'allocation régionale des ressources en santé publique au Québec', *Revue Canadienne de Santé Publique* 87(4), 280–285.

Geronimus, A.T., Bound, J., Waidmann, T.A., Colen, C.G. and Steffick, D. (2001) 'Inequality in life expectancy, functional status, and active life expectancy across selected black and white populations in the United States', *Demography* 38(2), 227–251.

Gispert, R. and Gutiérrez-Fisac, J.L. (1995) 'Health expectancy indicators: the report from Spain', in van de Water, H.P.A. and Perenboom, R.J.M. (eds) *Report of the First Meeting of the Euro-REVES Subcommittee: Policy Relevance and Conceptual Harmonization*. Leiden: TNO Prevention and Health.

Gutiérrez-Fisac, J.L., Gispert, R. and Solà, J. (2000) 'Factors explaining the geographical differences in disability free life expectancy in Spain', *Journal of Epidemiology and Community Health*, 54, 451–455.

Haynes, R. and Gale, S. (2000) 'Deprivation and poor health in rural areas: inequalities hidden by averages'. *Health and Place* 6, 1–11.

Idler, E.A. and Benyamini, Y. (1997) 'Self-rated health and mortality: a review of twenty seven community studies', *Journal of Health and Social Behaviour* 38, 21–37.

Jagger, C. (1996) 'Health expectancy calculation by the Sullivan method: a practical guide', NUPRI Research paper series, 68.

Lafontaine, P., Pampalon, R. and Rochon, M. (1991) 'L'espérance de vie sans incapacité en région au Québec', *Cahiers Québecois de Démographie* 20, 383–404.

Manuel, D.G., Goel, V., Williams, J.I. and Corey, P. (2000) 'Health-adjusted life expectancy at the local level in Ontario', *Chronic Diseases in Canada* 20(2), 73–81 (available via http://www.hc-sc.gc.ca/hpb/lcdc/publicat/cdic/cdic212).

Mathers, C.D. (1991) *Health Expectancies in Australia 1981 and 1988*. Canberra: Australian Institute of Health; AGPS.

Mayer, F., Ross, N., Berthelot, J-M. and Wilkins, R. (2001) 'Health expectancy by health region in Canada, 1996', Conference presentation REVES 13, Vancouver.

Mays, N., Chinn, S. and Mui Ho, K. (1992) 'Interregional variations in measures of health from the Health and Lifestyle Survey and their relation with indicators of health care need in England', *Journal of Epidemiology and Community Health* 46, 38–47.

Murray, C., Salomon, J. and Mathers, C.D. (2000) 'A critical examination of summary measures of population health', *Bulletin of the World Health Organization* 78 (8), 981–984.

Nayar, P.K.B. (1994) 'Kerala's low mortality and high morbidity: perceptual factors in health status', in Mathers, C., McCallum, J. and Robine, J.-M. (eds) *Advances in Health Expectancies*. Canberra, Australia: Australian Institute of Health and Welfare.

Pampalon, R., Duncan, C., Subramanian, S.V. and Jones, K. (1999) 'Geographies of health perception in Quebec: a multilevel perspective', *Social Science and Medicine* 48, 1483–1490.

Pampalon, R., Choinière, R. and Rochon, M. (2001) 'Healthy life expectancy and deprivation in Québec, 1996–1998', Conference presentation REVES 13, Vancouver.

Qiao, Z., Wilkins, R., Yang, M., Lan, Y., Chen, X., Xu, Y. and Ng, E. (1993) 'Health expectancy of adults in Xichang, China, 1990: autonomy in various activities of daily living', in Robine, J-M., Mathers, C.D., Bone, M. and Romieu, I. (eds) *Calculation of Health Expectancies: Harmonization, Consensus Achieved and Future Perspectives*. Montrouge, France: John Libbey Eurotext.

Regidor, E., Rodriguez, C. and Gutiérrez-Fisac, J.L. (1995) *Indicadores de Salud: Tercera evaluacion en Espana del programa regional europeo Salud Para Todos*. Madrid: Ministeriode Sanidad y Consumo.

Ritchie, K., Robine, J-M., Letenneur, L. and Dartigues, J.F. (1994) 'Dementia-free life expectancy in France', *American Journal of Public Health* 84, 232–236.

Robine, J-M. and Romieu, I. (1998) *Health Expectancies in the European Union: Progress Achieved*. Montpellier, France: REVES/INSERM (REVES Paper 319).

Robine, J-M., Colvez, A., Bucquet, D., Hatton, F., Morel, B. and Lelaidier, S. (1986) 'L'espérance de vie sans incapacité en France en 1982', *Population* 6, 1025–1042.

Robine, J-M., Cambois, E., Romieu, I. and Mormiche, P. (1998) *Variations régionales de l'espérance de vie sans incapacité en France entre 1982 et 1990: Report for Haut Comité de Santé Publique*. Montpellier, France: REVES/INSERM.

Ryan, J.S. (1992) 'Measuring the cultural inflation of morbidity during the decline in mortality', *Health Transition Review* 2(1), 79–89.

Van Oyen, H., Tafforeau, J. and Roelands, M. (1996) 'Regional inequities in health expectancy in Belgium', *Social Science and Medicine* 43(11), 1673–1678.

Victoria Department of Human Services, Health Outcomes Section (2001) Burden of Disease Estimates for LGAs of Victoria. Report and data available via http://www.dhs.vic.gov.au/phd/lgabod/index.htm

Wilkins, R. (1986) 'Health expectancy by local area in Montréal: a summary of findings', *Canadian Journal of Public Health* 77, 216–220.

Wilkins, R. and Adams, O.B. (1983) 'Health expectancy in Canada, late 1970s: demographic, regional, and social dimensions', *American Journal of Public Health* 73, 1073–1080.

Wilkins, R., Mayer, F., Ross, N. and Berthelot, J-M. (2001) 'Health expectancy by neighbourhood income in Canada using census disability data for 1996', Presented at REVES 13, Vancouver.

7

Cause-deleted Health Expectancies

COLIN D. MATHERS
WHO, Geneva, Switzerland

INTRODUCTION

Measures of the loss of health associated with disease, injury and health determinants are important for setting priorities, and for economic analyses of population-level health interventions for health planning. There is particular need for summary measures which combine the impact of mortality and morbidity since the loss of health due to the non-fatal disabling consequences of disease and injury is of increasing relative importance and public concern in low mortality populations.

In 1983, Colvez and Blanchet made the first attempt to develop such a measure, using the concept of the potential gain in disability-free life expectancy resulting from the elimination of a disease or injury (Colvez and Blanchet, 1983). This chapter reviews the subsequent development of these approaches, and the results of the major studies that have applied these methods to national health expectancy data.

At the 1992 REVES meeting in Montpellier, van de Water (1993) noted that

> The charm of the health expectancy indicator lies in its integral approach. As I see it, the development of the indicator as an all-embracing measure of health marks the transition to a new era of thinking about health and health related policies. When expansion of morbidity is the natural consequence of increasing life expectancies, society will see itself confronted with two main questions:
>
> - how does one diminish that burden of disease
> - how does one deal with the unavoidable consequences of the increasing burden of disease? (van de Water, 1993)

Determining Health Expectancies. Edited by J-M. Robine, C. Jagger, C.D. Mathers, E.M. Crimmins and R.M. Suzman.

To answer these questions requires that we go beyond a single global indicator of population health to measures that map consequences back to underlying diseases and from diseases back to determinants or causes. As van de Water (1993) said,

> One way or another we will have to find a method to help them link the results in ICIDH-terminology [impairments, disabilities, handicaps] to the ICD-terminology [diseases, injuries] and further down the line to determinants.

Various indicators of the impact of a health problem on the health of the population may highlight the importance of the area in terms of mortality, morbidity, health service use and costs. Commonly used measures include mortality measures, such as numbers of deaths or potential years of life lost (PYLL), and morbidity measures such as disease incidence or prevalence, or proxies for serious illness such as hospital admission rates. None of these measures is comprehensive in its coverage of the impact of a disease and used on its own may provide a distorted picture. Additionally, stakeholders and lobby groups are able to choose those indicators which present their interest area in the most favourable light.

In order to assist in addressing questions of priority setting and value for money in health, a summary measure of population health loss or gain must have the following properties:

- provide a common metric for fatal and non-fatal health outcomes;
- provide a common metric for estimating population health impact and assessment of cost-effectiveness;
- allow estimates of health impact to be mapped to causes (disease, impairment, risk factors, broader social determinants).

This chapter reviews various approaches which have been developed to obtain disease-specific measures of the burden of disease through calculating cause-deleted health expectancies and examines the extent to which they meet the criteria outlined above. They are also compared with health gap measures, such as the disability-adjusted life year or DALY, which was explicitly developed to address the same policy problems (World Bank, 1993; Murray and Lopez, 1996) (see Chapters 13 and 17).

An additional objective of some cause-deletion studies has been to examine whether elimination of specific diseases and injuries leads to a compression or expansion of morbidity and hence to understand the potential impact of prevention and treatment interventions on the evolution of population health. The hypotheses of compression and expansion of morbidity are discussed in Chapter 2. This chapter also examines the contribution of cause-deleted health expectancy analysis to this debate.

METHODOLOGICAL ISSUES

Colvez and Blanchet (1993) proposed that potential gains in life expectancy free of disability resulting from the elimination of disability and deaths from a particular cause were a useful tool for health planning. This approach has since been used for Australia (Mathers, 1992, 1996c, 1999), the United Kingdom (Bone *et al*, 1995) and the Netherlands (Nusselder *et al*, 1996). These studies all used Sullivan's method to calculate population health expectancies. The methods used for estimating cause-deleted health expectancies are described below. A Canadian study has examined a related measure, the attribute-deleted health expectancy, in which the contribution of various health dimensions or attributes (such as mobility or communication) to overall expected years with disability is examined through 'attribute-deletion'.

A related but somewhat different approach has been suggested by Hill *et al* (1996) based on a generalisation of the concept of entropy or elasticity of life expectancy, defined as the marginal change in life expectancy that results from a small (say 1%) decrease in mortality rates at all ages. This is also discussed below.

In this section, we also examine the major approaches developed so far for mapping disability to disease causes.

CALCULATING CAUSE-DELETED HEALTH EXPECTANCIES

The key to these methods is to estimate the contribution of specific diseases or disease groups to the prevalence of disability. The 'elimination' of a disease then reduces the overall prevalence of disability and also reduces mortality rates, resulting in an increase in disability-free or health-adjusted life expectancy.

The effect on health expectancies of eliminating a disease or injury is usually calculated assuming independence among causes of death and disability as follows:

(a) Cause-deleted probabilities of dying are estimated with cause-elimination life tables assuming independent causes of death (Tsai *et al*, 1978). Cause elimination is carried out for all age groups, including the final open-ended age group.
(b) Cause-deleted disability and handicap prevalences are calculated directly from the survey estimates by subtracting the cause-specific disability and handicap prevalences from the total prevalences.
(c) Cause-deleted health expectancies are calculated by Sullivan's method using the cause-deleted prevalences in the cause-elimination life tables.

Tsai *et al* (1978) derive the following formula for the effect of eliminating cause of death k on the life table probability q_i of dying in the age interval (x_i, x_{i+1}):

$$q'_i = 1 - (1 - q_i)^{(D_i - \pi_{ik} D_{ik})/D_i}$$

where D_i is the total number of deaths in the age interval (x_i, x_{i+1}), π_{ik} is the proportion of deaths from cause k that are eliminated $(0 \leqslant \pi_{ik} \leqslant 1)$, and D_{ik} is the total number of deaths from cause k in the age interval (x_i, x_{i+1}).

If the observed prevalence of disability in the age interval (x_i, x_{i+1}) is d_i, and d_{ik} is the prevalence of disability attributable to cause k, then the average expectation of life free of disability at age x_i after elimination of proportion π_{ik} of cause k may be calculated using Sullivan's method as:

$$DFLE_i = \sum_{i=x}^{w}(1 - \pi_{ik}d_i)L_i/l_x$$

where l_i and L_i are the life table functions for the number of persons surviving to exact age x_i and the total number of years lived in the age interval (x_i, x_{i+1}). These functions are calculated using the cause-eliminated probabilities of dying q'_i defined above.

Note that this method involves the hypothetical elimination of the disease or injury at all ages. Estimation of the change in a health expectancy due to elimination of a disease in a specific age range would require information on the duration or age of onset of the disability, since the disability may be the result of a disease or injury which occurred many years before (or prior to birth). Such information is only available in the Australian survey for injuries, but is in principle measurable in population surveys.

MAPPING DISABILITY TO DISEASE

In order to estimate gains in disability-free or handicap-free life expectancy resulting from the elimination of a disease or disease group, it is necessary to obtain estimates of the prevalence of disability and handicap attributable to the disease group. This is not straightforward because multiple health conditions are common, particularly for older people, but also for mental disorders at younger adult ages. In the UK Disability Surveys, up to 10 separate health conditions were recorded for disabled people and 78% of all disabled people cited multiple health problems as contributing to disability. Two main approaches have been used.

The first is to identify the principal cause of disability for each individual and attribute all disability for that individual to the principal cause. Thus elimination of that cause reduces the prevalence of disability by the number of people for whom that disability was a principal cause. This is the approach used by Mathers (1992) and Bone *et al* (1995).

The main limitation of the cause-deleted health expectancy approach is the problems with mapping disability to diseases and injuries. A significant proportion of respondents in most disability surveys that have asked about the causes of disability state that they do not know the main cause of their disability, and others undoubtedly give incorrect answers. Additionally, this approach does not take into account co-morbidity situations, where disability is the result of the interaction of a number of health problems. For older people particularly, a number of diseases and impairments may act interdependently to cause activity limitations. The approach taken by Bone (1992) and Mathers (1992) was to attribute all of a person's disability to the main health problem (as derived from respondents' self-reports) and to assume that elimination of the main health problem will result in elimination of the disability. There will be some persons for whom this will result in an overestimate of the health gain, since other conditions will cause residual disability. For others, this approach will underestimate health gain, since the health problem may be causing a proportion of their disability, even if not the main cause of disability. The effects of co-morbidity thus operate in both directions and the overall bias in estimated gain in health expectancy is unlikely to be very large.

The second approach, developed by Nusselder and co-authors (1996), uses multivariate modelling to estimate the proportion of disability prevalence associated with each of a number of chronic diseases. This approach holds considerable promise not only for addressing the issue of co-morbidity but also in analysing the contribution to disability of other causes such as aged frailty and risk factors. To date, it has not been feasible to carry out such an analysis of the Australian survey data, as the survey data available does not include sufficient information on health conditions.

ENTROPY OF HEALTH EXPECTANCIES

Most estimates of cause-deleted health expectancies have measured years gained from complete elimination of a disease or injury. A related approach has been suggested by Hill and co-authors (1996) based on a generalisation of the concept of entropy or elasticity of life expectancy. This is defined as the marginal change in life expectancy that results from a small (say 1%) decrease in mortality rates at all ages. Hill *et al* have derived formulae for the entropy of disease-free life expectancies with respect to changes in the incidence rates of the disease (which is assumed irreversible) and have given an example for dementia in Canada. Their approach does not provide a set of disease-specific elasticities for overall disability-free life expectancy and also does not include the effect of simultaneous change in disease-specific mortality on the health expectancy. In this regard, it follows an approach similar to that of Colvez and Blanchet (1983), who presented the first calculations of the potential gain in disability-free life expectancy from disease elimination in terms of separate estimates of the effects of mortality reduction and disability reduction. Hayward *et al* (1998) have also carried out a partial disease elimination analysis for the USA in which the effects of eliminating causes of death (but not disability) are analysed for active and inactive life expectancy.

In practice, the elimination of almost any disease or injury group will result in small changes in overall disability prevalence and mortality rates unless a very broad disease group is under consideration. Thus the cause-deleted approach discussed in this paper essentially provides estimates of the disease-specific entropies of health expectancies, if the gains are expressed in relative terms (as a percentage of the baseline health expectancy) rather than absolute terms (years).

Such entropies must be interpreted as the long-term consequences of the complete elimination of diseases, both in terms of mortality risk and disability risk. In general, there is little empirical evidence relating to the case-fatality rates for people with different severity levels of disability caused by a disease. Analysis of the long-term effects of partial elimination of disease, through a particular primary prevention programme for example, would ideally require information on the way in which that intervention alters the incidence, non-fatal disabling consequences, and corresponding case-fatality rates. It should be noted that the use of the prevalence-based Sullivan's method for estimation of cause-deleted health expectancies restricts the method to analysis of the long-term equilibrium consequences of disease elimination. Sullivan's method is not appropriate for modelling dynamic changes due to disease elimination, since it takes a long time for the age-specific prevalences of disability to reach the equilibrium values corresponding to the changed incidence rates (Mathers and Robine, 1997).

CAUSE DELETION AND COMPRESSION OR EXPANSION OF MORBIDITY

Cause elimination analysis provides an estimate of the gain in health-adjusted life expectancy and total life expectancy attributable to elimination of a disease or injury. However, interpretation of these results in terms of compression or expansion of morbidity is not always straightforward (Robine and Mathers, 1993). There are three possibilities:

1. Absolute compression of morbidity: the increase in health-adjusted life expectancy exceeds the increase in total life expectancy, reducing the 'lost' years of good health.

2. Relative compression of morbidity: health-adjusted life expectancy and 'lost' years of good health both increase, but health-adjusted life expectancy as a proportion of total life expectancy increases.
3. Relative expansion of morbidity: health-adjusted life expectancy and 'lost' years of good health both increase, but health-adjusted life expectancy as a proportion of total life expectancy decreases.

GAINS IN HEALTH EXPECTANCIES DUE TO DISEASE ELIMINATION – REVIEW OF STUDIES TO DATE

AUSTRALIA

Mathers (1992) used Australian disability survey data which included information on the main disabling health condition (as reported by the respondent) and the underlying cause (a range of disease and injury categories as well as other health determinants). For those disease groups which cause significant disability but little mortality, e.g. musculoskeletal conditions, there were significant gains in health-adjusted life expectancy (HALE) offset by comparable reductions in lost years of good health (LEH). For disease groups which cause relatively little prevalent disability but considerable mortality, e.g. neoplasms, there were significant gains in life expectancy (LE) and HALE. For disease groups such as circulatory conditions which result in significant mortality and disability, there were significant gains in LE and HALE.

Mathers (1996c, 1997) extended this approach to carry out a comprehensive analysis of potential gains in HALE due to elimination of specific diseases at chapter and subchapter level of the International Classification of Diseases (ICD-9), using population data from the Australian Survey of Disability, Ageing and Carers 1993 (Australian Bureau of Statistics, 1993). This survey allows disability to be classified into five levels of severity (based on the severity of handicap associated with the disability). These five levels are shown in Table 7.1. The severity weights shown in this table were chosen to be as consistent as possible with the order of magnitudes of the weights used in the Global Burden of Disease study (Murray and Lopez, 1996). They were also chosen to satisfy the criteria specified by Nord (1996), who gave guidelines for the appropriate preference weight ranges that could be associated with health states defined in terms of handicap severity.

The 1993 ABS Survey of Disability, Ageing and Carers contained two questions which were used to map disability to disease. These related to (a) the main disabling condition and (b) the cause of the main disabling condition. The main disabling condition was defined as the health condition (disease or impairment) that caused the most problems (in terms of activity restriction). If only one condition was reported by the respondent, it was considered the main

Table 7.1. Preference weights used for handicap severity states

Handicap severity	Definition	Weight
Disabled not handicapped	One or more of a set of disabling conditions or impairments which had lasted or were likely to last for six months or more but which did not limit ability to perform tasks in relation to one or more of the following five areas: self-care, mobility, verbal communication, schooling, and/or employment	0.02
Mild or not determined	Limited to some degree in ability to perform tasks in relation to self-care, mobility, verbal communication, schooling, and/or employment but no personal help or supervision required and no difficulty in performing the tasks, but the person uses an aid, or has difficulty walking 200 metres or up and down stairs	0.10
Moderate	No personal help or supervision required, but the person has difficulty in performing one or more of the tasks	0.25
Severe	Personal help or supervision sometimes required or the person is sometimes unable to perform one or more of the tasks	0.50
Profound	Personal help or supervision always required or the person is always unable to perform one or more of the tasks	0.75

disabling condition. The responses to this question were coded to categories based on a condensed ICD-9 3-digit classification of disease, but codes were also included for a range of impairments such as brain injury, blindness, amputated leg, joint problem, speech problem, etc.

Respondents were also asked the cause of the main disabling condition – and could specify a range of responses including accident/injury, working conditions, disease/illness/hereditary (around 30 disease categories coded), war, old age, present at birth, other and don't know.

Preliminary analysis of the survey data indicated that where a person gave a disease as their main disabling condition (e.g. arthritis, angina) they tended to give a 'determinant of disease' answer to the cause of condition question (e.g. stress, old age). Where a person gave an impairment as an answer (e.g. brain injury, blindness, amputation), they tended to give a disease or injury as the answer to the cause of condition (e.g. AIDS, diabetes). Injury and perinatal conditions were only coded as responses to the cause question, and were not available as categories for the principal condition question.

It was clear from the survey data that some of the people who specified a disease (such as cancer or heart disease) in response to the principal condition

Table 7.2. Estimated prevalence (%) of disability and handicap by severity, main health problem and sex, Australia, 1993

Main health problem[a]	Severe and profound handicap		Disability	
	Males	Females	Males	Females
Infectious and parasitic diseases	0.04	0.06	0.25	0.20
Neoplasms	0.07	0.11	0.38	0.33
Endocrine/nutritional/metabolic disorders	0.05	0.12	0.50	0.49
Blood disorders	0.00	0.01	0.01	0.05
Mental disorders	0.42	0.58	1.40	1.80
Nervous system/sense organ disorders	0.53	0.84	3.71	2.90
Circulatory system disorders	0.44	0.56	1.97	1.63
Respiratory system disorders	0.21	0.30	1.63	1.53
Digestive system disorders	0.03	0.04	0.36	0.25
Genito-urinary system disorders	0.01	0.04	0.06	0.14
Complications of pregnancy and childbirth	0.00	0.00	0.00	0.00
Skin and subcutaneous tissue disorders	0.01	0.01	0.07	0.12
Musculoskeletal disorders	0.58	1.32	2.93	4.66
Congenital anomalies	0.23	0.21	0.92	0.90
Perinatal conditions	0.01	0.02	0.02	0.02
Symptoms, signs and ill-defined conditions	0.06	0.04	0.34	0.24
Injury and poisoning	0.66	0.53	3.85	2.31
All causes	3.35	4.80	18.39	17.57

[a]Disease groups defined by chapters of ICD-9.

question also specified a disease or injury in response to the cause question and that some of these latter responses were inappropriate. For example, some respondents specifying cancer as the principal condition reported that it was caused by heart disease or motor vehicle accidents. For each major disease category, experts were consulted to determine which main disabling conditions could be causally associated with diseases or injuries in that group. This advice was used to assist in assigning disabled people to *main health problem* categories.

Table 7.2 shows the estimated prevalence of disability and handicap by main health problem in Australia in 1993. These prevalence data were used together with Sullivan's method to estimate the potential gains in HALE at birth due to elimination of disease and injury groups at ICD-9 chapter level and at subchapter level for specific diseases (Table 7.3). Figure 7.1 illustrates the results for males and females. The largest gains in HALE at birth are achieved by elimination of circulatory system diseases for males and cancers for females (with circulatory system disorders coming a close second). Following these disease groups are injury and poisoning for males and musculoskeletal conditions for females.

Table 7.3. Baseline and estimated change in life expectancy and health-adjusted life expectancy (HALE), at birth, due to elimination of disease and injury groups, Australia 1993

	Males			Females		
	LE (years)	HALE (years)	HALE/ LE (%)	LE (years)	HALE (years)	HALE/ LE (%)
At baseline	74.98	70.86	94.5	80.85	74.74	92.4
Change due to elimination of:						
Infectious and parasitic diseases	0.29	0.30	0.04	0.06	0.08	0.03
Neoplasms	3.46	2.84	−0.54	2.45	2.13	−0.16
Endocrine/nutritional/metabolic disorders	0.28	0.30	0.05	0.22	0.32	0.14
Blood disorders	0.03	0.02	0.00	0.02	0.03	0.01
Mental disorders	0.18	0.54	0.48	0.09	0.68	0.73
Nervous system/sense organ disorders	0.25	0.81	0.76	0.18	1.12	1.19
Circulatory system disorders	5.81	5.01	−0.60	2.48	2.67	0.45
Respiratory system disorders	0.86	0.92	0.14	0.44	0.65	0.30
Digestive system disorders	0.34	0.33	0.02	0.19	0.22	0.05
Genito-urinary system disorders	0.12	0.10	−0.01	0.09	0.13	0.05
Complications of pregnancy/ childbirth	0.00	0.00	0.00	0.00	0.00	0.00
Skin and subcutaneous tissue disorders	0.01	0.02	0.01	0.00	0.018	0.02
Musculoskeletal disorders	0.03	0.42	0.52	0.04	1.63	1.96
Congenital anomalies	0.19	0.27	0.12	0.18	0.23	0.08
Perinatal conditions	0.23	0.22	0.01	0.17	0.17	0.02
Symptoms, signs, ill-defined conditions	0.09	0.12	0.05	0.06	0.09	0.04
Injury and poisoning	1.47	2.05	0.86	0.50	1.02	0.68

Mathers (1999) used the same methods and data source to study the effects of cause elimination on compression or expansion of morbidity in older people.

Table 7.4 shows the changes in HALE resulting from the elimination in turn of each of the major disease groups. The baseline life expectancy and HALE of the population (with no disease elimination) are presented for comparison. Elimination of circulatory system disorders leads to the greatest gain in healthy years among both men and women, followed by neoplasms for men and musculoskeletal disorders for women. Figure 7.2 illustrates these potential gains in HALE for men and women aged 65 years.

For disease groups, such as musculoskeletal conditions and mental disorders, which cause significant disability but little mortality, there are small gains in life expectancy but large gains in HALE offset by comparable

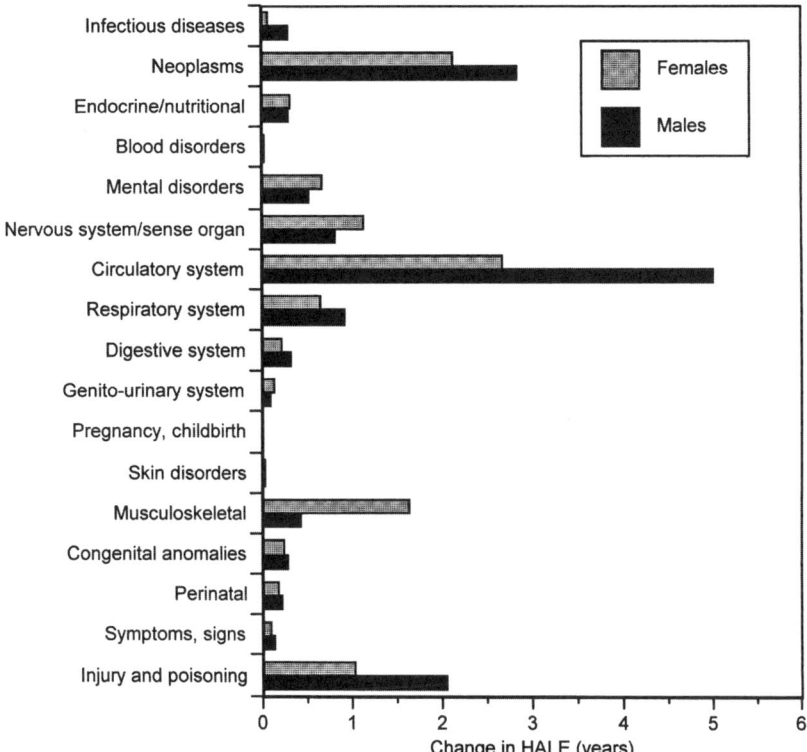

Figure 7.1. Change in health-adjusted life expectancy at birth (years) due to elimination of diseases and injuries, at ICD-9 chapter level, Australia 1993

reductions in lost years of good health. Elimination of these disease groups results in absolute compression of morbidity, where the 'lost' years of good health (total life expectancy minus HALE) decrease.

Where the 'lost' years of good health increase, but HALE also increases, this is referred to as a 'relative compression of morbidity'. In this case, HALE increases as a proportion of total life expectancy, although there is also an increase in the 'lost' years of good health. Relative compression of morbidity occurs for elimination of endocrine, nutritional and metabolic disorders, respiratory disorders and digestive disorders in men but only for neoplasms in women (Table 7.4).

Relative expansion of morbidity occurs when HALE and 'lost' years of good health both increase, but HALE as a proportion of total life expectancy decreases. For disease groups which cause relatively little prevalent disability but considerable mortality, such as neoplasms, there are significant gains in life expectancy with and without disability as those persons whose deaths are

Table 7.4. Baseline and change in life expectancy and health-adjusted life expectancy (HALE), at age 65, due to elimination of disease and injury groups, Australia 1993

	Males			Females		
	LE (years)	HALE (years)	HALE/ LE (%)	LE (years)	HALE (years)	HALE/ LE (%)
People aged 65 years at baseline	15.72	13.33	84.80	19.49	15.50	79.53
Infectious and parasitic diseases	0.06	0.08	0.18	0.02	0.03	0.07
Neoplasms	2.40	1.83	−1.15	1.07	0.91	0.29
Endocrine/nutritional/metabolic disorders	0.20	0.19	0.15	0.13	0.21	0.55
Blood disorders	0.02	0.02	−0.01	0.01	0.01	0.02
Mental disorders	0.10	0.29	1.30	0.06	0.48	2.23
Nervous system/sense organ disorders	0.16	0.58	2.76	0.08	0.83	3.90
Circulatory system disorders	5.35	4.42	−0.58	2.11	2.32	3.00
Respiratory system disorders	0.80	0.77	0.56	0.30	0.41	0.87
Digestive system disorders	0.21	0.19	0.09	0.11	0.13	0.22
Genito-urinary system disorders	0.12	0.09	−0.06	0.07	0.10	0.23
Skin and subcutaneous tissue disorders	0.01	0.02	0.05	0.00	0.01	0.05
Musculoskeletal disorders	0.03	0.51	3.04	0.03	1.34	6.72
Congenital anomalies	0.01	0.01	0.03	0.00	0.02	0.10
Injury and poisoning	0.15	0.45	2.08	0.05	0.40	1.83

averted live longer lives and experience disability from other causes. For men, but not women, this results in a relative expansion of morbidity for elimination of neoplasms, circulatory system disorders and genito-urinary conditions. There is no disease group whose elimination results in a relative expansion of morbidity among older women.

UNITED KINGDOM

Bone *et al* (1995) used the same approach as Mathers (1992) to calculate potential gains in disability-free life expectancy due to disease elimination for England and Wales in 1986. Disability data was derived from the Office of Population Censuses and Surveys (OPCS) Disability Survey and required that all individuals be classified according to principal cause of disability in terms of ICD-9 chapters. Bone *et al* discussed a number of possible approaches to this problem, given that up to 10 separate health conditions were cited in the disability surveys and 78% of all disabled people cited multiple health problems as contributing to disability. In the end, they used the same approach as Mathers (1992) to classify each individual according to the first-mentioned

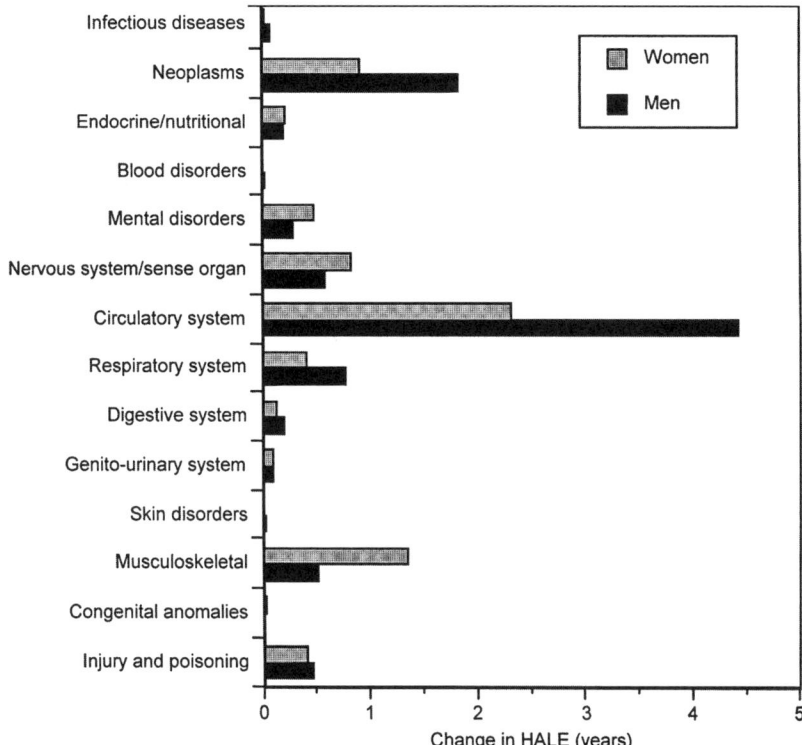

Figure 7.2. Change in health-adjusted life expectancy at age 65 (years) due to elimination of diseases and injuries, at ICD-9 chapter level, Australia 1993

condition as probably being the one of greatest concern. Clearly, depending on the exact form of the counterfactual disease elimination assumed, removal of the first-mentioned cause may not always result in complete elimination of the associated disability.

Figure 7.3 compares cause-deleted disability-free life expectancies (DFLE) for the UK in 1986 with those for Australia in 1988. The pattern of UK results corresponded closely to those for Australia, with the exception of gains in healthy life due to the elimination of injury, which were estimated as 6.1 years for men and 2.8 years for women, from birth. This difference is undoubtedly due to the way in which the Australian survey was handled; respondents were first asked if their disability was due to accident or illness before cause was investigated in detail. In the British survey, by contrast, self-reported causes were coded in such a way that it was not always possible to distinguish injury from illness.

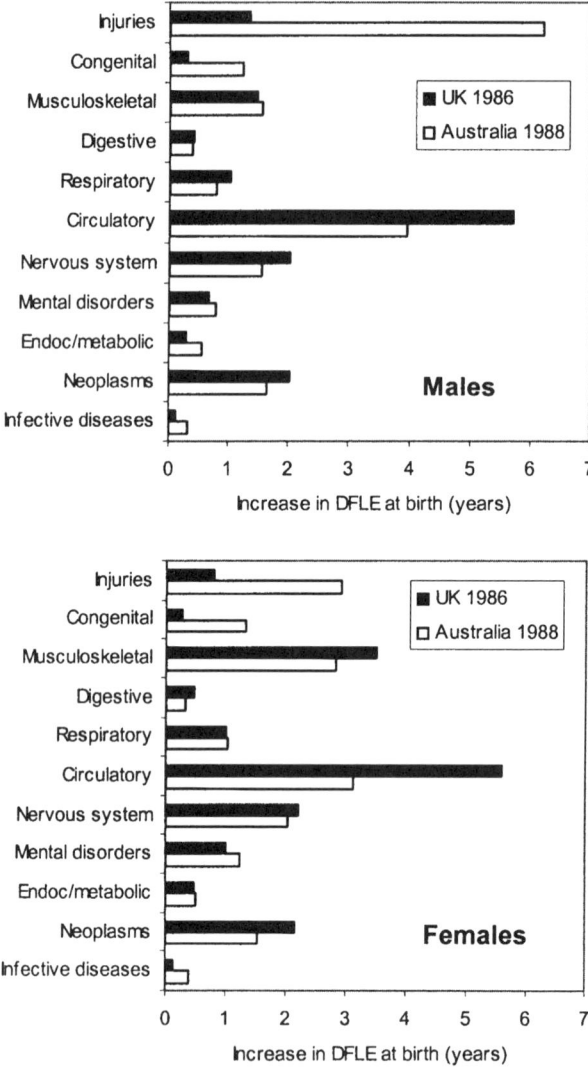

Figure 7.3. Increase in disability-free life expectancies (DFLE) at birth, after elimination of major disease groups, Australia 1988 and UK 1986

NETHERLANDS

Nusselder *et al* (1994, 1996) estimated cause-deleted DFLE for the Netherlands in 1987–1988 using multivariate methods for attributing disability to causes. Cross-sectional data on long-term disability and chronic diseases were derived from the Dutch National Survey of General Practice, conducted by the

Netherlands Institute for Primary Health Care in 1987–1988. Because virtually the entire non-institutionalised population of the Netherlands is registered with a general practitioner, after correction for non-response bias, the weighted sample can be regarded as representative of the entire non-institutionalised Dutch population.

The prevalence of long-term disability was measured in terms of ability to perform 11 activities including the ability to bend down and pick something up, to get in and out of bed, to dress and undress, to move between rooms, to walk 400 m, to carry a 5 kg object for 10 m, to read small letters in a newspaper, to have a conversation with another person, to follow a conversation in a group, and to go up and down stairs. Persons were considered disabled if they indicated that they needed help from another person or were unable to carry out without (great) difficulty one or more of the selected activities included in the indicator.

Prevalence of chronic conditions was assessed on the basis of a structured list comprising a broad spectrum of somatic disorders and conditions. The list did not cover all chronic conditions; for example, mental and sensory disorders, stroke, dementia and (hip) fractures were not included. A subset of conditions with high disease burden were chosen from the list for more detailed analysis. Persons living in health institutions were considered to have long-term disabilities and the numbers and disabilities of such persons were estimated using administrative data sources and surveys.

The effect of eliminating a chronic disease on DFLE was calculated using Sullivan's method by reducing the age-specific mortality rates accordingly and also reducing the age-specific prevalence of disability. A multiple logistic regression model was used to estimate cause-deleted disability prevalence, controlling for co-morbidity and age. The probability of disability was estimated using a logistic function which included age, seven disease clusters, and other diseases as independent variables. The effect of elimination was simulated by deleting the disease in the regression equation. The difference between the fitted total and cause-deleted disability prevalence was then attributed to the eliminated disease.

Table 7.5 shows the changes in life expectancy and DFLE resulting from elimination of each of the disease groups. The baseline health status of the population is shown for comparison. Elimination of heart disease and arthritis/back complaints leads to the greatest gain in DFLE. Ranking these diseases by impact differs between the two sexes: among men, heart disease has the largest impact while among women, arthritis/back complaints have the largest impact. For those diseases showing no significant change in total life expectancy (e.g. arthritis/back complaints and migraine/severe headache), the observed increase in DFLE leads to absolute compression of morbidity.

Elimination of chronic non-specific lung disease and diabetes mellitus among women reduces the number of years with disability, indicating an absolute

Table 7.5. Baseline[a] and change in total life expectancy (LE), disability-free life expectancy (DFLE), life expectancy with disability (LED), and percentage of life free of disability (% DLFE in LE) due to elimination of the specific disease, the Netherlands[b]

	LE (years)	DFLE (years)	LED (years)	% DFLE in LE[c]
Men at baseline[d] at age 15 years	59.3	47.5	11.7	80.2
Chronic non-specific lung disease	0.3	0.7	−0.4	0.7
Heart disease	4.0	2.5	1.6	−1.2
Cancer	3.8	1.7	2.1	−2.2
Diabetes mellitus	0.2	0.1	0.1	−0.1
Arthritis/back complaints	0.0	1.9	−1.8	3.1
Migraine/severe headache	0.0	0.4	−0.4	0.6
Other neurological diseases	0.2	0.2	0.0	0.1
Women at baseline[d] at age 15 years	65.6	45.6	20.0	69.5
Chronic non-specific lung disease	0.1	0.6	−0.5	0.8
Heart disease	2.9	1.4	1.5	−1.0
Cancer	3.3	1.1	2.2	−1.7
Diabetes mellitus	0.3	0.4	−0.1	0.3
Arthritis/back complaints	0.1	2.8	−2.7	4.2
Migraine/severe headache	0.0	0.5	−0.5	0.7
Other neurological diseases	0.2	0.2	0.0	0.1
Men at baseline[d] at age 65 years	14.2	6.9	7.3	48.9
Chronic non-specific lung disease	0.3	0.5	−0.2	2.3
Heart disease	3.1	1.5	1.6	0.0
Cancer	2.7	0.9	1.8	−2.3
Diabetes mellitus	0.1	0.0	0.1	−0.1
Arthritis/back complaints	0.0	0.7	−0.7	5.0
Migraine/severe headache	0.0	0.1	−0.1	0.4
Other neurological diseases	0.1	0.1	0.0	0.3
Women at baseline[d] at age 65 years	18.8	6.2	12.6	33.1
Chronic non-specific lung disease	0.1	0.2	−0.1	1.0
Heart disease	2.7	0.9	1.8	0.0
Cancer	1.9	0.4	1.5	−1.2
Diabetes mellitus	0.3	0.3	0.0	1.0
Arthritis/back complaints	0.1	1.0	−1.0	5.3
Migraine/severe headache	0.0	0.1	−0.1	0.4
Other neurological diseases	0.1	0.1	0.0	0.3

[a]Baseline figures are based on life tables for 1982 through 1991 and on disability prevalence for 1987–1988.
[b]Figures are rounded to 0.1 years and 0.1 percentage points.
[c]Change in percentage points.
[d]The baseline expectancies are based on the fitted age-specific prevalence.
Source: Nusselder *et al* (1996). Reproduced with permission.

compression of morbidity. No significant change is observed when other neurological conditions are eliminated. On the other hand, cancer, heart disease and diabetes mellitus among men show an increase in life expectancy with disability because the gain in DFLE is smaller than the gain in LE. This implies a relative expansion of morbidity. Similar results are found at age 65 (see Table 7.5) except for heart disease, where there is neither a relative expansion nor compression of morbidity.

Nusselder *et al* (2000) have also examined the gains in DFLE due to smoking elimination using multistate life table methods. This is the only example to date of a study that has examined the effect on a health expectancy indicator of the elimination of a disease risk factor as opposed to diseases.

They used a longitudinal study (GLOBE) of 27 000 Dutch nationals aged 15–74 years to derive incidence rates of disability, recovery rates from disability and mortality rates among non-disabled and disabled persons for the current mixed smoking–non-smoking population, using Poisson regression analysis. These transition rates were supplemented by estimates of transition rates among those aged 75 and over derived from the US Longitudinal Study of Aging (LSOA). Next, incidence, recovery and mortality rates among disabled and non-disabled persons were estimated for non-smokers in order to calculate life expectancy with and without disability after smoking elimination. Multistate life table methods were used to estimate DFLE for the mixed smoking–non-smoking population and for the non-smoking population (after eliminating smoking) in order to determine the change in DFLE resulting from elimination of smoking.

Nusselder and co-authors found that a non-smoking population on balance will spend fewer years with disability than a mixed smoking–non-smoking population. Although non-smokers have lower mortality risks and thus are exposed to disability over a longer period of time, their lower incidence of disability and higher recovery from disability yield a net reduction of the length of time spent with disability (0.9 years and 1.1 years in men and women aged 30, respectively) and increases in the length of time lived without disability (2.5 years and 1.9 years in men and women, respectively). They concluded that elimination of smoking will not only extend life and result in an increase in the number of years without disability, but will also compress disability into a shorter period. This implies that the commonly found trade-off between longer life and a longer period with disability does not apply in the case of smoking.

USA

Hayward *et al* (1998) have examined cause of death and active life expectancy in the older population of the United States. The primary focus of this study was on the differences in patterns of causes of mortality for disabled and non-disabled older Americans. Data from the Longitudinal Study on Aging were used to show

Table 7.6. Attribute-deleted HALE at age 25, by sex, Canada 1990–1992

	Attribute-deleted HALE (years)	HALE (years)	Difference (years)	Difference %
Men				
Overall			6.0	100
Sensory	46.7	44.9	1.8	30
Pain	46.4	44.9	1.5	25
Emotion	46.0	44.9	1.1	18
Cognition	45.7	44.9	0.8	13
Mobility	45.2	44.9	0.3	5
Dexterity	45.0	44.9	0.1	2
Residual[a]	–	–	0.4	7
Women				
Overall			8.4	100
Sensory	50.8	48.4	2.4	29
Pain	50.7	48.4	2.3	27
Emotion	49.7	48.4	1.3	16
Cognition	49.5	48.4	1.1	13
Mobility	49.2	48.4	0.8	10
Dexterity	48.6	48.4	0.2	2
Residual[a]	–	–	0.3	4

[a]Because the HUI is a multiplicative function, there is a residual, which is not the result of any attribute, but which is the combination of many attributes.
Source: Wolfson (1996). Reproduced with permission. Statistics Canada information is used with the permission of the Minister of Industry, as Minister responsible for Statistics Canada. Information on the availability of the wide range of data from Statistics Canada can be obtained from Statistics Canada's Regional Offices, its World Wide Web site at http://www.statcan.ca, and its toll-free access number 1-800-263-1136.

that there were few differences in the causes of death for the disabled and non-disabled population, despite differences in the length of life with and without disability. Disease elimination methods for causes of death (but not disability) were used together with multistate life table analysis to examine the gains in life expectancy as a result of reduction in mortality due to major diseases.

Their results showed that DFLE (active life expectancy) is least sensitive to mortality from cerebrovascular diseases and cancer, for both males and females. In the case of cerebrovascular diseases, their elimination results in only a marginal increase in overall life expectancy at age 70. Most of the gain for males is an increase in DFLE, whereas for females it is split roughly equally between DFLE and years with disability.

The elimination of heart disease mortality results in larger gains in total life expectancy (3 years for men and 4 years for women at age 70). Most of these gains are in DFLE at age 70, but there is a gradual shift with age, so that the elimination of heart disease mortality at the oldest ages adds more years with disability than without disability to life expectancy.

CANADA

Wolfson (1996) has calculated attribute-deleted health-adjusted life expectancies for Canada using population disability prevalence data as measured in the Health Utility Index (HUI) multi-attribute health state instrument together with measured utility weights for these health states. Table 7.6 shows the gains in health-adjusted life expectancy (HALE) that would occur through deletion of particular domains (attributes) of disability such as sensory disability, or cognitive disability. This is a related concept to disease (cause) elimination, but the attributes of disability (such as mobility limitation) are deleted as a way to show relative contribution of the various dimensions of disability to overall expected years lived with disability. No changes are made to mortality probabilities in this analysis so it is not comparable to the disease elimination studies where morbidity and mortality are simultaneously modified by disease elimination.

CAUSE ATTRIBUTION FOR SUMMARY MEASURES OF POPULATION HEALTH

Summary measures of population health (SMPH) are indicators that summarise the health of a population in a single number. Murray *et al* (2000) have classified SMPH into two broad families: health expectancies and health gaps. Health expectancies are measures of the area under the survival curve for a population. When a set of health state valuations are used to weight time spent in health states worse than ideal health, the health expectancy is referred to as a health-adjusted or disability-adjusted life expectancy (DALE). Another type of health expectancy is exemplified by disability-free life expectancy in which time spent in any health state categorized as disabled is assigned arbitrarily a weight of zero, and time spent in any state categorized as not disabled is assigned a weight of one (i.e., equivalent to full health).

In contrast to health expectancies, health gaps quantify the *difference* between the actual health of a population and some stated norm or goal for population health. Years of life lost measures are all measures of a mortality gap, or the area between the survivorship function and some implied target survivorship function. The best-known health gap that includes morbidity as well as mortality is the disability-adjusted life year or DALY (Murray and Lopez, 1996), discussed in more detail in Chapter 13.

CAUSAL DECOMPOSITION OF SMPH

There are two dominant traditions in widespread use for causal attribution: categorical attribution and counterfactual analysis. In categorical attribution, an event such as death is attributed to a single cause according to a defined set of rules. In counterfactual analysis, the contribution of a disease, injury or risk factor is estimated by comparing the current and future levels of a summary measure with the levels that would be expected under some alternative hypothetical scenario (Murray and Lopez, 1999). There has been little discussion of their advantages and disadvantages or of the inconsistency of using both approaches in the same analysis. An example of the latter is provided by the Global Burden of Disease 1990 Study (Murray and Lopez, 1996). Burden attributable to diseases and injuries has been estimated using categorical attribution whereas burden attributable to risk factors or diseases such as diabetes, which act as risk factors, has been estimated using counterfactual analysis.

In categorical attribution, an event such as death or the onset of a particular health state is attributed categorically to one single cause according to a defined set of rules. Categorical attribution is familiar in population health statistics relating to cause of death and principal diagnosis for health system encounters. In cause-of-death tabulations, for example, each death is assigned to a unique cause according to the rules of the International Classification of Diseases (ICD), even in cases of multi-causal events. For example, in ICD-10, deaths from tuberculosis in HIV-positive individuals are assigned to HIV. This categorical approach to representing causes is the standard method used in published studies of health gaps such as the Global Burden of Disease 1990 (Murray and Lopez, 1996).

For data relating to health system encounters, there are a similar set of rules for identifying the principal diagnosis. These rules may relate to the 'underlying reason' for the health system encounter in a similar way to the cause-of-death rules, or may relate to the diagnosis responsible for the most resource use during the health system encounter.

Because health expectancies are positive measures of health integrated across the life span, they combine the effects of all causes acting at each subsequent age and categorical attribution is not possible. The disease elimination approach discussed in this chapter is a form of counterfactual analysis in which the hypothetical scenario is that the disease has been eliminated in the distant past so that all disability and mortality associated with that disease are absent. Note that this method involves the hypothetical elimination of the disease or injury at all ages. Estimation of the change in a health expectancy due to elimination of a disease in a specific age range would require information on the duration or age of onset of the disability, since the disability may be the result of a disease or injury which occurred many years before (or prior to birth).

The disease elimination approach taken by Bone (1992) and Mathers (1992, 1999) attributes all of a person's disability to the main health problem (as derived from respondents' self-reports) and assumes that elimination of the main health problem will result in elimination of the disability. The mutivariate modelling approach developed by Nusselder and co-authors (1996) in principle could be used to estimate counterfactual prevalences resulting from the elimination of each chronic disease separately; then the full disease elimination analysis of the health expectancy could be carried out consistently using counterfactual methods. This has not yet been attempted.

COMPARISON OF CAUSE ATTRIBUTION FOR HEALTH EXPECTANCIES AND HEALTH GAPS

Mortality gaps have generally been categorically attributed to underlying cause of death using ICD rules. Health gaps such as DALYs also have generally used categorical attribution for disease and injury causes. The YLD (years lived with disability) component is calculated in terms of the loss of health (quantified by the disability weight) associated with each of the disease stages, severity levels and sequelae caused by the disease. DALY calculations start from information on diseases and injuries (incidence, prevalence and duration) and use categorical attribution to estimate the associated impairments, disability and mortality. Using counterfactual methods discussed above, it is also possible to estimate the attributable burden of specific risk factors or health determinants.

Mathers *et al* (1999) carried out the first national burden of disease study for Australia and estimated DALYs for a comprehensive set of disease and injury categories. Table 7.7 compares the changes in HALE at birth resulting from the elimination of specific diseases and injuries in 1993 with the total DALYs for the same cause in 1996 (expressed as a percentage of total DALYs due to all causes). The top 25 diseases and injuries for men and women are separately ranked in descending order of HALE increase. Elimination of ischaemic heart disease leads to the greatest gain in HALE for both men and women (1.9 years and 1.1 years, respectively), followed by cerebrovascular disease and other vascular diseases for men and osteoarthritis and cerebrovascular disease for women. DALY ranks shown in Table 7.7 are generally similar for most leading causes of loss of health, with the exception of vascular diseases, falls and hypertensive heart disease, which are ranked much more highly by the HALE gain measure. Among the top 20 causes of DALYs in Australia, benign prostatic hypertrophy (ranked 10th for males) is not identified as a cause in the HALE analysis, and lower respiratory tract infection (ranked 19th for males and 15th for females) is also not identified as a cause of disability in the HALE analysis.

Figure 7.4 compares the changes in HALE at birth resulting from the elimination of disease groups defined by ICD-9 chapters with DALYs (as a percentage of total) for males and females. As for specific diseases, the two sets of estimates give a generally similar pattern of rankings. The main exceptions are mental disorders, which are given much greater weight in the DALY

Table 7.7. Ranking of 25 leading causes of loss of health, HALE gain at birth through disease elimination 1993, and total DALY rankings 1996, Australia

Males	HALE gain (years)	DALY rank	Females	HALE gain (years)	DALY rank
1. Ischaemic heart disease	1.93	1	1. Ischaemic heart disease	0.92	1
2. Cerebrovascular disease	0.65	2	2. Osteoarthritis	0.85	10
3. Vascular disease	0.52	18	3. Cerebrovascular disease	0.57	2
4. COPD	0.51	4	4. Alzheimer's disease	0.50	3
5. Lung cancer	0.43	3	5. Vascular diseases	0.30	20
6. Alzheimer's disease	0.31	5	6. Eye disorders	0.25	8
7. Prostate cancer	0.29	6	7. COPD	0.19	4
8. Osteoarthritis	0.28	12	8. Diabetes	0.18	9
9. Colorectal cancer	0.22	7	9. Falls	0.18	18
10. Diabetes	0.15	8	10. Hearing loss	0.16	12
11. Hearing loss	0.14	9	11. Hypertensive disease	0.15	13
12. War	0.14	n.a.	12. Colorectal cancer	0.15	6
13. Hypertensive disease	0.13	26	13. Lung cancer	0.14	7
14. Parkinson's disease	0.12	11	14. Breast cancer	0.13	5
15. Lymphoma	0.09	17	15. Asthma	0.11	24
16. Falls	0.09	28	16. Rheumatoid arthritis	0.10	34
17. Eye disorders	0.09	23	17. Road traffic accidents	0.09	49
18. Asthma	0.07	36	18. Parkinson's disease	0.09	11
19. Stomach cancer	0.07	14	19. Osteopathies/deformities	0.09	45
20. Pancreas cancer	0.07	16	20. Lymphoma	0.06	16
21. Nephritis/nephrosis	0.06	25	21. Depression	0.05	32
22. Road traffic accidents	0.06	39	22. Ovary cancer	0.05	17
23. Bladder cancer	0.06	21	23. Pancreas cancer	0.05	14
24. Skin cancers	0.06	13	24. Nephritis/nephrosis	0.05	19
25. Inflammatory heart disease	0.06	15	25. Inflammatory heart disease	0.04	21

COPD, chronic obstructive pulmonary disease.
Sources: Mathers (1996c, 1999) adapted.

estimates, and musculoskeletal disorders for women, which are given greater weight by the HALE gain measure. It is likely that mental disorders, benign prostatic hypertrophy and some other types of conditions are under-reported in population disability surveys. Differences between the HALE gains and DALY estimates may also reflect limitations in the use of average weights for broad handicap severity categories in the estimation of HALE gains.

The main limitations of the HALE gain approach relate to the use of self-report data to map disability to diseases and injuries. Apart from the underreporting of some classes of conditions, a significant proportion of respondents state that they do not know the main cause of their disability, and others undoubtedly give incorrect answers. Co-disability also complicates the identification of underlying cause and, in this circumstance, the concept of a

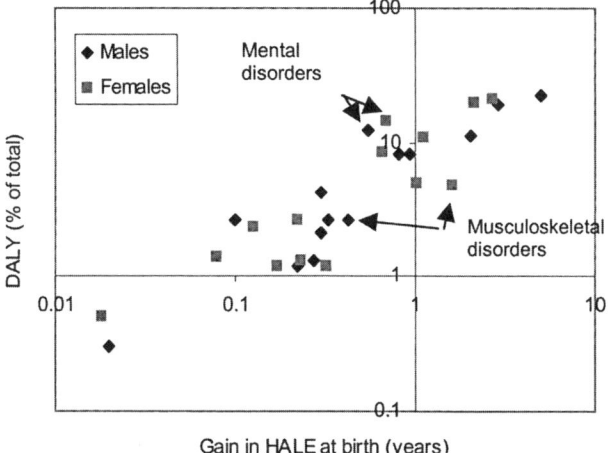

Gain in HALE at birth (years)

Figure 7.4. Comparison of DALYs and HALE gains for disease and injury groups at ICD-9 chapter level, Australia

main health problem may break down since a number of diseases and impairments may act interdependently to cause activity limitations. As discussed above, Nusselder *et al* (1996) addressed this issue using multivariate methods.

It is also important to note that analysis of gains in disability-free life expectancy, such as those carried out previously (Mathers, 1992; Nusselder *et al*, 1996), can give a considerably different picture to that based on health-adjusted life expectancy. Those diseases which result in relatively more disability at the lower end of the severity scale will rank more highly in terms of gains in disability-free life expectancy, which weights all disability equally, than in terms of gains in health-adjusted life expectancy.

CRITERIA FOR CAUSAL DECOMPOSITION OF HEALTH EXPECTANCIES

Murray *et al* (2000) proposed a set of desirable properties for evaluating summary measures of population health (SMPH) based on commonsense notions of population health. These included two attributes based on practical considerations of policy usefulness:

1. Summary measures should be comprehensible and feasible to calculate for many populations. Comprehensibility and complexity are different. Life expectancy at birth is a complex abstract measure but is easy to understand. Health expectancies are popular because they are also easily understood.

2. Summary measures should be linear aggregates of the summary measures calculated for any arbitrary partitioning of subgroups. Many decision-makers, and very often the public, desire information that is characterised by this type of additive decomposition. In other words, they would like to be able to answer what fraction of the summary measure is related to health events in the poor, in the uninsured, in the elderly, in children, and so on. Additive decomposition is also often appealing for cause attribution.

Most health expectancies satisfy the first attribute. However, they cannot be additively decomposed in respect of causes or population subgroups. Disability-adjusted life expectancies are additively decomposable into health expectancies for specified levels of disability severity. This form of decomposition may be useful in understanding which levels of disability severity are contributing most to changes in population health. In general, health gaps can be decomposed into the contribution of various causes in a more intuitive and easily communicated fashion than health expectancies. DALYs are additive across causes to give the total health gap for a population. Disability-adjusted life expectancy and a health gap measure such as the DALY thus fulfil different needs for SMPH to summarise and report on trends and achievements in population health across countries.

CONCLUSIONS

Measures of disease impact are of considerable importance for identifying the major health problems contributing to loss of healthy life and as inputs to priority setting processes, economic analyses and health planning. This chapter has reviewed the use of cause-deleted health expectancies as disease-specific population measures that combine information on mortality and morbidity, and compared them with health gaps.

Gains in health-adjusted life expectancy due to elimination of diseases can directly identify whether compression or expansion of morbidity is likely to occur as a result of public health and medical interventions. For example, elimination of neoplasms and circulatory system disorders in Australian males would result in a relative expansion of morbidity, whereas relative expansion occurs only for neoplasms in females. Elimination of smoking in the Netherlands would result in an absolute compression of morbidity.

The studies reviewed in this chapter have demonstrated the potential usefulness of health expectancies to evaluate the likely long-term effects of health interventions on the healthfulness of life as well as the length of life. For further development of this approach, it will be important to develop multivariate techniques to more appropriately take account of the effects of co-morbidity and to develop empirical methods for defining, measuring and valuing disability states according to severity.

If complete data on the distribution of disability associated with incident cases of disease or injury were available for a population, then health expectancies and gaps due to specific diseases could be calculated in a manner consistent with each other. They could then be appropriately used to complement each other in describing the health of a population and the contribution of specific conditions and health determinants to loss of health.

REFERENCES

Australian Bureau of Statistics (1993) *Disability, Ageing and Carers: Summary of Findings*. Canberra, Australia: ABS (ABS Cat. No. 4430.0).

Bone, M.R. (1992) 'International efforts to measure health expectancy', *Journal of Epidemiology and Community Health* 46, 555–558.

Bone, M.R., Bebbington, A.C., Jagger, C., Morgan, M. and Nicolaas, G. (1995) *Health Expectancy and Its Uses*. London: HMSO.

Colvez, A. and Blanchet, M. (1983) 'Potential gains in life expectancy free of disability: a tool for health planning', *International Journal of Epidemiology* 12(2), 224–229.

Hayward, M., Crimmins, E. and Saito, Y. (1998) 'Cause of death and active life expectancy in the older population of the United States', *Journal of Aging and Health* 10(2), 192–213.

Hill, G.B., Forbes, W.F. and Wilkins, R. (1996) 'The entropy of health and disease: dementia in Canada', in 9th meeting REVES, Rome, 11–13 December 1996.

Mathers, C.D. (1992) 'Estimating gains in health expectancy due to elimination of specified diseases', in 5th meeting REVES, Ottawa, 19–21 February 1992.

Mathers, C.D. (1996a) 'Issues in the measurement of health status', in 9th Meeting REVES, Rome, 11–13 December 1996.

Mathers, C.D. (1996b) 'Trends in health expectancies in Australia 1981–1993', *Journal of the Australian Population Association* 13(1), 1–16.

Mathers, C.D. (1996c) 'Applications of health expectancy methodology to measurement of the burden of disease in Australia 1993', in 9th meeting REVES, Rome, 11–13 December 1996.

Mathers, C.D. (1997) 'Gains in health expectancy from the elimination of disease: a useful measure of the burden of disease?', in 10th meeting REVES, Tokyo, 9–11 October 1997.

Mathers, C.D. (1999) 'Gains in health expectancy from the elimination of diseases among older people', *Disability and Rehabilitation* 21(5–6), 211–221.

Mathers, C.D. and Robine, J.M. (1997) 'How good is Sullivan's method for monitoring changes in population health?' *Journal of Epidemiology and Population Health* 51(1): 80–86.

Mathers, C.D., Vos, T. and Stevenson, C. (1999) *The Burden of Disease and Injury in Australia*. Canberra: AIHW.

Murray, C.J.L. and Lopez, A.D. (eds) (1996) *The Global Burden of Disease: a comprehensive assessment of mortality and disability from diseases, injuries and risk factors in 1990 and projected to 2020*. Harvard: Harvard School of Public Health.

Murray, C.J.L. and Lopez, A. (1999) 'On the comparable quantification of health risks: lessons from the Global Burden of Disease Study', *Epidemiology* 10(5), 594–605.

Murray, C.J.L., Salomon, J.A. and Mathers, C.D. (2000) 'A critical examination of summary measures of population health', *Bulletin of the World Health Organization* 78(8), 981–994.

Nord, E. (1996) 'Health status index models for use in resource allocation decisions: a critical review in the light of observed preferences for social choice', *International Journal of Technology Assessment in Health Care* 12, 31–44.

Nussdelder, W.J., van der Velden, J., Lenior, M.E., Sonsbeek, J.L.A. and van den Bos, G.A.M. (1994) 'The effect of elimination of selected chronic diseases on disability-free life expectancy: compression or expansion of morbidity? Preliminary results', in Mathers, C.D., McCallum, J. and Robine, J-M. (eds), *Advances in Health Expectancies: Proceedings of the 7th Meeting of the International Network on Health Expectancy (REVES)*. Canberra: Australian Institute of Health and Welfare.

Nusselder, W.J., van der Velden, K., Sonsbeek, J.L.A., *et al* (1996) 'The elimination of selected chronic diseases in a population: the compression and expansion of morbidity', *American Journal of Public Health* 86(2), 187–193.

Nusselder, W.J., Looman, C.W., Marang-van de Mheen, P.J. and Mackenbach, J.P. (2000) 'Smoking and the compression of morbidity', *Journal of Epidemiology and Community Health* 54(8), 566–574.

Robine, J-M. and Mathers, C.D. (1993) 'Measuring the compression or expansion of morbidity through changes in health expectancy', in Robine, J-M., Mathers, C.D., Bone, M.R. and Romieu, I. (eds) *Calculation of Health Expectancies, Harmonization, Consensus Achieved and Future Perspectives*. Montrouge: John Libbey Eurotext.

Tsai, S.P., Lee, E.S. and Hardy, R.J. (1978) 'The effect of a reduction in leading causes of death: potential gains in life expectancy', *American Journal of Public Health* 68, 996–971.

van de Water, H.P.A. (1993) 'Policy relevance and the further development of the health expectancy indicator', in Robine, J.-M., Mathers, C.D., Bone, M.R. and Romieu, I. (eds) *Calculation of Health Expectancies: Harmonization, Consensus Achieved and Future Perspectives*. Montrouge/Montpellier: Colloque INSERM/John Libbey Eurotext Ltd, pp. 23–31.

Wolfson, M.C. (1996) 'Health-adjusted life expectancy', *Health Reports* 8(1), 41–45. Statistics of Canada.

World Bank (1993) *World Development Report 1993: Investing in Health*. New York: Oxford University Press.

8

Mental Health Expectancy

KAREN RITCHIE and CATHERINE POLGE

INSERM, Montpellier, France

Kramer's prediction in 1980 of a 'coming pandemic of mental disorders and associated chronic diseases and disabilities' has been an important underlying impetus for the calculation of health expectancies. However, despite the emphasis placed by Kramer on psychiatric illness, the first health expectancy calculations were confined exclusively to states of physical health largely due to concerns that definitions of mental health states were likely to be particularly problematic. Since 1989 the mental health subcommittee of REVES (Ritchie, 1991, 1992) has attempted to convince colleagues of the potential importance of mental health expectancy calculations, given that mental disorder is currently estimated to be responsible for 60% of all disabilities (WHO, 1984). Moreover, in public health terms, persons with mental illness constitute a particularly vulnerable subgroup; they are at increased risk from death due to accidents and natural causes, are at increased risk of physical and mental abuse, and engender high rates of morbidity in care-givers.

Case detection of mental illness remains a central problem (Kay, 1990, 1993). There have been significant advances in recent decades in our understanding of the biological mechanisms underlying mental disorder. However, research designed to isolate specific biological markers remains both inconsistent and inconclusive. At a clinical level competing conceptualizations of mental illness and reliance on non-specific behavioural indicators of dysfunction have led to considerable disagreement at the levels of nosology, differential diagnosis and management. Psychiatric illness in Europe is both underdiagnosed and undertreated. The World Health Organization and the American Psychiatric Association have made significant contributions towards the standardization of nomenclature and diagnostic criteria through the development of two international classification systems: the International Classification of Diseases (ICD) and the Diagnostic and Statistical Manual of the American Psychiatric

Determining Health Expectancies. Edited by J-M. Robine, C. Jagger, C.D. Mathers, E.M. Crimmins and R.M. Suzman.
© 2003 John Wiley & Sons, Ltd

Association (DSM). As a result, research applying these algorithms shows greater consistency even across cultures. Attempts are also presently being made conjointly by the US National Institutes of Health and WHO to better adapt the International Classification of Impairments, Disabilities and Handicaps (ICIDH) to the problems of mental illness. The development of cross-cultural population indicators of mental health such as health expectancies is now widely considered to be feasible provided workers in this area are prepared to adhere to these common classification systems (Ritchie, 1994; Roelands and Van Oyen, 1994).

At the general level of public health, mental health expectancies may contribute in at least three ways: (a) indicating the *consequences* of mental disorder by calculating the number of years expected to be lived by a population in a specific state of mental ill-health and thus permitting the planning of service needs; (b) showing *trends over time* thus facilitating the evaluation of changing methods of care; and (c) providing *international comparisons* which may highlight social inequalities and cross-cultural differences in attitudes to mental health. In order to establish priorities for the calculation of health expectancies in the mental health area, the mental health subcommittee of REVES conducted a world-wide census in 1990 to establish mental health priorities in both developed and developing countries (Ritchie, 1990). The results of this survey indicated that the problems of ageing-related cognitive change (notably the dementias), depression, schizophrenia, mental retardation and suicide are currently considered priority areas in most countries. Concern was also expressed regarding the mental health consequences of social upheaval: notably war, unemployment, urban violence. It has thus been suggested that mental health expectancies should aim to focus on these areas.

The first calculations of mental health expectancy have concerned the senile dementias. These disorders have been given priority as the condition most likely to reach epidemic proportions as average life expectancy continues to rise. Ineichen (1987), warning of a 'rising tide' of dementia in Britain, predicted a 5 to 17% increase in dementia prevalence by the year 2001. In Australia, Henderson (1983) referred to a coming epidemic of dementia, estimating a 91% increase in the number of cases by the year 2001. Applying a linear model of the relationship of dementia to age derived from a meta-analysis of epidemiological studies which have used DSM-III diagnostic criteria to recent population projections, Ritchie and Robine (1994) have shown that between 1990 and 2020 the French population will increase by 58% but the prevalence of dementia is estimated to increase by 89%. The average life expectancy of an elderly person with early senile dementia is around eight years. This time is spent in a state of progressive dependency for both activities of daily living and decision-making functions. A change in the number of dementia-free years lived by a given population will thus have a

Table 8.1. Life expectancy (LE), dementia-free life expectancy (DemFLE) and life expectancy with dementia (DemLE) at the age of 65 years by sex and country

Country	LE at 65 years		DemFLE at 65 years		DemLE at 65 years		% DemFLE/LE	
	Men	Women	Men	Women	Men	Women	Men	Women
France	15.4	19.7	14.8	18.8	0.6	0.9	96.4	95.4
UK (Liverpool)	13.1	17.1	12.6	15.9	0.5	1.2	96.2	93.1
UK (3 cities)	14.4	19.7	13.7	17.8	0.7	1.9	94.6	89.9
Belgium	14.0	18.3	13.4	16.7	0.6	1.6	95.7	91.3
Ireland	13.5	16.9	13.0	15.7	0.5	1.2	96.5	93.1
Netherlands	14.5	19.0	14.0	17.7	0.5	1.3	96.4	93.2
United States	18.11	21.48	16.9	19.6			93.5	91.4
Switzerland (Zurich)	16.9	21.0	16.2	18.4	0.7	2.6	96.0	88.0

significant impact on the demand for both domiciliary and institutional services (Ledésert et al, 1994).

Calculations of dementia-free life expectancy have now been made for France (Ritchie et al, 1994), the United Kingdom (Ritchie et al, 1993), Belgium (Roelands and Van Oyen, 1994), the Netherlands (Perenboom et al, 1995; Perenboom and van de Water, 1997), Ireland (Eire) (Jagger et al, 1998), Switzerland (Herrmann and Michel, 1996), Australia (Ritchie et al, 1993, 1994). All of these studies have been based on large-scale epidemiological studies of ageing and have used diagnostic criteria for senile dementia compatible with DSM algorithms, in conjunction with national mortality tables. Dementia-free life expectancy has been calculated in all studies using Sullivan's method. The results of these studies are given in Table 8.1 with the exception of Australia, for which estimates are only available after age 70. Australian values at this higher age are similar, being only slightly lower than those found for France and the UK. These small differences are unlikely to be statistically significant (Ritchie et al, 1994). Tentative estimates are also given for the United States (Sauvaget et al, 1997). However, these results must be considered apart from the others as they are based on a population belonging to a health maintenance organization, rather than deriving from a general, representative population study.

At age 65 life expectancy in Western countries is seen to vary between 13 and 18 years for men and 17 and 21 years for women, the lowest life expectancy being found in Ireland, and the highest in Switzerland. Despite these differences, the different studies show surprisingly similar results for men with regard to mental health expectancies with DemFLE as a proportion of life expectancy being between 95 and 96.5% for all countries. For women there is greater variability between countries, ranging from 90% in the UK to 95.4% in France. Dementia-free life expectancy for both men and women is highest in Switzerland and France and lowest in Ireland.

For all countries studied, life expectancy with dementia (DemLE) for both sexes combined remains stable at approximately one year. That is, beyond age 65 all survivors may expect to live one year of life with dementia. In terms of service provision, this implies that one year of care must be provided for every member of a given population over 65 years. There is a clear sex difference in this respect with DemLE estimates being around double for women compared to men in all countries. The burden of care is twice that for women (half a year of care will be necessary for each man in the community and slightly over one year for each woman). The proportion of demented survivors in relation to the total number in the initial cohort increases steadily in all countries from around age 70 to reach its highest point at around age 85. Taking into account the dual trends with age of an increase in dementia prevalence and a decrease in the number of survivors, we find that in all countries the greatest number of persons with dementia will be between 80 and 85 years. Thus while dementia prevalence increases exponentially with age, to reach around 40% at 95 years, the greatest number of persons requiring care will be in their early eighties. This point has important implications for health service planning as health profiles and service requirements change with age.

Results from dementia-free life expectancy calculations have demonstrated that such a measure is both feasible and useful in a public health context provided that internationally recognized diagnostic algorithms and case-detection methods are used. Criteria based on the ICD and the DSM are the most widely adopted. Studies which have used other forms of case identification, in particular unstandardized clinical examinations or screening instruments, have been shown to give aberrant values (Ritchie *et al*, 1994). Calculations should also be confined to moderate and severe forms of dementia, as error rates in the screening of mild dementia are presently too high for meaningful analysis. Given that persons with mild dementia are still generally functionally independent, there is also little immediate practical use in making estimates with this group in terms of health policy.

With regard to other mental health indicators, some early data is available. A first calculation of depression-free life expectancy has been made for the Netherlands (Deeg *et al*, 1996). Depression-free life expectancy was estimated to constitute 19.4% and 22.4% of life expectancy at age 55 for men and women respectively. This estimate has been carried out using a short depression screening test, without prior validation of the cut-off point within the Dutch population, and should therefore only be considered a preliminary finding. Further work needs to be carried out with this indicator to standardize case identification procedures based on more robust criteria such as the research criteria established by ICD and DSM.

Table 8.2. Life expectancy (LE), life expectancy in good mental health (MHLE) and life expectancy in good mental health as a proportion of life expectancy (%MHLE/LE) at the age of 65 years in Bulgaria and Catalonia by sex

	Catalonia			Bulgaria		
	LE	MHLE	MHLE/LE	LE	MHLE	MHLE/LE
Men	16.4	14.1	86.0	12.7	5.1	39.7
Women	20.5	16.5	80.5	15.3	4.3	28.4

Three studies have attempted to assess general mental health. In Denmark case-identification was achieved by the 5-item Mental Health Inventory (Bronnum-Hansen and Rasmussen, 1994) and in both Spain and Bulgaria, by the General Health Questionnaire (Gispert *et al*, 1998; Mutafova *et al*, 1999). The results of these studies show that while the overall prevalence of poor mental health appears to increase with age, the percentage of life years with poor mental health remains relatively stable, with the gains being made by women in terms of life expectancy being partly 'lost' in overall poor mental health. A comparison of the Spanish and Bulgarian studies, which have both used the same instrument to measure mental health, show quite different mental health expectancy values (Table 8.2). As the studies used different age cohorts, only the age group over 65 is comparable.

The differences are striking. While case identification methodology is similar, the sampling frame in the two studies is different and the case probability estimates used are derived from the Catalonia study without prior re-validation in Bulgaria. Such differences are, however, insufficient to account for the very great differential. There may be cultural differences in degree of complaint, but almost certainly the lower values of mental health expectancy in Bulgaria are significantly related to the stress of civil unrest in eastern Europe, and thereby underline the potential utility of such a method in drawing attention to time changes in mental health due to social change.

Early experience with mental health indicators has above all underlined the necessity to standardize instruments, as this risks being the principal cause of variability. This implies use of the same instrument followed by validation against clinical judgement within each population under study, as mental health problems are commonly measured by scales, and the cut-off points may not be the same across population groups. The census of European surveys of mental health carried out by the Euro-REVES mental health subcommittee has identified 67 mental health population studies, many of which have used common indicators (Hibbett *et al*, 1999). Thus a large pool of data presently exists from which further calculations may be made and from which meta-analyses may be constructed to examine health states with low prevalence. A database, SIGMUND, has been established which incorporates information gained from the census, and provides information on protocols, sampling, instruments and data availability (Polge, 1997).

Calculations of mental health expectancy to date have been almost exclusively by the Sullivan method using national life tables and age-specific disease prevalence data. The multistate method is perhaps better adapted to the problem of mental disorder as such states are commonly fluctuating over time. This type of calculation requires longitudinal data to enable estimation of transition rates between mental health states and between each health state and death. The number of longitudinal studies which have been registered in SIGMUND suggests that it is now possible to undertake cross-national multistate calculations of mental health expectancies. Transition estimates from different degrees of cognitive impairment towards death, dementia and recovery from the National Long Term Care Survey in the United States (Hayward *et al*, 1994), although based only on a brief screening test for dementia rather than internationally acceptable diagnostic algorithms, none-theless provide an interesting first example of this type of methodology.

Finally, at a conceptual level it is envisaged that two classes of mental health calculation should be developed: *disease-specific life expectancies* such as depression-free life expectancy and dementia-free life expectancy, and calculations relating to the *consequences of mental disorder*, such as life expectancy in good perceived mental health, life expectancy without social isolation or handicap-free life expectancy in the face of a given disorder. At the present time efforts have focused on the first type of calculation, and it is hoped that in the coming years the second will also become a subject of interest, as it is increasingly recognized by health providers that the consequences of mental ill-health may continue to handicap individuals long after the underlying cause has been addressed through clinical intervention.

REFERENCES

Bronnum-Hansen, H. and Rasmussen, N. (1996) 'Mental health expectancy calculation. Denmark', in 2nd Euro-REVES meeting, London.

Deeg, D.J.H., Westendorp, D.E. and Serrière, M. (1994) *Autonomy and Well-being in the Aging Population. I. Report from the Longitudinal Aging Study Amsterdam 1992–1993*. Amsterdam: VU University Press.

Gispert, R., Ritchie, K., Rajmil, L., Rué, M., Glutting, J.P. and Roset, M. (1998) 'Mental health expectancy: an indicator to bridge the gap between clinical and public health perspectives of population mental health', *Acta Psychiatrica Scandinavica* 98, 182–186.

Hayward, M.D., Crimmins, E.M. and Friedman, S. (1994) 'Cognitive functioning changes among the chronically impaired elderly in the United States', in Mathers, C.D., McCallum, J. and Robine, J-M. (eds) *Advances in Health Expectancies*. Canberra: Australian Institute of Health and Welfare, AGPS.

Henderson, A.S. (1983) 'The coming epidemic of dementia', *Australian and New Zealand Journal of Psychiatry* 17, 117–127.

Herrmann, F.R. and Michel, J.P. (1996) 'Dementia free life expectancy in Switzerland: comparison between expected and observed estimates', in 9th Work-group meeting REVES, Rome.

Hibbett, M.J., Jagger, C., Polge, C., Cambois, E. and Ritchie, K. (1999) 'Cross-European mental health indicators. A dream or a reality?' *European Journal of Public Health* 9, 285–289.

Ineichen, B. (1987) 'Measuring the rising tide: how many dementia cases will there be by 2001?', *British Journal of Psychiatry* 150, 193–200.

Jagger, C., Ritchie, K., Bronnum-Hansen, H., Deeg, D., Gispert, R., *et al* (1998) 'Mental health expectancy – the European perspective', *Acta Psychiatrica Scandinavica* 98, 85–91.

Kay, D.W. (1990) 'Psychiatric and cognitive functional considerations', in 2nd Work-group meeting REVES, Geneva.

Kay, D. (1993) 'Ageing and cognition: approaches to the diagnosis of dementia in the community', in Robine, J-M., Mathers, C.D., Bone, M.R. and Romieu, I. (eds) *Calculation of Health Expectancies; Harmonization, Consensus Achieved and Future Perspectives* (*Calcul des espérances de vie en santé: harmonisation, acquis et perspectives*). Paris: John Libbey Eurotext.

Kramer, M. (1980) 'The rising pandemic of mental disorders and associated chronic diseases and disabilities', *Acta Psychiatrica Scandinavica* 62, 282–297.

Ledésert, B., Ritchie, K. and Touchon, J. (1994) 'Disability due to dementia', in Mathers, C.D., McCallum, J. and Robine J-M. (eds) *Advances in Health Expectancies*. Canberra: Australian Institute of Health and Welfare, AGPS.

Mutafova, M., Van de Water, H., Maleshkov, C., Tonkova, S., Perenboom, R. and Boshuizen, H. (1999) 'Attempt for the assessment of the mental health of the population in Bulgaria', in Egidi, V. (ed.) *Towards an Integrated System of Indicators to Assess the Health Status of the Population*. Rome: ISTAT.

Perenboom, R.J.M. and van de Water, H.P.A. (1997) 'Mental health expectancy in the Netherlands, 1989–1995', in 10th Work-group meeting REVES, Tokyo.

Perenboom, R.J.M., van de Water, H.P.A. and Boshuizen, H.C. (1995) 'Dementia-free life expectancy in the Netherlands, 1993', in 8th Work-group meeting REVES, Chicago.

Polge, C. (1997) 'Sigmund: A European database of mental health surveys', *European Journal of Psychiatry* 12, 268–269.

Ritchie, K. (1990) 'Report of the Committee on Mental Deterioration', in 2nd Work-group meeting REVES, Geneva.

Ritchie, K. (1991) 'Report of the Committee on Mental Deterioration', in 4th Work-group meeting REVES, Noordwijkerhout.

Ritchie, K. (1992) 'Life-expectancy without cognitive deterioration: theoretical and methodological difficulties', in Robine, J-M., Blanchet, M. and Dowd, J.E. (eds) *Health Expectancy*. London: HMSO.

Ritchie, K. (1994) 'International comparisons of dementia-free life expectancy: a critical review of the results obtained', in Mathers, C.D., McCallum, J. and Robine, J-M. (eds) *Advances in Health Expectancies*. Canberra: Australian Institute of Health and Welfare, AGPS.

Ritchie, K. and Robine, J-M. (1994) 'Senile dementia in France: estimating the current burden and projecting future trends', *Médecine Sciences* 10, 680–686.

Ritchie, K., Jagger, C., Brayne, C. and Letenneur, L. (1993) 'Dementia-free life expectancy: preliminary calculations for France and the United Kingdom', in Robine,

J-M., Mathers, C.D., Bone, M.R. and Romieu, I. (eds) *Calculation of Health Expectancies; Harmonization, Consensus Achieved and Future Perspectives* (*Calcul des espérances de vie en santé: harmonisation, acquis et perspectives*). Paris: John Libbey Eurotext.

Ritchie, K., Robine, J-M., Letenneur, L. and Dartigues, J.F. (1994) 'Dementia-free life expectancy in France', *American Journal of Public Health* 84, 232–236.

Roelands, M. and Van Oyen, H. (1994) 'Mental and social variables as operationalisation of health in the calculation of health expectancy', in Mathers, C.D., McCallum, J. and Robine, J-M. (eds) *Advances in Health Expectancies.* Canberra: Australian Institute of Health and Welfare, AGPS.

Sauvaget, C., Tsuji, I., Haan, M.N. and Hisamichi, S. (1997) 'Trends in dementia-free life expectancy among the elderly in the United States of America', in 10th Workgroup meeting REVES, Tokyo.

World Health Organization, Scientific Group on the Epidemiology of Ageing (1984) *The Use of Epidemiology in the Study of the Elderly.* Geneva: World Health Organization (Technical Report Series No. 706).

PART III

Measurement, Collection and Calculation Problems

Introduction

CAROL JAGGER

University of Leicester, Leicester, UK

A key part of the work of REVES and each of its meetings has been the development and dissemination of the methodology behind health expectancies and their relationship to other health indicators. Although consensus is impossible to reach on all issues, REVES has encouraged constructive criticism of methods and these have been disseminated in a balanced way for researchers both inside and outside the network.

This section focuses on the main methodological issues in health expectancy calculation. Methodology here includes not only the variety of methods of calculating health expectancies, which depends on the type of data available be it cross-sectional or longitudinal, but also two other issues that impact on the comparability of estimates, the major goal of REVES. Chapter 9 addresses the role of data collection methods in the comparability of health expectancies both between countries and within countries over time. It emphasises the need to ensure that the underlying concepts of the definition of health used for the health expectancies are in agreement, rather than expecting that the exact same question form or measurement instrument will behave identically across cultures or over time. This is developed further in Chapter 10, which concentrates on the measurement of disability since disability-free life expectancy is the health expectancy that has been most calculated across the world but for which we still have few truly comparable estimates. The major contribution made by REVES in understanding disability and the ageing process is also discussed.

When the REVES network first began, longitudinal data on morbidity were relatively rare and the focus on calculation was therefore on the method that incorporates health information from prevalence surveys with population mortality data. This method, known as the Sullivan method (Sullivan, 1971), has been widely discussed during the REVES meetings and its properties, limitations and advantages in monitoring trends over time have been well

Determining Health Expectancies. Edited by J-M. Robine, C. Jagger, C.D. Mathers, E.M. Crimmins and R.M. Suzman.

described (Mathers, 1991; Mathers and Robine, 1997; van de Water *et al*, 1995). A major advance in educating researchers world-wide to the basic methodology of health expectancy has been the work of the European arm of REVES, Euro-REVES. During the project establishing this sub-network and aiming specifically at harmonisation of concepts, methods and analysis of health expectancies across the European Union, a calculation guide on the Sullivan method was established. This has been successfully used in training workshops in Asia and more detailed materials have now been developed to enable further workshops to be easily run.

Although prevalence data may allow the first calculations of health expectancy for a country, longitudinal data that explicitly contain the transitions to morbidity and death and to recovery are preferable and allow a much wider exploration of the ageing and health processes. More recently, further advances have been made with calculation methods for longitudinal data, with readily available software enabling a wider audience to be able to use these more complex methods. These innovative methods that in particular allow optimal use of subjects with missing data and less well-balanced study designs with unequal intervals between waves are described in Chapter 11 along with other health expectancy calculation methods.

Health expectancies as described above calculate life spent in discrete health states. A further variant of this form of health expectancy weights health states to arrive at a single indicator, a health-adjusted life expectancy. The major exponents of these methods have been the Canadian teams and Chapter 12 describes the advantages and limitations of these methods. Other health indicators such as the disability-adjusted life year (DALY) and the disability-adjusted life expectancy (DALE) have been promoted by the World Health Organization. These too have their supporters and critics and they have been represented at REVES meetings. Chapter 13 describes the original DALY, and critically reviews its progress together with its health expectancy equivalent, DALE.

REFERENCES

Mathers, C.D. (1991) *Health Expectancies in Australia 1981 and 1988*. Canberra: Australian Institute of Health; AGPS. (Technical report)

Mathers, C.D. and Robine, J.M. (1997) 'How good is Sullivan's method for monitoring changes in population health expectancies', *Journal of Epidemiology and Community Health* 51, 80–86.

Sullivan, D.F. (1971) 'A single index of mortality and morbidity', *HSMHA Health Reports* 86, 347–354.

van de Water, H.P.A., Boshuizen, H.C., Perenboom, R.J., Mathers, C.D. and Robine, J.M. (1995) 'Health expectancy: an indicator for change?', *Journal of Epidemiology and Community Health* 49, 330–331.

9

Data Collection Methods and Comparability Issues

VITTORIA BURATTA and VIVIANA EGIDI
ISTAT, Rome, Italy

With increased survival of populations has come a growing need to develop measurements of population health status together with the necessity to develop common methods and instruments to make comparative analyses both between and within countries. A major problem in achieving comparability has been that indicators have used many different health information sources. Despite progress made as to definitions to be adopted and instruments for measurement, the methods of data collection also impact on comparability. This chapter will review how different survey designs (cross-sectional, longitudinal), questionnaire design, mode of data collection (face-to-face interview, telephone interview, postal survey) as well as issues of proxy response and timing of data collection can affect the prevalence of health states and consequently comparability of health indicators.

CONCEPTS, PROCEDURES AND METHODS: THE SOURCES OF INCOMPARABILITY

It is a good strategy to establish comparability wherever possible. One could be tempted to think that this aim can be achieved simply by standardising instruments and measurements. However, believing that rigid definitions, identical survey procedures, questions and methods of processing and estimating the indicators will automatically assure comparability is incorrect. Indeed, standardisation may even have an adverse effect on comparability. Health questions formulated in the same manner, for example, may obtain differing responses in different population groups according to culture, level of

Determining Health Expectancies. Edited by J-M. Robine, C. Jagger, C.D. Mathers, E.M. Crimmins and R.M. Suzman.
© 2003 John Wiley & Sons, Ltd

education or even the frequency and quality of contact with doctors as well as individuals' sensitivity toward health issues. A better solution is the harmonisation of the underlying health concepts, of survey instruments and of processing methods which, within the context of a clearly defined and fully agreed upon conceptual framework, would enable each country to have a relatively free hand in experimenting with the information collection methods most appropriate for the requirements and characteristics of their country. This strategy, precisely because it is less efficient from the point of view of availability of directly comparable data, may prove to be more efficacious as a means of controlling and counteracting a number of factors that hinder comparability.

CONCEPTS AND DEFINITIONS

Undoubtedly, the first step in designing a harmonised system of measurement of population health status is to clarify the exact meaning of *good* or *poor* health status. Many of the difficulties involved in evaluation and comparison of measurements can be attributed to the extreme complexity of this topic. Good or, alternatively, poor health is a vaguely defined condition that cannot be precisely defined. It is therefore difficult to pinpoint a moment of transition – i.e. when an individual is no longer (or feels he or she is no longer) healthy. Generally speaking, each health condition must therefore be considered as transient, a 'grey area' which may have a positive outcome (recovery) or a negative one (progressing by degrees of severity toward death). It goes without saying that, given such a complex concept, where so many factors must be considered, the definitions of 'health' to be adopted operationally must be as precise as possible and all relevant aspects must be taken into consideration. We shall attempt to describe these aspects to arrive at a reference grid.

   The first aspect of concern is the approach adopted in evaluating the health status of an individual (Bowling, 1993). In essence this is whether a *subjective* approach is adopted, i.e. based on the individual's self-assessment, or if the approach is *objective*, 'unhealthiness' indicated on the basis of the presence of morbidity. With a *subjective* approach individuals are requested to assess their own state of health by means of an ordinal scale (with usually four or five categories), ranging from excellent to very poor. The basic idea here is that, if precise diagnostic categories are not of interest, individuals, rather than health professionals, will serve as a reliable and significant source of information for the assessment of personal health status. Comparisons carried out with such indicators have both the advantage and the disadvantage of allowing the individual to take into account all the variables (cultural, economic, social, environmental and health-related) which influence health and which render the perceptions of each individual different from the next, even when prevailing conditions are the same. It is worth noting, in fact, that the evaluation provided

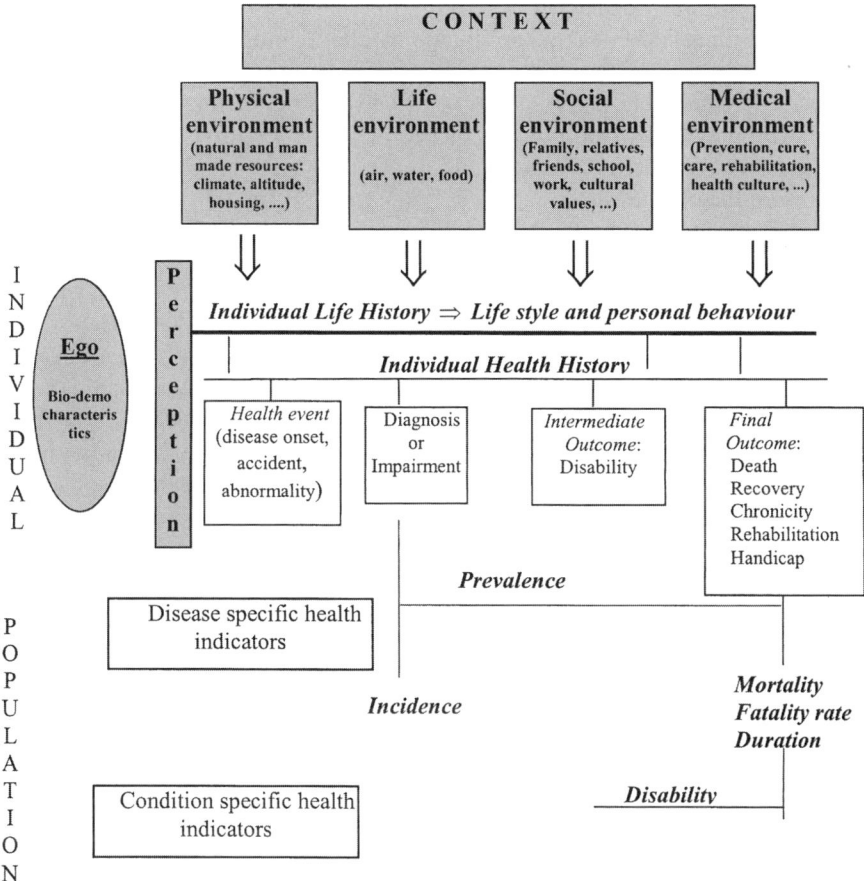

Figure 9.1. A conceptual framework for health analysis and demand indicators. *Source:* Egidi and Buratta (1995)

by the respondent during the interview is not only the outcome of the perception of the particular individual but is also conditional upon willingness to state the situation perceived. Each of these factors (actual health status, perception, willingness to declare) contributes to the theoretical complexity of the indices produced by subjective definitions of health conditions. However, these factors provide important information, over and above all the influences, about situations as they are directly experienced by individuals and used by individuals to determine behaviour patterns and make decisions. Significantly, such indicators have attracted a great deal of attention over the last few years since they have proved to be consistently predictive of survival, especially among older populations (Figure 9.1).

Even if we limit ourselves to the *objective* view of health, considered as an 'absence of illness', the task of coming up with a definition is still difficult. First illness and disease are processes involving time (duration) and their course may not be fully completed: onset may take place years before diagnosis. Moreover the outcome is defined only when such outcome is negative (death). Positive outcome (recovery), on the other hand, is often only the result of a progressive disappearance of symptoms not easily pinpointed in time. Furthermore, some illnesses or diseases may become chronic – and this may bring with it significant developments as to the risk of death due to other causes.

Diseases and illnesses determining states of poor health may be reported by individuals (irrespective of whether diagnosis has actually taken place) or by clinical diagnosis at the time of the interview. In both cases the diseases may be identified according to the International Classification of Diseases (ICD).

Poor health may be characterised by varying degrees of severity and these degrees of severity may have different repercussions on the individual's psychological and physical capacities. In other words the state of poor health in question may have consequences for the capacity of individuals to carry out activities and may provoke a transient or permanent limitation on carrying out activities considered essential for everyday life. Chapter 10 discusses the most widely used disability measures based on the consequences rather than on the presence of poor health.

It is still a matter of debate whether it is preferable in household based surveys to present respondents with a checklist of questions covering the main chronic conditions or to present them with open-ended questions. Adopting either of these strategies influences results considerably and may contribute significantly to the incomparability of indicators.

Furthermore, one illness may combine with others, either similar or dissimilar; for example, one infection combines with another chronic infection, or two chronic diseases may coexist in the same patient. This will affect the progress of any given disease or illness and its outcome, not to mention, of course, possible consequences in terms of disability.

The different role of individual perception should be considered within the context of the distinction between the subjective and the objective approach. This is evident where individuals are asked to assess their own state of health, but it cannot be ignored even when poor health is described by the actual presence of morbidity (irrespective of whether medical diagnosis has been carried out). The readiness of individuals to perceive the first signs of the disease or illness, their willingness to seek health services, their ability to choose from the range of available resources the most appropriate structure for diagnosis and treatment of a given pathological state, and last but not least, the availability of suitable structures, are all factors which affect measurement of the object of study. Moreover, behaviour patterns vary with regard to therapeutic treatment (once more, a subjective element) and these, and all the previous factors contribute to the progression of poor health. Often, differentials between groups including the sexes may be explained in terms of factors such as these. Non-household based survey methods aimed at evaluating the health of individuals through doctors, for instance disease registers, are also affected by perception-linked subjective factors. Here, the source of information changes and, perhaps the arbitrariness of perception is reduced, although problems relating to diagnostic techniques remain.

In summary, as the basis for the construction of comparable indicators, the definition of morbidity states should include consideration of the issues discussed above. Having addressed concepts and definitions, we now move to the role of different methods of data collection.

DATA COLLECTION METHODS

Methods of collecting data on the health and morbidity conditions of the population may be grouped under two general headings: those based on interview surveys (cross-sectional or longitudinal) and those based on the more routine data collection of events (hospital statistics, administrative statistics, disease registers).

For both cross-sectional and longitudinal surveys, much of the incomparability in health indicators between countries and over time may be attributed to methodological and organisational survey procedures. Here, we shall list some of the main aspects and, where appropriate, illustrate them from the Italian experience.

SURVEY SIZE

The size of the surveys may vary considerably from country to country. In some cases, small samples mean that it is impossible to work on data at subpopulation levels.

SAMPLE STRUCTURE

The target population is made up of all individuals who are in a given area at a given time and who live in households, or who live in institutions (hospitals, hostels, homes for the elderly, prisons). People living in private households form the basis of most surveys, but it is necessary to widen this to include those who live in institutions more often since, particularly in older populations, the health of those living in institutions is worse than those in households. Comparison between countries may be adversely affected by differences in the proportions in institutions compared to the whole population and this may itself be a result of differing definitions of institutions between countries.

Table 9.1. Persons bathing only with help, by age, Italian Health Survey (ISTAT, 1994)

Age group	Rate (per 100)
6–14	2.9
15–24	0.1
25–34	0.2
35–44	0.3
45–54	0.5
55–64	1.8
65–74	4.7
75+	22.9
All ages	*2.6*

Another biasing factor may be the elimination of homeless respondents who are not included in either household or institution based surveys and whose health conditions in general may be considered worse than those of persons of the same age residing in a household. This requires further attention by most surveys.

The importance of an appropriate target population is shown by an example using help with bathing to define disability in the daily life of children (ISTAT, Italian Health Survey, 1994). For children a positive answer to incapacity may arise because the functional disability is temporary and, most importantly, tied to the age of the child. A child of six years is 'not yet' able to take a bath alone, while a person aged 70 years may 'no longer' be able to do so. Thus, the motives are different and, so are the consequences: temporary incapacity in the first instance, permanent disability in the second. Since the specific objective of a health survey is normally to investigate permanent disabilities, a not wholly appropriate reference target creates bias in the estimates (Table 9.1).

STRATIFICATION OF SECOND LEVEL SAMPLE UNITS

The choice of variables defining the strata and the stratification procedures of the countries concerned may vary considerably.

REPLACEMENT PROCEDURES FOR NON-RESPONSE

Some countries permit sample replacement at the second level (territorial unit) and first level (household) units whilst others determine sample size so that the units which have been 'dropped' (and which are not replaced) will not result in the sample size falling below the threshold necessary for the significance of estimates.

QUESTIONNAIRE DESIGN

A fundamental phase in determining comparability between surveys is the questionnaire structure. The presence of open or structured questions, filters, particular sequences, the registration adopted, the structure of the scales of measurement, the response categories and also the design of the questionnaire all play a central role in the collecting of information.

Confusion in the respondent can also arise from the wording of the questions. One example is questions dealing with *need for assistance in activities of daily life*. The aim of these questions is to determine whether a person with a disability caused by illness or injury needs assistance and not to explore the total self-sufficiency of the individual in everyday life activities. This difference is most evident when thinking about the self-sufficiency of older men in cooking or in other home activities. They may be completely unable to perform these activities despite having no health problems.

Sometimes the *order of the questions* can affect results. For example, questions such as those concerning perceived health should precede the entire battery of items aimed at exploring the objective state of health in more detail, for instance acute illness, chronic illness and disabilities; otherwise the respondent may be influenced in the evaluation of health by the answers given to previous questions. Additionally, the sequence of items in any standardised list of questions should have a constant order of response categories. For example, the list of items on people's functional disabilities, which are repetitive, could create confusion. The respondent is asked 'Are you able to do A?', 'Are you able to do B?', etc. The sequence of response items (for example, 'no', 'yes, with assistance', 'yes, by myself') should be in the same order. In fact, an interviewer effect can be found as well as a respondent effect, since both expect to find 'not being able' in the first position, and so on. An example of this is given by the 1990 and 1994 Italian health surveys where the question on locomotion 'What is the furthest distance you can walk on your own without stopping and without severe discomfort?' was the same in both years. The order of the response options in 1990 was: Only a few steps/More than a few steps, but less than 200 metres/More than 200 metres; whilst in 1994 the order was: More than 200 metres/More than a few steps, but less than 200 metres/Only a few steps. As can be seen in Table 9.2, a large decrease was observed in 1994 in the level of walking disability; other aspects of disability did not reflect these differences.

The use of a nominal scale rather than a numerical scale of response items may also provide different results. In Italy, two different surveys ask the question 'How is your health generally?': an annual survey on 'Different aspects of daily life', which uses a numerical scale, from one (worst) to five (best) points, and the health interview survey, which uses a word scale ranging from 'very bad' to 'very good' with five qualitative levels.

Table 9.2. Percentage of people without walking disability (able to walk more than 200 metres), by age, Italian Health Survey 1990 and 1994 (ISTAT, 1990, 1994)

Year	All ages	6–14	15–24	25–34	35–44	45–54	55–64	65–74	75+
				Age groups					
1990	87.4	91.8	92.3	93.5	90.3	86.2	83.6	80.2	54.2
1994	91.6	95.8	97.5	97.5	97.3	95.2	90.3	81.3	52.8

Table 9.3. Persons by self-perceived health, Italian Health Survey (ISTAT, 1994)

Nominal scale	Very good	Good	Fair	Bad	Very bad	D.K.
	20.7	43.8	26.3	6.9	1.5	0.7
Score scale	5	4	3	2	1	D.K.
	49.2	24.8	15.5	5.3	2.8	2.4

In the numerical scale there is a greater concentration on the most positive and negative items than in the word scale (Table 9.3). In the case of the word scale the respondent need not translate the point into a state of well-being and this reduces the risk of subjectivity in the interpretation. As was evident from the two surveys in 1994, it is easier for a respondent to answer that his or her health is worth 5 rather than that he or she feels 'very good' (Table 9.3).

REFERENCE PERIOD

For health interview surveys, the reference period over which health is rated may have a considerable effect on the estimates of health problems and the options employed by each country and, within the same country on different occasions, have been found to vary considerably. At present there seems to be a general move towards having a single reference period for the self-rating of health conditions and for the occurrence of events such as accidents, illnesses or use of health services. It must be remembered, however, that collecting data with a short reference period on phenomena that are important but relatively 'rare', in the sense that they do not occur frequently in a person's life (for example, a stay in the hospital, or an accident at home or at work), may lead to overestimation, because the person tends to insert it in the reference period, even if it occurred outside (the so-called, telescoping effect). One solution to this problem could be to precede the actual question with another question relative to a longer period. For example, 'Did this happen to you in the last year' followed by 'with reference to that event, did it happen to you in the last three months?'. Following this criterion, estimates on the occurrence of different events can be improved, as can be seen in Table 9.4. The number of

Table 9.4. Persons (millions) having had a hospital admission (ISTAT, 1994)

Source	Question reference period		
	3 months	Last 12 months	1 year estimate
Health interview survey (1994)	2.5		10
Everyday life survey (1994)		7.5	7.5

hospital admissions in one year provided by hospital discharge was 10 million cases in 1994, reflected in the health interview survey result where the three-month reference period was adopted.

ACCEPTANCE OF PROXY RESPONSE

It is well known that the response of individuals rating their own health differs from the response of others (proxies) rating the health of that individual. The allowance or not of proxy responses and the proportion of such responses considerably affect morbidity estimates. This is not an easy problem to solve but the decision is usually confined to the very elderly or young or those with mental disorders since such people are more often not able to answer for themselves. But this effect can also be seen in other populations, as is seen in Table 9.5 where the proportion of ex-smokers is underestimated by proxy responses.

METHODS OF DATA COLLECTION

Methods of data collection adopted during surveys may vary greatly from country to country. The task of health evaluation may be delegated to a medical team with appropriate diagnostic instruments (health examination surveys), or this task may be carried out by means of questionnaires (health interview surveys). In the latter case, traditional face-to-face interviews may be conducted or the respondents may fill in questionnaires (self-completion method), which may be preferable for sensitive questions. Face-to-face

Table 9.5. Persons by smoking habits, Italian Everyday Life Survey (ISTAT, 1994)

	Direct response	Proxy response
Smokers	25	26
Ex-smokers	20	16
Non smokers	52	57
No response	1	1
Total	100	100

interviews may use computers (CAPI) rather than paper questionnaires or interviews may be carried out initially or successively by telephone (CATI). Data collected by these different methods have the capacity to reflect specific cultural characteristics of the population examined and are crucial aspects of measurement quality and comparability. Questions put in the same way may be answered differently using different data collection methods.

Also of importance are the characteristics of the *data collection network*, that is the characteristics and training of data collectors. Professional, specifically trained interviewers are the best solution. Often, however, interviewers are not specifically trained and are often not professionals. Differences in terms of data quality among countries depend to a great extent on this aspect, and comparability may therefore also be greatly affected.

TIMING OF INTERVIEWS

In some countries, the survey design includes interviews at various times of the year (often on a quarterly basis) to monitor season-specific development of morbidity. In other countries interviewing is not repeated, and carried out on a specific date. Often chronic disease prevalence data collected by a health interview survey are affected by seasonality because the symptoms of the disease may be more evident in different seasons and therefore influence an individual's perception. Thus, an annual survey performed in winter tends to overestimate chronic illnesses that grow more acute in the period of reference of the survey, while, at the same time they may underestimate the illnesses that become acute in spring. As an example, consider the result on two classes of illness obtained from the two Italian surveys of 1994: the annual survey on 'Aspects of daily life', carried out in November, and the quarterly survey on 'Health condition'. The effect of the 'temporal correlation' on the estimate is evident (Table 9.6). When such a correlation does not exist, collecting data over a longer period (one year) or shorter period (quarterly), at one time of the year rather than another, has little effect on the accuracy of the estimates. However, when this correlation does exist, it is preferable either to divide up the data collection period or re-proportion the estimate with weights that remove the seasonality.

CORRECTION PROCEDURES FOR MISSING AND INCONSISTENT RESPONSES

Various compatibility plans and correction systems based on deterministic or probabilistic models are adopted by different countries. Assessment of the impact of these various methods of correction on the comparability of the measurements obtained requires attention.

Table 9.6. Persons affected by arthritis and allergy (%) (ISTAT, 1984)

	Source			
	Annual survey 1994 (November)		Health survey 1994 (quarterly)	
Illness	Male	Female	Male	Female
Arthritis	18.9	27.7	14.8	22.6
Allergy	5.9	5.8	8.3	9.0

The nature of the disease and its duration (more or less than six months) are key elements for the identification of suitable reference periods. A preliminary distinction is between *acute and chronic diseases*. Recommended instruments to measure chronic conditions are not yet available but, generally speaking, household based surveys would appear to be particularly suitable for the measurement of the diffusion of long-duration diseases, such as chronic diseases, and diseases for which mortality is low. However, it remains a moot point whether it is preferable to provide respondents with a checklist of questions on the main chronic conditions or open-ended questions. Certain checks may be included in cross-sectional surveys to attempt to capture accurately diseases of brief duration. Often, for example, the reference period considered includes a period of varying length before the survey itself (Has the respondent contracted a disease over the last x weeks?), with a view to facilitating surveys of diseases of briefer duration. Choice of the most suitable period must in any case also consider uncertainty deriving from loss of memory and recall, this varying with the type of event and when it took place. Furthermore, for certain high mortality diseases (e.g. malignant tumours) or diseases considered socially unacceptable, health interview surveys, as an instrument, are much less suitable. Respondents are often not aware of their real state or, if they are aware of it, they are unwilling to declare it.

Although there are good arguments in favour of longitudinal as opposed to cross-sectional surveys, especially if a causal rather than descriptive approach is required or when transitions between health states are of interest, the problems outlined above are further magnified in longitudinal research. In addition, there are other factors such as length of survey, interval between interviews, differential response in units of the second or first stratum in successive series of surveys, that make true comparison between countries and over time more problematic. The WHO project 'Determinants of Healthy Ageing', involving a number of both developed and developing countries, may turn out to be useful for experimenting with international collaboration on these questions and for gaining a better idea of the advantages and disadvantages of longitudinal vis-à-vis cross-sectional health surveys. We now outline the additional aspects of longitudinal studies that can interfere with comparability.

INTERVIEW SPACING

This is probably the most important factor in determining the structure of responses. Choosing the interval length between two interviews depends on many factors including the nature of the phenomenon that determines meaningful duration in which changes can be expected in the observed variables, the budget of the survey, problems of telescoping or omissions, problems of panel effects which occur when the response given in the interview depends on the response given in the last interview and the tracking of mobile or migrant respondents.

RESPONDENT SELECTION

This plays a fundamental role and is even more important than in cross-sectional studies. In fact the choice of respondent at different points of time may be aimed at self-response, proxy or response on behalf of the household. The strategy adopted can significantly influence the response quality.

MODE OF INTERVIEW

The administration technique adopted can determine the degree of respondents' cooperation in the first interview and in the follow-up but can also affect the ability to trace people and determine movements and migration, as well as the data quality.

In addition to cross-sectional and longitudinal surveys, data may be collected through routine statistics since most countries have registration systems for many events such as births and deaths, hospital admissions, morbidity registers and many health care activities. In these cases the quality of comparability depends on factors such as the source of information (a statistical institute or department, or an administrative department) the classifications in use, the registration technique (computer assisted or manual registration), the coverage (a sample of events, partial registration, or integral registration), the definitions adopted (the official definition of a hospital sometimes includes institutions for long-term care) and the periodicity of the data collection.

In general, comparability of hospital statistics is better than that for health interview surveys. This kind of data system generally has a long history. Hospital statistics are based on medical diagnoses that are more comparable than self-perceptions. In addition, hospital cases will tend to be the more severe cases of disease. Thirdly, information on certain technical procedures is available only through the hospitals because they are performed exclusively there, for example major surgery which itself now has an international system of coding.

Registers are also used to collect information for various diseases, for example cancer, cardiovascular diseases and other chronic diseases including mental disorders. They have the advantage of continuity, but are usually costly to maintain and often limited in geographic coverage.

WHICH STRATEGY?

Given the extreme complexity of the concept of health, the provision of an exhaustive definition acceptable for the variety of conditions contained in the concept is an impossible goal. Furthermore, it would not be appropriate to make such definitions without being aware of the many aspects considered above that add considerable complexity (Danish Ministry of Health, 1994; Jacobson *et al*, 1990; Laaser, 1996). Indeed adopting a few standardised measurements may well oversimplify information to such an extent that it would not be possible to truly assess health differentials observable across time or between countries. The strategy to be adopted might therefore turn out to be that of *not* succumbing to the ideal of a universally acceptable definition and, instead, concentrating on definitions that are clearly directed toward specific aims, and which acknowledge who is the user of the data, therefore providing the answers to the relevant questions.

The aims of a morbidity study may, in fact, vary greatly and may include: assessment of quality of survival for scientific and forecasting purposes; studying the changes in quality of survival and monitoring of the direction taken by countries towards Health for All targets; assessment of the impact of specific actions of health policy; and health planning and assessment of resource adequacy and the costs involved in reaching specified goals. It is not necessarily the case that the same indicators will serve a variety of ends: health expectancy, mortality by cause, hospital morbidity, incidence, prevalence, duration, disability, medical consumption, finance, manpower (Patrick and Guttmacher, 1993; RIVM, 1994; van de Water and van Herten, 1996). Each measure is concerned with particular issues but, taken together, they outline the position with regard to health of a given country. This requires acknowledgement of the nuances and interconnections to be able to construct an ideal integrated system of health measures. Only a system such as this would permit true comparisons between countries, in other words capable of simultaneously taking into consideration all the various factors involved.

A starting point, perhaps, is recognition of the fact that our knowledge of this field is still highly limited and we are a long way from being in a position to know and to control the innumerable variables which influence health states and differentials of the population. Given this, much circumspection is required when moving towards a gradual harmonisation of concepts and measurements, with an assessment of the costs and benefits of each change made to definitions adopted and survey methods on a regular basis (OECD, 1996a, 1996b).

A separate discussion of analyses conducted for investigative purposes is required, that is to say analyses aimed at the identification of determinants of the state of health and of its differentials. In cases such as these, comparability is absolutely necessary and this will affect all aspects of the approach. Indeed, occasionally, one is tempted to bypass the problem by adopting a standardised survey protocol for various countries and, in the case of household interview surveys, to adopt a common interview module. It should be stressed that for non-experimental sciences, the condition upon which verification of hypotheses is based is the homogeneity of populations or groups with respect to uncontrolled variables (as if the units were attributed to the various groups in a totally random manner) (Caselli *et al*, 1990). This discourages consideration of populations that differ excessively among themselves *a priori*. Interpretative analysis and, even more so, causal analysis involve adoption of a correct reference population as well as, of course, a set of hypotheses and the correct study design. In this sense, one should not aim at the standardisation of analyses or, as occasionally happens, attempt standardised supranational surveys at the expense of furthering in-depth surveys and analysis based on harmonised methods and working hypotheses.

An important step towards the comparability of morbidity measurements would be the wide distribution of metadata on morbidity surveys carried out in various countries. For example, information on health surveys conducted within each country should be readily available in such a way as to permit immediate understanding of the data and its characteristics. Systematic study of the roles played by methodological and organisational survey procedures on measurements might lead to a more optimal choice on the part of the various countries. In the same manner, the adoption of a variety of definitions of health for each country might enhance comparison by the addition of aspects that would otherwise be neglected.

The challenge is now to continue along the road we have taken and broaden the field to include other instruments and indicators, to analyse their characteristics and their efficiency under various conditions, and to encapsulate those factors impeding progress towards a satisfactory level of international comparability. Identification and removal (or, at least, control) of such elements will increase comparability of indicators without thereby requiring us to sacrifice specificity of information. Obviously, this is clearly a difficult task – as may be noted on considering the not always successful efforts made – but it is a task which must be faced up to if a measurement system is to be constructed permitting truly comparative evaluation of the health conditions of populations and, in the longer term, providing guidelines for social and health policy makers in monitoring their progress towards Health for All by the year 2000 (World Health Organization, 1981a, 1981b, 1981c, 1990, 1994).

REFERENCES

Bowling, A. (1993) *Measuring Health*. Philadelphia, Milton Keynes: Open University Press.

Caselli, G., Duchene, J., Egidi, V., Santini, A. and Wunsch, G. (1990) *A Matter of Life and Death. Methodologies for the life history analysis of adult mortality*, Louvain-la-Neuve: Editions Academia (Institut de Démographie, Université Catholique de Louvain, Working Paper no. 151).

Danish Ministry of Health, The life expectancy committee (1994) *Lifetime in Denmark*.

Egidi, V. and Buratta, V. (1995) *Towards a Harmonized Morbidity Indicators System*. Urgup, Turkey: EAPS working Group on morbidity and mortality.

Jacobson, B., Smith, A. and Whitehead, M. (1990) *The Nation's Health: A Strategy for the 1990s*. London: King Edward's Hospital Fund for London.

Laaser, U. (ed.) (1996) *Perspectives for a European Public Health Information System*. Düsseldorf, Germany: NRW.

Organisation for Economic Co-operation and Development (OECD) (1996a) *OECD Health Data 96*. Paris: OECD.

Organisation for Economic Co-operation and Development (OECD) (1996b) *The German health information system A possible means to improve the international comparison of health care data?* Paris: OECD. (Document for the Working party on social policy.)

Patrick, D. and Guttmacher, S. (1993) 'Socio-political issues in the use of health indicators', in Culyer A.J. (ed.) *Health Indicators*. Oxford: Martin Robertson.

RIVM (National Institute of Public Health and the Environment) (1994) *Public Health Status and Forecasts*. The Hague: RIVM.

van de Water, H.P.A. and van Herten, L.M. (1996) *Bull's Eye or Achilles' Heel*. The Hague: TNO Prevention and Health.

World Health Organization (1981a) *Global Strategy for Health for All by 2000*. Geneva: WHO.

World Health Organization (1981b) *Developing Indicators for Monitoring Progress Towards Health for All by the Year 2000*. Geneva: WHO.

World Health Organization (1981c) *The Use of Health Indicators: How to Make Statistics Talk*. Copenhagen: WHO.

World Health Organization (1990) *Implementation of Global Strategy for 'Health for All by the Year 2000' Eighth report on their world health situation*. Geneva: WHO.

World Health Organization (1994) *Concern for Europe's Tomorrow*. Copenhagen: WHO.

10

Disability Measurement

DORLY J.H. DEEG, LOIS M. VERBRUGGE* and CAROL JAGGER†
Vrije University, Amsterdam, The Netherlands, *University of Michigan, Ann Arbor,
MI, USA and †University of Leicester, Leicester, UK

INTRODUCTION

Disability-free life expectancy is the most common health expectancy. Its constituents are rates of disability and mortality. Disability is the inability to perform usual daily activities. This seemingly simple definition conceals the multiplicity of definitions that have been used among research groups and among nations. This is due partly to differences in conceptual frameworks, partly to availability of data. It is therefore not surprising that during the first years of the existence of REVES, a lot of effort was spent on conceptualizing disability in the larger framework of health and disablement. These efforts ran parallel to, and were informed by, the revision of the International Classification of Impairments, Disabilities and Handicaps (ICIDH) by the World Health Organization (WHO, 1980), and now newly revised into the International Classification of Functioning, Disability and Health (WHO, 2001). In addition to conceptual issues, other issues relate more directly to the measurement of disability. These include validity, range, sensitivity to change, and specificity to the environment. Because the natural focus of REVES is international comparability, measurement issues have always been in the foreground of discussions.

This chapter first describes the distribution of disability in the population. It then proceeds to review briefly the conceptual models that have been discussed in REVES. After a description of the various disability measures used, it embarks on a discussion of pertinent measurement issues. The chapter finishes with some recommendations for the use of disability measures in the calculation of active life expectancy.

Determining Health Expectancies. Edited by J-M. Robine, C. Jagger, C.D. Mathers, E.M. Crimmins and R.M. Suzman.
© 2003 John Wiley & Sons, Ltd

DISABILITY LEVELS ARE NOT UNAMBIGUOUS

The prevalence of disability shows large differences across socio-demographic subgroups. Numerous studies from a wide range of countries show that the prevalence of disability increases with age, that women are more often disabled than men, and that unmarried, lower educated, and poor persons have greater chances of being disabled (Albrecht and Verbrugge, 2000). Although disability may emerge at all ages, prevalence reaches substantial levels only at ages 65 years and above. This is probably the reason that most contributions to REVES on disability deal with the older population.

The basic building blocks of disability in older people have been the ability to perform personal care activities, the so-called activities of daily living (ADLs), and household activities, instrumental activities of daily living (IADLs). As an example, Sauvaget and Tsuji and colleagues (Sauvaget *et al*, 1999) showed for Japan that both prevalence and incidence of different aspects of disability rose sharply with age, with highest rates for needing help with IADLs and lower rates for needing help with mobility activities and with ADLs. Although women had generally higher rates of prevalence and incidence than men, the proportion of their remaining life spent in disability did not differ. At age 65, total life expectancy was 16.0 years for Japanese men, and 22.4 years for Japanese women. For both men and women life expectancy with disability in ADL and mobility was 11% each, and life expectancy with disability in IADL was about 26% of total life expectancy. While these percentages are more favorable than in other developed countries (Romieu and Robine, 1994), these findings highlight that disability measures based on more complex activities such as IADLs, produce higher numbers of years spent in disability than disability measures based on simpler activities.

Many studies described in the literature so far have made use of measures of disability defined in terms of assistance needed or received. As Verbrugge (1994a) has noted, however, the use of assistance is meant to reduce existing disability, and therefore is not a measure of disability itself. Carrière and Légaré (2000), for Canada, studied this issue by defining *gross* disability as a measure based on perceived need of assistance ignoring any social interventions, and *net* disability as a measure based on perceived needs of assistance that are not met. The latter indicator thus takes into account the gap between the expressed need for assistance and the assistance actually received. Expressed in years spent with disability in IADLs and ADLs, the net disability amounts to 16% of remaining life expectancy at age 60, increasing to 25% of remaining life expectancy at age 80. For women the gap is greater than for men (18–26% vs. 13–21%). In comparison, the percentage of life expectancy spent with disability for which the need for assistance was met ranged from 11% at age 60 to 16% at age 80.

Another issue related to the definition of disability in terms of need for assistance with IADLs is the traditional division of tasks between the sexes. Sex differences in responses to IADL questions may be partly attributable to sex role differences rather than to true differences in disability. Deeg (1993) defined the concepts of *functional* and *situational* disability, where situational disability stems from the fact that an activity has never been learned and thus is never done, or that doing an activity is not necessary because someone else in the household routinely performs it. Based on a scale of a sex-balanced selection of IADL items, in the Dutch population ages 55 and over, 21% of the total assistance needed in women, and 33% in men, was attributable to situational disability. Even greater percentages were found in an American sample of cancer patients (Allen *et al*, 1993). For both men and women, disability-free life expectancy at age 55 would increase by 3.5 years if situational disability were eliminated in the Netherlands (Deeg, 1993).

CONCEPTUAL THINKING ABOUT DISABILITY

Part of the ambiguity in the prevalence of disability, and thus in estimates of disability-free life expectancy, stems from the use of data that were designed on the basis of different conceptual models. In this section, some elements of conceptual models, proposed by REVES members, are reviewed.

During early REVES meetings, the International Classification of Impairments, Disabilities and Handicaps (ICIDH) was adopted as the basic model for future work. The ICIDH was developed by the WHO (1980) in order to clarify the concepts of impairment, disability and handicap as consequences of disease, and to allow comparable presentation of data. This classification describes a progression of consequences following a disease event: a pathological change leads to impairment of structure or function, which may lead to disability. Disability is defined as a modification or loss of the individual's ability to carry out certain activities. The disability may interact with the person's environment in such a way as to reduce the capacity to fulfill the role expected of this individual, thus creating a handicap (Robine *et al*, 1997; Thuriaux, 1989).

Colvez (1992) focused on the goal of inter-cultural comparability, and stated that a measure of disability should be meaningful to the older population, and should be free of cultural norms and sex bias. Taking a functionalist approach, that is, analyzing the consequences of diseases on human behavior rather than morbidity itself, Colvez defined 'survival' roles as those activities for which a reduction in performance leads to a disadvantage regardless of the social or cultural context. From the ICIDH, ADL independence and mobility proved to be best suited to these criteria.

Thuriaux (1989) supported the functionalist approach for the work of the WHO. In his view, cross-national comparability is particularly important for comparison between developed and developing countries, because the pattern of disability in developing countries is different from that in developed countries, and is likely to change rapidly. Thuriaux emphasized the importance of regular data collection at specific time intervals to monitor change. Therefore, an important criterion for an indicator of survival roles is its sensitivity to change.

According to Thuriaux (1989, 1993), the ICIDH has a wide range of use and of types of users. It had facilitated communication between categories of professionals in health care and policy on such various topics as early identification, intervention, rehabilitation, entitlements and insurance. However, the ICIDH met with some criticism: (1) there were problems of boundaries between disability and handicap; (2) explicit attention needed to be paid to the relationship between the concepts, and the role of time; (3) not enough attention was given to gradation of severity; (4) definitions of disability were in terms of what people cannot do, rather than what people can do; (5) more emphasis on the effect of the environment was needed; (6) recent insights in biological mechanisms should be incorporated; (7) culture- and gender-specific definitions and examples needed correcting.

In the 1990s, definitions of disability were modified to emphasize the environmental component. For example:

> [Disability] is the outcome of conflict between an individual's functional incapacity or deficiency and demands of the situation/environment. (Flores *et al*, 1992)

The onset of disability occurs when an individual can no longer do something despite any compensation strategy. Flores and colleagues (1992), in a French community, attempted to measure disability directly by tests of performance, i.e. by observation of the functions of ambulation, grasping and communication. The role of the environment was measured by varying the difficulty of the tests. For example, the ability to climb three steps was measured with two versions of a test: one version had steps of height 35 cm (as in a bus), the other of 15 cm (as in the home). The percentage with disability rose at an earlier age for the 35 cm steps as compared to the 15 cm steps, starting at age 45 and 65, respectively. However, the environment-induced differential between the two step heights decreased with age: for women already at age 45, for men at age 65. After these ages, the functional deficiency outweighed the extent of environmental demand. Translated to disability-free life expectancy, the differential amounted to as many as 8.5 years for women at age 10, and as few as 1.2 years for women at age 80. These findings are a good illustration of the role of the environment, and of the biases that may occur when ignoring this role.

The process of revision of the ICIDH has produced renewed concepts, in particular neutral or positive terms where the first model only included negative terms. For example, efforts to reach a better reflection of the environment proposed the term 'facilitators' in addition to the term 'obstacles'. These concepts and terms should facilitate research on the relative impact of personal and environmental factors on the disablement process. In turn, such research should lead to interventions that achieve more equity in society (Bolduc, 1993).

Although the ICIDH conceptual model was the one most discussed among REVES participants, other conceptual models of health were considered. Verbrugge and Jette's (1994) disablement process model extended the ICIDH by redefining 'disability' and 'handicap' as the better delineated 'functional limitations' and 'disability', respectively, and by including risk factors and personal and environmental characteristics that may influence the process. Minaire (1992) reviewed three models in addition to the ICIDH: (1) the biomedical model, (2) the situational model, and (3) the quality of life model. Each meets with critique, particularly because they are useful for limited purposes, but nevertheless are often misused. According to Minaire, the ICIDH model is the clearest, most consistent, most cross-disciplinary model. However, Minaire had doubts about its usefulness for the study of incidence instead of prevalence. He proposed that the combination of the four models would serve best the identification of factors that modify the sequence of the disablement process. This combination could also serve to classify disability-free life expectancy.

A WIDE RANGE OF DISABILITY MEASURES

Cross-national comparability has already been stated as an important goal when monitoring the health of national populations. However, this goal is very hard to reach without extra pressure on those who decide on survey designs. In the 1980s, the World Health Organization launched the program Health for All 2000 (WHO, 1981), with the purpose of reducing the inequalities in health between and within countries. The program defined a series of health indicators to measure the differences in health in and between countries. To evaluate the attainment of the goal, the progress in health was quantified in terms of these indicators. The countries that adopted the program were to report on this progress every three years. However, according to a 1990 questionnaire by the Netherlands Central Bureau of Statistics (NCBS) in countries of the European Region, North America, Japan, and Australia (Evers, 1991), the survey data available to substantiate the indicators varied widely across countries in number, selection, wording, and coding. Italy and the United Kingdom had the most indicators available, 24 each. Ireland and Turkey had less than 10. Also, the number of countries using a specific indicator varied. The most widely used indicators were self-perceived health and the proportion of non-smokers (23 out of 26 countries each). Any specific disability indicator was available for only 21 or fewer countries. The NCBS questionnaire was directed at national statistical offices. If a similar questionnaire had included surveys carried out by research institutes such as universities, the variety would have been even greater. The results of the questionnaire illustrate the disparities in availability and usability of health indicators, and thus, the need for harmonization.

Five years after the NCBS questionnaire, in 1995, an inventory by REVES (Robine *et al*, 1999) concluded that despite the frameworks recommended by international organizations, still each country pursued its own, often existing, health policy with its own concepts, objectives and indicators. Moreover, there appeared to be a discrepancy between references to concepts and their application in surveys and reports. For example, the ICIDH was increasingly quoted in reports, but only rarely applied. Only in countries which had recently become involved in monitoring public health, such as Spain, did the indicators used correspond to the recommendations.

SOME WIDELY USED MEASURES OF DISABILITY

The most widely used indicator of disability is the ability to perform ADLs related to self-care. Disability-free life expectancy often has been calculated based on this indicator. Katz and colleagues (1963) were the first to propose a set of ADL questions. This set included bathing, dressing, going to the toilet, getting from a bed to a chair, continence, and feeding oneself. Since 1963, however, questions on additional activities were introduced, and selections were made from the pool of all possible questions. As a consequence, no two surveys have exactly the same set of ADL questions, thus hampering mutual comparability. When measured in a survey setting, ADLs are asked in the form of questions with the response categories: without difficulty, with difficulty, only with help from another person, and unable. Variations on these categories include: with some difficulty, with a lot of difficulty, difficulty but no assistance, equipment assistance, and personal assistance. Alternatively, respondents to surveys can be observed while they actually perform the activity, but there are only very few examples of this mode of data collection (e.g. Kuriansky and Gurland, 1976). If individuals are not able to engage in self-care activities such as bathing or getting out of bed by themselves, they are severely limited, and thus the ADL indicator measures severe disability. In ICIDH terminology, this indicator in fact corresponds to handicap, because self-care is a role that is expected of every healthy person.

Ability to perform instrumental activities of daily living (IADL) is an almost equally widespread indicator, measuring more complex activities that are required to live independently (Lawton and Brody, 1969). The original set included using the telephone, shopping, preparing a meal, cleaning the house, doing the laundry, using transportation, taking medication, and handling finances. IADLs are almost always asked with the same response format as ADLs. Most of these activities have a cognitive component. In ICIDH terminology, again, they, in fact, indicate handicap.

The ICIDH concept of disability is more closely measured by functional limitations, which is the inability to perform actions that are needed to carry out an activity. Such actions are not activities in themselves. Examples are walking stairs, carrying a weight, or reaching above one's shoulder. As in the case of ADL and IADL, this indicator of disability is mostly measured using questions, with response formats asking about difficulty or inability (Nagi, 1976). Actions, however, lend themselves better than activities to measurement by observation. Since the late 1980s, an increasing number of surveys have incorporated tests of physical performance (Guralnik *et al*, 1989, 1994). A recent criticism of performance tests is that they measure 'experimental' ability, rather than actual ability in daily life (Glass, 1998).

Handicaps indicate restrictions in role functioning, and in some surveys are conceived to include occupational and social activities (Evers, 1991; Fougeyrollas *et al*, 1998; Koyano *et al*, 1991; Wiersma *et al*, 1988). Questions on these activities cover a great variety of activities, yet any one survey covers only a narrow selection of all possible activities. In a few cases, healthy life expectancy has been calculated based on social functioning (Roelands and Van Oyen, 1994). An attempt at general coverage of restrictions in role functioning is made as a part of the Medical Outcomes Study Short Form (Stewart *et al*, 1988). Six questions ask about health-related limitations in specified daily activities, followed by a question on how long the limitation has lasted.

Several indicators that are often stated to measure disability in ICIDH terminology actually cover impairment. They measure perception, incontinence, and cognitive and emotional functioning. Health expectancies based on each of these, as well as on combinations, have been calculated for some countries. The OECD questionnaire (McWhinnie, 1981) includes widely used questions on difficulty with near and distant vision, and difficulty with hearing in a conversation with a group of four or more persons and with hearing in a conversation with one other person. Incontinence is sometimes included with ADL questions (Katz *et al*, 1963), but more often is asked separately. For cognitive function, the most widely used measurement instrument is the Mini-Mental State Examination (Folstein *et al*, 1975), which covers orientation in time and place, memory and learning, attention and language. This test includes 23 items. Shorter tests are available, such as the Short Portable Mental Status Questionnaire (Pfeiffer, 1975), and the Katzman test (Katzman *et al*, 1983). All tests build on the early work of Wechsler, who designed the Wechsler Memory Scale and the Wechsler Adult Intelligence Scale (Wechsler, 1945,

1955). For the measurement of depressive symptoms, there is no single scale that is most widely used. In many recent studies, both in the US and in Europe, the Center for Epidemiologic Studies Depression scale (Radloff, 1977) has been chosen. Somewhat less often, the Geriatric Depression Scale (Yesavage *et al*, 1983) is used. However, in Europe there are traditions of other scales, including the General Health Questionnaire (Goldberg, 1972), the Geriatric Mental State schedule (Copeland *et al*, 1976), and the Hospital Anxiety and Depression Scale (Zigmond and Snaith, 1983). All of these questionnaires of cognitive and emotional functioning are screening tests; a diagnosis of dementia or depression can only be obtained in a second phase with more in-depth interviews and tests.

A widely used indicator of general health is self-perceived health. This indicator consists of a question that asks the subject to rate her/his own health, either in general or (less often) in comparison with age peers. Although this indicator does not measure disability, nor any other concept in the ICIDH, it has the advantages of having a fairly standard format and of being easily obtained in surveys. This is why its use in the calculation of health expectancy had been increasing. However, in addition to reflecting general health rather comprehensively (Golini and Calvani, 2001), it also reflects norms and standards about health that are determined by time and culture (Deeg, 1999), thus limiting its use for international comparison.

THE CHOICE OF MEASURE IS CONSEQUENTIAL

Ideally, policy makers and researchers first define their goals, then decide on the disability measures included in their surveys. With regard to important public health issues, four general goals may be identified (Bone *et al*, 1994): (1) monitoring health trends, (2) comparing the health of populations and subgroups, (3) assessing health outcomes of intervention strategies, and (4) predicting health service needs. Health expectancies may be useful tools to address the first, second, and fourth goals in particular. For the purposes of this chapter, health will be substituted with disability.

Regarding the first goal, Jagger (1996) showed that conclusions can differ depending on the measure of disability used: using limiting long-standing illness, an increase of disability over time was apparent. By contrast, using inability to perform ADLs, disability appeared to have decreased over time. These contrasting trends suggest that a definition in terms of limiting long-standing illness taps different dimensions of disability than a definition in terms of inability to perform ADLs.

The goal of monitoring health trends is especially pertinent for the older population, in view of the debate on the question whether their longer survival is accompanied by lower disability rates, or conversely by a rise in disability.

(See Chapter 2.) For the population of 75 years and over, Jagger and Clarke (1991) studied changes in the level of disability from 1981 to 1988. From the same set of ADL items, they constructed two dependency scores, one based on the intensity of assistance received (mild/moderate disability: either use of appliance or help from another person; severe disability: use of both appliance and help from another person), and the other based on the pervasiveness of the disability (the number of ADLs for which help from another person was received). Whereas the first indicator showed substantial decline across the seven-year period, the second indicator showed no change. Thus, their findings were ambiguous with differing conclusions depending on the disability score used.

Addressing the second goal of comparison between subgroups in the population, Laditka and Jenkins (2001) also started from the same set of six ADL items, and constructed four scales, ranging from a broad to a narrow definition of disability. The broadest definition was based on the number of activities for which any difficulty was reported, and the narrowest definition, on the number of activities for which assistance for most of the time was reported. The prevalence of moderate disability, defined as a scale score of 1 or 2, was 3.5 times greater when the broadest definition rather than the narrowest definition was used. The prevalence of severe disability, defined as a scale score of 3 or higher, was 3.9 times greater. This general finding contained two noteworthy variations in detail. First, the various ADL items showed differing sensitivities to the definition of disability used. Walking and transferring showed the largest variation, amounting to prevalences in the broadest definition that were 10.5 and 4.6 times greater, respectively, than in the narrowest definition of disability. Bathing had the smallest sensitivity, its prevalence being 1.9 times greater in the broad definition of disability than in the narrow one. Second, various subgroups in the population differed in their sensitivity to the definition of disability used. Black and white unmarried women with low education showed the largest variation in disability prevalence: in the broadest definition, the prevalence was 4.9 times greater than in the narrowest definition, whereas for married women with high education the prevalence differed only by a factor 2.0 (in black women) and 3.1 (in white women).

Further findings of Laditka and Jenkins (2001) pertain to the fourth public health goal of predicting health service needs. Considering the fact that unmarried women with low education are the greatest users of long-term care services, and eligibility for these services is based mainly on disability estimates, Laditka and Jenkins (2001) demonstrate that the specific selection of ADL items, and the disability scale made up of them, can make very substantial differences in the volume of long-term care services that is to be made available to the subgroup most in need of these services.

With regard to health policy planning in general, Thuriaux (1991) argued that goals using healthy life expectancy should not be stated in terms of *increasing* life expectancy in *good* health, but of *decreasing* life expectancy in *poor* health. In developing countries, disability rates are low, implying that the ratio of healthy life expectancy over total life expectancy is high. In consequence, gains in healthy life expectancy will not be substantial even with great reductions in disability, e.g. at younger ages. Goals could be stated more appropriately, for instance reducing disability rates differentially across age groups, or postponing the onset of disability by five years in all age groups.

DATA COLLECTION ISSUES

It was argued in the previous section that the selection and definition of disability items is consequential for policy decisions and comparability across surveys. This section makes the same argument for the way the data are collected. The questionnaire to OECD countries performed by the NCBS in 1990 paid attention not only to what items were available, but also to the survey design. The conclusion was that if the survey data for one specific indicator were available, the methods of data collection still differed widely with respect to frequency, sample definition, mode of data collection (in-person or telephone interview, or mailed questionnaire), use of proxies, and non-response (Evers, 1991). Several validity issues related to the data collection method are discussed below in more detail.

First, the *sampling frame* of national surveys often includes only community dwelling persons, because it is based on households. To obtain estimates of disability that also include the institutionalized population, data from other sources need to be combined with data from the community sample. For this exercise, assumptions need to be made on comparability of measures (if disability measures for the institutionalized are available), or on the proportion of the institutionalized population that is actually disabled (if disability measures for the institutionalized population are not available) (Van Ginneken *et al*, 1991). Exclusion of the institutionalized population is especially problematic when the older population is the focus of research. Moreover, cross-national comparability is hampered because the role of institutions in national health care systems differs substantially (Jamieson, 1989). On the other hand, inclusion of the institutionalized population creates the problem of sensitivity of the disability scale used. For community living subjects, the scale needs to have sufficient variation at the positive end (mild disability). Including IADL items helps accomplish this. By contrast, for subjects in institutions, the scale needs to have variation at the negative end (severe disability). Here, ADL items are the measure of choice (Barberger-Gateau, 1990). Moreover, IADL measures may be irrelevant when residents no longer perform these tasks.

Second, the use of *proxy respondents* influences prevalence estimates of disability. A proxy respondent may be used when the sample member is not at home, but more often a proxy is interviewed when the sample member is too frail to respond to a questionnaire. Because proxies tend to be family members who care for the sample member, they may exaggerate their role by overestimating the disability of the subject. Vice versa, the subjects may underestimate their disability, especially when questions are phrased in terms of 'can you do an activity' and the subject does not perform the activity any more (Barberger-Gateau, 1990; Kelly-Hayes *et al*, 1992).

Third, disability may be more or less *central* to a survey. If it is less central, or if time constraints are very strict, the number of disability questions may be reduced. Reduction of the number of items implies selection. However, responses to particular items may differ across cultures, implying that cross-cultural comparability may be aided by inclusion of a wide range of activities, in order to compensate for excessive influence of single items. It is important to note that the number of items included affects the prevalence estimates, in particular in the common approach to construct a scale based on the count of the number of activities for which difficulty (or need of assistance) is reported (Wiener *et al*, 1990). The more activities are included, the greater the chance for a particular subject to report difficulty with one activity, and thus the greater the prevalence estimate.

A further issue is whether a scale constructed from any number of items measures one single construct (*unidimensionality*). The inclusion of activities that are sensitive in the community dwelling population as well as activities that show sufficient variation in the institutionalized population increases the heterogeneity of the items that constitute a scale, and may be in conflict with the goal to achieve a unidimensional scale. A debate is still continuing as to whether ADL and IADL items form a hierarchical (and thus unidimensional) scale, or if multiple, non-hierarchical dimensions of disability should be distinguished (Barberger-Gateau *et al*, 2000; Kempen *et al*, 1995; Ferrucci *et al*, 1998; Spector and Fleishman, 1998; Thomas *et al*, 1998). In the case of hierarchy, a scale is more likely to measure one concept than if there is no hierarchy. The hierarchy issue is especially pertinent if a scale is dichotomized, for example to calculate disability-free life expectancy (Barberger-Gateau, 1990).

CRITERIA FOR HARMONIZATION OF DISABILITY MEASURES

Despite the numerous measurement issues involved, the first step toward harmonization of disability measurement is the choice of one disability indicator. An indicator that is most feasible for inclusion in national surveys should be as brief as the global measure of self-rated health. In other words, it should measure disability with parsimony (Verbrugge *et al*, 1995). The indicator should serve the three purposes of description, explanation and screening. Verbrugge (1994b) described the following 10 desirable characteristics of a global disability indicator.

1. Content: it should cover social dysfunctions that are protracted and health-related.
2. Demographic scope: it should be relevant for all ages, both genders, and diverse race/ethnic groups.
3. Words: it should make sense to respondents on first hearing.
4. Dimensions: among the various dimensions (difficulty, inability, performance or non-performance, use of personal or equipment assistance, need for assistance, satisfaction with performance) it should select those that suit the survey's scientific or public health purposes.
5. Response range: it should cover the full range of best to worst functioning with several gradations between.
6. Response metric: the response categories should distinguish people by severity of disability.
7. Qualifiers: the question should be brief and not cluttered with qualifiers.
8. Comparisons: the question should also be free of comparisons, such as with age peers.
9. Number of items: the fewer the better.
10. Measurement qualities: it should be valid and show short-term reliability.

As data from longitudinal studies became increasingly available during the 1990s, the importance of sensitivity of disability measures to changes over time was recognized (Barberger-Gateau, 1990). Thus, sensitivity to change should be considered an eleventh desirable characteristic. Verbrugge (1994b) provided an inventory of candidate global disability indicators based on North American surveys, listed the methodological issues related to the 10 desirable characteristics that have not yet been solved, and described the cognitive and methodological research that needs to be done to address these issues.

One approach to address these issues is to select from existing surveys those that include a global disability indicator along with a range of detailed disability items. Alternatively, one can construct a global indicator from detailed items, or one can reduce the number of detailed items with minimal loss to analytic value. Then, one can examine the performance of the global indicator in terms of: (1) its relation with the detailed items, to determine its included and excluded content; (2) its relation with global morbidity, to examine its non-redundancy; (3) its relation with chronic conditions to assess its health-relatedness; and (4) its unique predictive ability for subsequent outcomes. Verbrugge and colleagues (1995) used data from three different surveys to address these questions. They concluded that a global disability indicator had a greater association with chronic diseases than detailed items; that it was distinct from global morbidity as measured by the self-rated health item; and that it covered longer-term disability from essential activities (such as paid work and housework). Verbrugge *et al*'s recommendation for population surveys is to include four or five items covering all domains of disability, i.e. functional limitations, ADL and IADL disability, with response categories measuring one dimension, preferably difficulty doing the activities.

Building upon this work, in 1996 a selection of candidate global disability items was sent out to REVES members and other professionals with an interest in disability indicators. Their opinions about content and question structure were queried. Their replies were presented at the ninth REVES meeting (Verbrugge *et al*, 1996). This has now been developed further as part of a European project 'Setting up a coherent set of health indicators for the European Union'. The global disability question is now called the Global Limitations Indicator (GALI) and is one of three global health questions (the others being self-perceived health and chronic morbidity) contained in the Minimum European Health Module. This module is being recommended for inclusion in all future European health surveys and has to date been included in the French and Belgian surveys.

CONCLUSIONS

The feasibility of international comparisons of disability-free life expectancies will depend crucially on the way disability is measured. This chapter described the measurement of disability from the point of view of using disability measures in the calculation of active life expectancy. Because the monitoring of active life expectancy is a tool in developing public health policy of nations, much attention was paid to international comparability. Amongst others, it was recommended that population surveys should include a valid and reliable disability indicator that covers the whole range of severity observed in the general population. It was pointed out that disability indicators should measure dysfunction itself, and not interventions aimed at reducing dysfunctions, such as assistance. Furthermore, in addition to disability, population surveys should include a set of socio-demographic characteristics to address disability in pertinent subgroups of the population. The conceptual models developed in the early 1990s may serve as a framework for judging the comparability of various national disability measures. Measurement issues related to data collection were reviewed, and criteria for the selection of a global disability indicator were described. In summary, this review of the work of REVES members of 12 years hopefully informs and stimulates the ongoing efforts to reach harmonization of disability measurement.

REFERENCES

Albrecht, G.L. and Verbrugge, L.M. (2000) 'The global emergence of disability', in Albrecht, G.L., Fitzpatrick, R. and Scrimshaw, S.C. (eds) *The Handbook of Social Studies in Health and Medicine*. London/Thousand Oaks/New Delhi: Sage.

Allen, S.M., Mor, V., Raveis, V. and Houts, P. (1993) 'Measurement of need of assistance with daily activities: Quantifying the influence of gender roles', *Journal of Gerontology: Social Sciences* 48, S204–211.

Barberger-Gateau, P. (1990) 'Conceptual and operational definitions of the disability process in population studies: Epidemiologic and geriatric consideration [In French]'. Presented at REVES 2nd meeting, Geneva.

Barberger-Gateau, P., Rainville, C., Letenneur, L. and Dartigues, J.F. (2000) 'A hierarchical model of domains of disablement in the elderly: A longitudinal approach', *Disability and Rehabilitation* 22(7), 308–317.

Bolduc, M. (1993) 'For a conceptual model that better reflects the environment', in Robine, J-M., Mathers, C.D., Bone, M.R. and Romieu, I. (eds) *Calculation of Health Expectancies; Harmonization, Consensus Achieved and Future Perspectives* (*Calcul des espérances de vie en santé: harmonisation, acquis et perspectives*). Paris: John Libbey Eurotext.

Bone, M., Bebbington, A.C. and Nicolaas, G. (1994) 'Policy relevance and comparability problems of health expectancy indicators', in Mathers, C.D., McCallum, J. and Robine, J-M. (eds) *Advances in Health Expectancies*. Canberra: Australian Institute of Health and Welfare, AGPS, pp. 309–324.

Carrière, Y. and Légaré, J. (2000) 'Unmet needs for assistance with ADLs and IADLs: A measure of healthy life expectancy', *Social Indicators Research* 51/1, 107–123. Presented at REVES 8th meeting, Chicago, October 1995. REVES paper 207.

Colvez, A. (1992) 'Classification of observed disability for a number of survival roles at three levels: Expectancy of life free from severe, moderate or slight disability', in Robine, J-M., Blanchet, M. and Dowd, J.E. (eds) *Health Expectancy*. London: HMSO.

Copeland, J.R.M., Kelleher, M.J., Kellett, J.M., Gourlay, A.J., Gurland, B.J., Fleiss, J.L. and Sharpe, L. (1976) 'A semistructured clinical interview for the assessment of diagnosis and mental state in the elderly: The Geriatric Mental State Schedule. I. Development and reliability', *Psychological Medicine* 6, 439–449.

Deeg, D.J.H. (1993) 'Sex differences in IADL in the Netherlands: Functional and situational disability', in Robine, J-M., Mathers, C.D., Bone, M.R. and Romieu, I. (eds) *Calculation of Health Expectancies; Harmonization, Consensus Achieved and Future Perspectives* (*Calcul des espérances de vie en santé: harmonisation, acquis et perspectives*). Paris: John Libbey Eurotext.

Deeg, D.J.H. (1999) 'Self-rated health: Does it measure health as well as we think it does?', Presented at REVES 11th meeting, London. REVES paper 322.

Evers, S. (1991) 'Health For All indicators in health interview surveys: The measurement of disability related indicators', Presented at REVES 4th meeting, Noordwijkerhout (Leiden) REVES paper 73.

Ferrucci, L., Guralnik, J.M., Cecchi, F., Marchionni, N., Salani, B., Kasper, J., Celli, R., Giardini, S., Heikkinen, E., Jylhä, M. and Baroni, A. (1998) 'Constant hierarchic patterns of physical functioning across seven populations in five countries', *The Gerontologist* 38, 286–294.

Flores, J.L., Minaire, P., Cherpin, J. and Weber, D. (1992) 'Measuring disability and environmental characteristics: Influence on calculating disability-free life expectancy', in Robine, J-M., Blanchet, M. and Dowd, J.E. (eds) *Health Expectancy*. London: HMSO.

Folstein, M.F., Folstein, S.E. and McHugh, P.R. (1975) 'Mini-Mental State. A practical method for grading the cognitive state of patients for the clinician', *Journal of Psychiatric Research* 12, 189–198.

Fougeyrollas, P., Noreau, L., Bergeron, H., Cloutier, R., Dion, S.A. and St-Michel, G. (1998) 'Social consequences of long term impairments and disabilities: Conceptual approach and assessment of handicap', International Journal of Rehabilitation Research 21, 127–141.

Glass, T.A. (1998) 'Conjugating the "tenses" of function: Discordance among hypothetical, experimental, and enacted function in older adults', *The Gerontologist* 38, 101–112.

Goldberg, D. (1972) *The Detection of General Illness by Questionnaire*. Maudsley: OUP. Monograph no. 21.

Golini, A. and Calvani, P. (2001) 'Relationship between perceptions of health, chronic diseases and disabilities'. Tokyo: Nihon University Population Research Institute. NUPRI Research Paper Series No. 73. Presented at REVES 10th meeting, Tokyo.

Guralnik, J.M., Branch, L.G., Cummings, S.R. and Curb, J.D. (1989) 'Physical performance measures in aging research', *Journal of Gerontology: Medical Sciences* 44, M141–146.

Guralnik, J.M., Simonsick, E.M., Ferrucci, L., Glynn, R.J., Berkman, L.F., Blazer, D.G., Scherr, P.A. and Wallace, R.B. (1994) 'A short physical performance battery assessing lower extremity function: Association with self-reported disability and prediction of mortality and nursing home admission', *Journal of Gerontology: Medical Sciences* 49, M85–94.

Jagger, C. (1996) 'Improving measures of health status – a range of measures for a range of questions', Presented at REVES 9th meeting, Rome.

Jagger, C. and Clarke, M. (1991) 'The changing disability profile of the elderly', Presented at REVES 4th meeting, Noordwijkerhout (Leiden). REVES paper no. 57.

Jamieson, A. (1989) 'A new age for older people? Policy shifts in health and social care', *Social Science and Medicine* 29, 445–454.

Katz, S., Ford, A.B., Moskowitz, R.W., Jackson, B.A. and Jaffe, M.W. (1963) 'Studies of illness in the aged: the index of ADL: A standardized measure of biological and psychosocial function', *Journal of the American Medical Association* 185, 914–919.

Katzman, R., Brown, T., Fuld, P., Peck, A., Schechter, R. and Schimmel, H. (1983) 'Validation of a short orientation-memory-concentration test of cognitive impairment', *American Journal of Psychiatry* 140, 734–739.

Kelly-Hayes, M., Jette, A.M., Wolf, P.A., D'Agostino, R.B. and Odell, P.M. (1992) 'Functional limitations and disability among elders in the Framingham Study', *American Journal of Public Health* 82, 841–845.

Kempen, G.I.J.M., Myers, A.M. and Powell, L.E. (1995) 'Hierarchical structure in ADL and IADL: Analytical assumptions and applications for clinicians and researchers', *Journal of Clinical Epidemiology* 48, 1299–1305.

Koyano, W., Shibata, H., Nakazato, K., Haga, H. and Suyama, Y. (1991) 'Measurement of competence: reliability and validity of the TMIG Index of Competence', *Archives of Gerontology and Geriatrics* 13, 103–116.

Kuriansky, J.B. and Gurland, B.J. (1976) 'The performance test of activities of daily living', *International Journal of Aging and Human Development* 7, 343–352.

Laditka, S.B. and Jenkins, C.L. (2001) 'Difficulty or dependency? Effects of measurement scales on disability prevalence among older Americans', *Journal of*

Health and Social Policy 13/3: 1–15. Presented at REVES 12th meeting, Los Angeles, March 2000.

Lawton, M.P. and Brody, E.M. (1969) 'Assessment of older people: Self-maintaining and instrumental activities of daily living', *Gerontologist* 9, 179–186.

McWhinnie, J.R. (1981) 'Disability assessment in population surveys: Results of the OECD common development effort', *Revue Epidémiologie et Santé Publique* 29, 413–419.

Minaire, P. (1992) 'Disease, illness and health: Theoretical models of the disablement process', *Bulletin of the World Health Organization* 70/3: 373–379. Presented at REVES 2nd meeting, Geneva, 1990; REVES 3rd meeting, Durham, 1990; REVES 4th meeting, Noordwijkerhout (Leiden), 1991.

Nagi, S.Z. (1976) 'An epidemiology of disability among adults in the United States', *Milbank Memorial Fund Quarterly* 54, 439–468.

Pfeiffer, E. (1975) 'A short portable mental status questionnaire for the assessment of organic brain deficit in elderly patients', *Journal of the American Geriatric Society* 23, 433–441.

Radloff, L.S. (1977) 'The CES-D scale: a new self-report depression scale for research in the general population', *Applied Psychological Measurement* 1, 385–401.

Robine, J-M., Ravaud, J.F. and Cambois, E. (1997) 'General concepts of disablement', in Hamerman, D. (ed.) *Osteoarthritis. Public Health Implications for an Aging Population*. Baltimore/London: The Johns Hopkins University Press.

Robine, J-M., Romieu, I. and Cambois, E. (1999) 'Health expectancy indicators', *Bulletin of the World Health Organization* 77(2), 181–185. Presented at REVES 8th meeting, Chicago, October 1995.

Roelands, M. and Van Oyen, H. (1994) 'Mental and social variables as operationalisation of health in the calculation of health expectancy', in Mathers, C.D., McCallum, J. and Robine, J-M. (eds) *Advances in Health Expectancies*. Canberra: Australian Institute of Health and Welfare, AGPS. Presented at REVES 7th meeting, Canberra, February 1994.

Romieu, I. and Robine, J-M. (1994) 'World atlas on health expectancy calculations', in Mathers, C.D., McCallum, J. and Robine, J-M. (eds) *Advances in Health Expectancies*. Canberra: Australian Institute of Health and Welfare, AGPS. Presented at REVES 7th meeting, Canberra, February 1994.

Sauvaget, C., Tsuji, T., Aonuma, T. and Hisamichi, S. (1999) 'Health-life expectancy according to various functional levels', *Journal of the American Geriatrics Society* 47(11), 1326–1331. Presented at REVES 10th meeting, Tokyo, October 1997.

Spector, W.D. and Fleishman, J.A. (1998) 'Combining activities of daily living with instrumental activities of daily living to measure functional disability', *Journal of Gerontology: Social Sciences* 53B, S46–S57.

Stewart, A., Hays, R. and Ware, J. (1988) 'The Medical Outcome Study short form general health survey', *Medical Care* 26, 724–733.

Thomas, V.S., Rockwood, K. and McDowell, I. (1998) 'Multidimensionality of instrumental and basic activities of daily living', *Journal of Clinical Epidemiology* 51, 315–321.

Thuriaux, M.C. (1989) 'Life expectancy free from disability (LEFD) and the international classification of impairments, disabilities and handicaps (ICIDH): Two working tools for the WHO', Presented at REVES 1st meeting, Quebec. REVES paper 25.

Thuriaux, M.C. (1991) 'Possible health policy uses of healthy life expectancy', REVES 4th meeting, Noordwijkerhout (Leiden). REVES paper 77.

Thuriaux, M.C. (1993) 'The international classification of impairments, disabilities, and handicaps (ICIDH): Current status and development', in Robine, J-M., Mathers,

C.D., Bone, M.R. and Romieu, I. (eds) *Calculation of Health Expectancies; Harmonization, Consensus Achieved and Future Perspectives* (*Calcul des espérances de vie en santé: harmonisation, acquis et perspectives*), Paris: John Libbey Eurotext. [*Also published as:* Thuriaux MC (1995) The ICIDH – Evolution, status and prospects. *Disability and Rehabilitation* 17(3–4), 112–118.]

Van Ginneken, J.K.S., Dissevelt, A.G., Van de Water, H.P.A. and Van Sonsbeek, J.L.A. (1991) 'Results of two methods to determine health expectancy in the Netherlands 1981–1985' *Social Science and Medicine* 32, 1129–1136. Presented at REVES 1st meeting, Quebec.

Verbrugge, L.M. (1994a) 'The experience and measure of disability', in Mathers, C.D., McCallum, J. and Robine, J-M. (eds) *Advances in Health Expectancies*. Canberra: Australian Institute of Health and Welfare, AGPS. Presented at Reves 7th meeting, Canberra, February 1994.

Verbrugge, L.M. (1994b) 'A global disability indicator: Companion to self-rated health', in Schechter, S. (ed.) *Proceedings of the 1993 NCHS Conference on the Cognitive Aspects of Self-reported Health Status*. Hyattsville, MD: Office of Research and Methodology, National Center for Health Statistics. (Cognitive methods staff, Working Paper Series no. 10.) [*Also published as:* Verbrugge, L.M. (1997) 'A global disability indicator', *Journal of Aging Studies* 11(4), 337–362.]

Verbrugge, L.M. and Jette, A. (1994) 'The disablement process', *Social Science and Medicine* 38, 1–14.

Verbrugge, L.M., Merrill, S.S. and Liu, X. (1995) 'Measuring disability with parsimony', in *Proceedings of the 1995 Public Health Conference on Records and Statistics*, Hyattsville, MD: National Center for Health Statistics. [*Also published as:* Verbrugge, L.M., Merrill, S.S. and Liu, X. (1999) 'Measuring disability with parsimony', *Disability and Rehabilitation* 21(5–6), 295–306.] Presented at REVES 8th meeting, Chicago, October 1995.

Verbrugge, L.M., Van den Bos, T. and Van der Water, H. (1996) 'A REVES enterprise: Developing a global disability indicator', Presented at REVES 9th meeting, Rome. REVES paper 280.

Wechsler, D. (1945) 'Standardized memory scale for clinical use', *Journal of Psychology* 19, 87–95.

Wechsler, D. (1955) *WAIS Manual: Wechsler Adult Intelligence Scale*. New York: Psychological Corporation.

Wiener, J.M., Hanley, R.J., Clark; R. and Van Nostrand, J.F. (1990) 'Measuring the activities of daily living: Comparisons across national surveys', *Journal of Gerontology: Social Sciences* 45, S229–237.

Wiersma, D., De Jong, A. and Ormel, J. (1988) 'The Groningen Social Disabilities Schedule: Development, relationship with ICIDH, and psychometric properties', *International Journal of Rehabilitation Research* 11, 213–224.

World Health Organization (1980) *International Classification of Impairments, Disabilities and Handicaps*. Geneva: World Health Organization.

World Health Organization (1981) *Development of Indicators for Monitoring Progress towards Health for All by the Year 2000*. Geneva: WHO. Health for All Series, No. 4.

World Health Organization (2001) *International Classification of Functioning, Disability and Health*. Geneva: World Health Organization.

Yesavage, J.A., Brink, T.L., Rose, T.L., Lum, O., Hunag, V., Adey, M. and Leirer, V.O. (1983) 'Development and validation of a geriatric depression screening scale: A preliminary report', *Journal of Psychiatric Research* 17, 37–49.

Zigmond, A.S. and Snaith, R.P. (1983) 'The Hospital Anxiety and Depression Scale', *Acta Psychiatrica Scandinavica* 67, 361–370.

11

The Evolution of Demographic Methods to Calculate Health Expectancies

SARAH B. LADITKA and MARK D. HAYWARD*

State University of New York Institute of Technology, NY, USA and
*Pennsylvania State University, University Park, PA, USA

In this chapter, we discuss methods used to calculate estimates of total life expectancy, healthy (e.g. no functional problems or disability) life expectancy, and unhealthy life expectancy. To frame this discussion, we distinguish between models or rates used to estimate the parameters of life expectancy processes, such as the probability of becoming impaired or the probability of recovery, and methods that use the parameters (estimates) produced by these models to calculate summary indices of total, healthy, and unhealthy life. Approaches estimating the parameters of healthy life are those based on either prevalence or incidence rates. Methods that have been used to compute summary indices of healthy life include prevalence-based life tables, multistate life tables, and microsimulation. In the next section, we provide an overview of the underlying model structure of healthy life expectancy processes, and describe how the models and life table calculation methods are related. In the two sections that follow, we examine the development of these models and methods using an evolutionary framework, reviewing each in the order in which it was introduced to the research community.

MODEL STRUCTURE AND A COMPARISON OF COMPUTATIONAL APPROACHES

To date, almost all healthy life expectancy research has implicitly assumed that age-related changes in health are governed by a Markov process. Under the

Determining Health Expectancies. Edited by J-M. Robine, C. Jagger, C.D. Mathers, E.M. Crimmins and R.M. Suzman.
© 2003 John Wiley & Sons, Ltd

Markov assumption, an unhealthy male or female at any age has at least some probability of returning to the healthy state. The probability of recovery is independent of either the duration of the current episode of poor health or the occurrence of prior episodes of poor health. Useful descriptions and representations of Markov chains and processes are provided in Cinlar (1975).

Although the Markov model is common to healthy life expectancy models, the parameters of the health process have relied on two different rates, i.e., prevalence and incidence rates, which measure two different phenomena (Crimmins *et al*, 1993). Parameters based on prevalence rates capture information about the current population structure; parameters based on incidence rates contain information about the life cycle implications of current health and mortality conditions. When the observed prevalence of poor health is used it is not possible to infer specific changes in mortality and morbidity transitions. In contrast, using incidence rates permits researchers to compute the life table prevalence of health status, which is implied by the current level of health and mortality transitions. The most recent innovation in incidence-rate-based parameter estimation is to recover the parameters of the embedded Markov process, which we call estimating embedded Markov parameters.

Prevalence life tables, exemplified by the Sullivan (1971) method, and multistate life tables typically provide only measures of central tendency (expected values). We refer to these two methods as macrosimulation. The macrosimulation methods treat the calculation of healthy life as deterministic, ignoring the random nature of vital events. A recent innovation in calculating healthy life expectancy is microsimulation. This method permits the distribution of life sequences to be generated for each person in a starting population (i.e., individual-level biographies), and these sequences underlie the calculation of expected values. Macrosimulation and microsimulation also differ in how the random nature of the process (variance) is handled. Variance estimates permit researchers to identify statistical differences in the life course experiences of population subgroups. Jagger (1999) describes how to calculate variance estimates of state life expectancies for prevalence-based life tables. Measures of variance have been theoretically developed using multistate methods (Rendall, 1991), but have only recently been calculated (Lee and Rendall, 1998). In contrast, microsimulation explicitly models the random nature of the process and permits two important sources of stochasticity to be readily calculated: the variability in state life expectancies as well as the sampling error attributable to the model's parameters (Wolf and Laditka, 1997).

Microsimulation generally allows researchers to incorporate covariate information more easily than macrosimulation approaches. Traditional life table models have used stratification as the primary means to evaluate population subgroup differences in life course experiences. Recently, multi-variate multistate life table models have been used as a way of modeling variability based on observed covariates in complex life cycle processes such as health and retirement (e.g. Crimmins *et al*, 1996; Hayward and Grady, 1990; Land *et al*, 1994). Microsimulation complements and extends multivariate multistate life table methods by allowing for a fuller and more flexibly defined combination of outcome-state and covariate history. In summary, indicators of healthy life produced by microsimulation methods are explicitly informed by individual-level analyses of events and relationships, and thus bridge demographic models of population processes and individual-level analyses of behaviour.

METHODS USED TO COMPUTE SUMMARY INDICES OF HEALTHY LIFE

PREVALENCE-BASED LIFE TABLE

The prevalence-based life table method represents the earliest technique to calculate healthy life expectancy. Developed originally in the 1930s to examine how long individuals could be expected to work in their lifetimes, the approach has been applied for almost three decades to calculate healthy life expectancy. The underlying stochastic process governing moves between health states is relatively uncomplicated. In this model, life is assumed to follow an evolutionary process from good health to poor health to death. Transitions out of good health, the origin health state, are assumed to occur because of the onset of health problems or death. Once an individual becomes unhealthy, the model assumes that no recovery is possible. Typically, because of data limitations rather than anything inherent in the approach, mortality rates are assumed to be the same for all individuals, regardless of health status. These basic assumptions hinder the modeling of a realistic profile of functioning changes over the life cycle to the extent that recovery from poor health occurs.

The Sullivan method offers many advantages. It is straightforward to apply. REVES meetings have featured workshops and a manual on calculating the Sullivan method (Jagger, 1999). Data from cross-sectional studies, which are less costly and more readily available than panel surveys, can be used to estimate the model. Many countries have cross-sectional surveys in place, which provide regular estimates of population health. Moreover, the sample sizes of these health surveys produce highly reliable estimates of age-specific prevalence rates. Further, prevalence-based methods are less influenced by survey design and analytic strategies than methods relying on longitudinal data (Saito *et al*, 1992).

Although the Sullivan method will continue to be a popular method of calculating healthy life indices, it has several drawbacks. The method's assumptions constrain the portrayal of the expected life cycle or functional status histories of persons who are exposed to current mortality and morbidity conditions. Further, once individuals have experienced a health problem, it does not permit recovery. Under conditions in which individuals experience both the onset of health problems and recovery, the Sullivan method will yield an inaccurate portrayal of the timing and volume of a cohort's health experiences. The Sullivan method also can produce what appears to be a counter-intuitive relationship between changes in prevalence rates of health status and healthy life expectancy. During periods of rapidly declining mortality, calculations of healthy life based on the Sullivan method remain fairly stable relative to the growth in overall life expectancy (e.g. Bebbington, 1991; Crimmins *et al*, 1997). This is because the health composition of the population, represented by prevalence rates, is not strongly affected by mortality changes (e.g. Crimmins *et al*, 1993; Preston, 1982). Crimmins *et al* (1994) carried out a series of simulation exercises using a multistate life table model, demonstrating that falling mortality rates and falling morbidity rates increase the years of healthy life. Falling mortality unaccompanied by falling morbidity, however, led to an increase in the expected years of poor health. The results of Sullivan-based models thus are consistent with a method that takes account directly of the underlying dynamics of health.

A large number of studies presented in the REVES network have employed the Sullivan method to calculate estimates of healthy life expectancy (e.g. Bebbington, 1988, 1991; Mathers, 1991; Wilkins and Adams, 1983, 1989). Using the Sullivan method, Robine *et al* (1997) calculated disability-free life expectancy for over 30 countries. This method was also used to examine trends in disability-free life expectancy in France in the period 1981 to 1991 (Robine *et al*, 1998), with the conclusion of an increase in the proportion of life lived free from significant disability – conclusions similar to those of Crimmins *et al* (1997), who used data from the United States. Also using the Sullivan method, Hayward and Heron (1999) found substantial differences in total and healthy life expectancy across racial groups in the United States.

Bebbington (1992) used a modification of the Sullivan method and data from Great Britain to calculate quality-adjusted life years based on several levels of disability. Bebbington relaxed the commonly made assumption of equal mortality rates across the health states, and concluded that Sullivan's method gives a lower estimate of disability than the double-decrement life table model, a finding consistent with that of Rogers *et al* (1990), who compared the results of various methods of calculating healthy life expectancy using data from the United States. Canada-Vicinay (1996), using the Sullivan method and data from Spain and France, examined the effects of acute and chronic disease on morbidity, and developed estimates of healthy-state life expectancy and 'disease-ridden' life expectancy, concluding that observed disease prevalence generally declines from age 70 for both males and females. The prevalence decline patterns for specific diseases, however, differed substantially by gender.

MULTISTATE LIFE TABLE

The development of multistate life table methods in the 1970s (Rogers, 1975; Schoen, 1975; Schoen and Woodrow, 1980) provided demographers with a means to model the dynamics of health change in the population in a more realistic fashion than the Sullivan approach. A key component of the multistate life table is its relaxation of the assumption of unidirectional health changes over the life course. This method allows individuals, as they age, to experience onset of and recovery from health problems. Further, people need not traverse between 'adjacent' health states, and can experience multiple and recurrent health problems over their lives. Individuals' health experiences are assumed to be governed by incidence rates (or life table transfer rates). Theoretically, the age-specific rates refer to movements in a time period, not persons moving, and the number of movements a person can make in any time period is not restricted (Schoen, 1988).

The multistate life table method provides estimates of years an average individual of a particular age can expect to spend in good and poor health. The method can also provide estimates of the expected number of transitions over one's lifetime or within a specified period of time. Thus, researchers can gain some sense of the health trajectories experienced by persons in the population. Moreover, given a set of disability and mortality incidence rates, one is able to determine the age structure of health for a stationary population; i.e., for a stationary population, the levels of disability arising from the interaction of disability and mortality processes over the life course.

The major strength of the multistate life table method is its ability to capture the implications of age-related declines and improvements in health. This provides a more accurate assessment of the expected life cycle health experiences for an average person in the population. Moreover, this method allows the explicit assessment of how disability and mortality processes contribute to the structure of population health, or the changing prevalence of health problems associated with age (e.g. Crimmins *et al*, 1994). These strengths have prompted some scholars to urge the adoption of the multistate life table method as the methodological 'standard' means of calculating healthy life expectancy. We urge caution for a number of theoretical and methodological reasons.

Methodological Issues

The multistate method is totally dependent on the availability of longitudinal data. These data are required to calculate incidence rates – the input to the multistate life table. Most countries, however, do not have registries providing population estimates of incidence rates. This has fostered the use of large, nationally representative surveys to calculate incidence rates; but the availability of surveys of this type is highly circumscribed in terms of historical coverage. Further, these surveys are concentrated in a handful of countries (primarily the United States, France, and recently Canada). In addition, the design of longitudinal surveys and measurement of health are generally not explicitly motivated by a conceptual model of the underlying stochastic processes of morbidity onset and recovery (Crimmins and Hayward, 1997). For example, interviews are often separated by one or two years and sometimes as much as four to five years (e.g. the National Long Term Care Survey in the United States). When panel data are the basis of calculating incidence rates, individuals' health changes are usually inferred by comparing health status measured at the time of each interview. The lack of direct observation of health changes leads to the common assumption that individuals experience only one transition within a given time period, for example, a one-year or two-year interval (e.g. Crimmins *et al*, 1994). To the extent that individuals experience multiple health events within an interval, the multistate method underestimates the expected number of lifetime transitions.

The sample sizes of longitudinal surveys also are rarely large enough, given the rarity of health events, to calculate reliable age-specific occurrence/exposure rates. This has fostered the use of statistical models to estimate health status transitions, which we think is a positive development (e.g. Hayward and Grady, 1990; Crimmins *et al*, 1994, 1996; Land *et al*, 1994; Laditka and Wolf, 1998). However, the absence of vital registries hampers the assessment of the accuracy of sample-based estimates. This points to the importance of calculating indices of healthy life for multiple surveys. As yet, the multiplicity of health status definitions and survey designs has constrained these types of comparisons. In addition, the multistate calculation of healthy life indices has been hampered by the absence of standardized and widely available software. The development of multistate life table software would aid considerably in establishing this method as part of the demographer's tool kit.

Theoretical Issues

Although longitudinal data are used to define incidence rates reflecting the underlying stochastic processes, these data generally reference health changes for relatively short time periods for a synthetic cohort. Longitudinal data for an actual birth cohort are not available at this time. Dramatic cohort changes have occurred in old age mortality, resulting in unknown selectivity in cross-sectional estimates of incidence rates. In addition, cohort differences in socioeconomic achievement are also reflected in our cross-sectional estimates of incidence rates. Thus, the assumption of unchanging rates over time is a difficult one.

These methodological and theoretical considerations notwithstanding, the multistate life table method has been widely used for the calculation of healthy life expectancy for the United States (Crimmins *et al*, 1994, 1996; Hayward *et al*, 1998; Land *et al*, 1994; R.G. Rogers *et al*, 1989; A. Rogers *et al*, 1990). Crimmins *et al* (1994) have also used the multistate method to simulate the implications of changes in morbidity and mortality processes for healthy life expectancy and the age structure of morbidity prevalence in the population. Hayward *et al* (1998) used multistate life table methods to calculate healthy life. In this research, mortality was defined in terms of specific causes of death. This allowed the assessment of relative causes of death associated with healthy life expectancy and the implications of declines in specific fatal diseases for healthy life expectancy. (For a different approach to the problem of the effects of disease elimination, see Manton and Stallard, 1990.)

Indices of healthy life have also been calculated for major American subgroups using multistate life table methods. The results show: females live longer lives and spend more of their lives disabled than males (Crimmins *et al*, 1996; Hayward *et al*, 1998; Land *et al*, 1994); whites live longer than blacks and have a more compressed period of disability (Crimmins *et al*, 1996); and more educated persons live longer than less educated persons, and spend fewer years with a disability (Crimmins *et al*, 1996; Land *et al*, 1994). Indices of healthy life produced by multistate life tables are less common for other countries. This is due to the relative paucity of longitudinal data. Multistate life tables are available for Japan (Liu *et al*, 1995) and France (Brouard and Robine, 1992), although, to our knowledge, no research has examined population heterogeneity in healthy life within a population other than that of the United States. Taking account of population heterogeneity in healthy life estimates is important when making international comparisons because population compositional differences can lead to disparate estimates. Moreover, cross-national comparisons are important to validate the influence of sex and socioeconomic conditions on healthy life.

MICROSIMULATION OF HEALTHY LIFE

The most recent innovation to calculate summary indices of healthy life is microsimulation, which is a sampling approach (Laditka and Wolf, 1998). The basic approach can be thought of as a random experiment for each person in a population. In a survey, the population can refer to replicates of each individual in the survey. Laditka and Wolf (1998) took a slightly different approach by defining the population as a standard population (i.e., life table cohorts of males and females of 100 000). Each person in the population is subjected to a given probability of an event (e.g. the probability of the onset of disability). Among those persons who experience the onset of disability, another set of random experiments is conducted to determine whether the individuals experience the cessation of disability or some other possible event in the state space, such as recovery. The end result of these experiments is that each individual in the population has a simulated healthy life biography, thereby approximating the distribution of lifetime outcomes for a given set of starting conditions. The simulated process is inherently random in that the model produces both expected (mean) values and estimates of variation around the expected value arising both from the real distribution of health events in the population, and from sampling variability that impacts the precision of the transition rate estimates.

Wolf and Laditka (1997) examined sources of variability within healthy life. Variation around expected values was benchmarked in terms of the standard deviations for state life expectancies as well as the frequency distribution of remaining years of life in each health state. Variability in years of healthy life was found to be quantitatively significant. In addition, the frequency distributions of healthy and unhealthy life showed that the distributions were quite skewed, especially for the unhealthy states. Investigation of the variability in the model's parameters showed the uncertainty related to sampling error was quite small.

DATA/MODELS USED TO ESTIMATE HEALTH EXPECTANCY PARAMETERS

PREVALENCE RATES

In terms of data, the Sullivan method typically combines current mortality incidence rates with the age-specific proportions of the population that are in the health states. The prevalence estimates of health status are often derived from large cross-sectional surveys or population censuses and thus provide a measure of the health status of an observed population. The health composition of the observed population is then used to divide the life table population into subpopulations, e.g. a healthy population and an unhealthy population.

The basic input to this method, the observed prevalence of health, is determined by the population's history of health and mortality. Mortality incidence rates, although dynamic in a definitional sense, typically refer to the current mortality experiences of a cross-section of the population, whose survival also is determined by a lifetime history of health and mortality. Placed in the prevalence-based life table model, mortality rates define the survival experience of a synthetic population, i.e., a population in which the rates of 'today' are assumed to span the lifetime of individuals alive at this point. The

Sullivan method thus reflects the current health composition of a real population adjusted by the mortality of a synthetic population.

INCIDENCE RATES

Actuarial Rates

The inputs into the multistate life table model are incidence rates denoting the movements between states (e.g. from healthy to unhealthy life). Ideally, age-specific life table transfer rates are used as the inputs. Transfer rates, say from state i to state j, $d_{ij}(x,n)$, are the number of moves from state i to j between the ages of x and $x+n$ divided by the person-years lived in state i between the ages of x and $x+n$, L_i. The rates refer to actual moves, not persons moving, within an age interval.

Typically, incidence rates of morbidity change are calculated using data from large nationally representative surveys of older persons. In the United States, for example, researchers have frequently used the 1984–1990 Longitudinal Study of Aging (LSOA) (e.g. Crimmins *et al*, 1994, 1996; R.G. Rogers *et al*, 1989), a four wave panel data set, to estimate incidence rates of disability onset and recovery. Brouard and Robine (1992) also used panel data to calculate disability incidence rates for France. These panel data were somewhat more limited than the LSOA, having only two waves of data collection. Similar to Brouard and Robine, Liu *et al* (1995) used panel data from two interview waves to estimate incidence rates for Japan.

Longitudinal surveys of health seldom collect complete histories on the exact timing and nature of each health status event. Instead, health transitions are inferred by comparing an individual's health status across interview waves. Researchers faced with this problem have generally relied on survivorship proportions or transition probabilities to estimate the multistate life table. An example of this type of transition probability is the proportion of persons in state i at exact age x who are in state j one year (or two years) later (A. Rogers *et al*, 1989, 1990). Typically, these types of probabilities are smoothed using data smoothing or graduation smoothing (e.g. exponential smoothing) to eliminate effects of sampling fluctuations. A similar approach is the use of Markov-based event history methods and panel regression models to statistically estimate transition rates using panel data (e.g. Guilkey and Rindfuss, 1989; Hayward and Grady, 1990). This approach assumes that transition rates are a function of the state a person is in at a particular age, and duration dependence is ignored. In addition, transition rates are assumed to be constant within an age interval. These approaches offer the advantage of specifying parametric functions to predict transition rates, thereby smoothing the rates across ages. Moreover, exposure within an age interval can be adjusted to produce 'central' rates or rates that are adjusted for competing risks and censoring (e.g. Hayward and Grady, 1990; Trussell and Hammer-slough, 1983).

Embedded Markov Parameters

The most recent innovation to estimate incidence rates is to recover parameters of the embedded Markov process or chain. Liu (1995) provides a theoretical discussion of this approach. Using a community-based sample of older persons in North Carolina, Land *et al* (1994) estimated parameters (i.e., transition intensities) of a continuous time, discrete state Markov model of functional status using a panel regression model. Their approach shares the advantages of other regression-based approaches (e.g. Hayward and Grady, 1990); for example, it smoothes the transition intensities, thereby reducing sampling fluctuations. This framework, however, also imposes constraints. For example, observations are assumed to have a uniform time interval between successive measures of health status. The transition intensities must be treated as constant within the interval between successive measures; this is a relatively weak assumption if the interval width is small. Further, this approach is sensitive to the number of non-absorbing states (i.e., the number of states is generally limited to two) in addition to death.

Laditka and Wolf (1998), using data from the 1984–1990 LSOA, used a discrete approximation, and recovered the transition matrix of a Markov chain. The analytic strategy underlying this model of monthly functional status transitions is to identify the transition matrix of a Markov chain that most closely reproduces observed data. Laditka and Wolf used a maximum likelihood approach that expresses the probability of an observed individual-level transition in terms of underlying model parameters, analogous to the continuous-time approach developed by Kalbfleisch and Lawless (1985). The model assumes that month-to-month transitions within the set of discrete states are described by a first-order Markov chain.

The major methodological innovation in the approach used by Laditka and Wolf (1998) is that it allows for any pattern of unrecorded intervening functional status transitions, thereby permitting the relaxation of the assumption that no more than one transition occurred between interviews. This approach accommodates long, as well as varying, time intervals between recorded functional statuses. Such interval characteristics are common in survey data (e.g. the National Long Term Care Survey in the United States). Further, this approach imposes no theoretical upper limit on the number of absorbing states. A practical consideration of this approach is that to produce robust parameter estimates, a sufficient number of observed transitions between health states are required. In addition, this approach has yet to be replicated widely by researchers; however, software developed by Brouard and

Lievre (2001) designed to replicate the estimation approach of Laditka and Wolf (1998) may aid researchers in the use of this method.

CONCLUSIONS

This chapter has examined the three major methods that have been used to calculate indices of healthy life, and several approaches used to estimate parameters of the health process. We have framed the discussion by distinguishing between methods used to calculate indicators of healthy life and models used to estimate parameters used in these methods. We suggest it is useful for researchers to differentiate between the calculation and estimation processes. Further, we have highlighted ways in which these calculation methods and estimation models are related.

Indicators of healthy life expectancy will increasingly be used to monitor changes in population health, develop health care policy, and forecast service use and costs. Thus, it is vital for policy makers to have information about the length of total, healthy, and unhealthy life, and when possible, the degree of variability and uncertainty associated with these estimates. To address this goal, we therefore recommend that researchers make use of all parameter estimation approaches and calculation methods that are at their disposal. Pragmatically, the absence of longitudinal data, and technical difficulties in estimating parameters using regression smoothing of transition rates and estimating embedded Markov parameters, points to the importance of using prevalence rates and the Sullivan method to calculate summary indices of healthy life. These summary indices can be used to benchmark historical changes in healthy life, and they are a useful basis on which to make cross-country comparisons. At the present time, Sullivan-based methods offer the best means to gauge population health both internationally and historically.

We suggest, as a future direction, that more researchers explore micro-simulation as a method to calculate indices of healthy life. Microsimulation permits researchers to identify the frequency of specific types of health trajectories. To the extent that trajectories are clustered together, this may point to future theoretical or substantive research to understand what sort of sociological, economic, or even biological factors differentiate one health pathway from another. Further, the ability of microsimulation to simulate the entire frequency distribution of time individuals in a population spend in each health status may aid researchers and policy makers to better address issues of equity and efficiency in the financing and provision of health care and other services. Microsimulation also permits the investigation of uncertainty in estimates of healthy life expectancy that can be traced to sampling variability. Sampling error is likely to introduce non-negligible uncertainty into the resulting estimates of healthy life expectancy. Measuring this uncertainty has important implications. If policy makers use estimates of healthy life expectancy to quantify the value of future financial obligations for a large population, even small variations in values of key healthy life process parameters may result in differences of many millions of program dollars. An improved understanding of uncertainty may also assist researchers to develop better models of healthy life.

ACKNOWLEDGMENT

We thank Douglas Wolf for valuable comments on an earlier version of this chapter.

REFERENCES

Bebbington, A.C. (1988) 'The expectation of life without disability in England and Wales', *Social Science and Medicine* 27, 321–326.

Bebbington, A.C. (1991) 'The expectation of life without disability in England and Wales', *Population Trends* 66, 26–29.

Bebbington, A.C. (1992) 'Expectation of life without disability measured from the OPCS disability surveys', in Robine, J-M., Blanchet, M. and Dowd, J.E. (eds) *Health Expectancy*. London: HMSO.

Brouard, N. and Lievre, A. (2001) Computing Health Expectancies using IMaCh. INED and EUROREVES. Available at http://sauvy.ined.fr/imach. Accessed 25 July 2001.

Brouard, N. and Robine, J-M. (1992) 'A method of calculation of health expectancy from longitudinal surveys on the elderly people in France', in Robine, J-M., Blanchet, M. and Dowd, J.E. (eds) *Health Expectancy*. London: HMSO.

Canada-Vicinay, J.A. (1996) 'Mortality and lethality bias in estimates of health expectancy: A cross sectional approach using national health survey', in 9th Workgroup meeting REVES, Rome.

Cinlar, E. (1975) *Introduction to Stochastic Processes*. Englewood Cliffs, NJ: Prentice Hall.

Crimmins, E.M. and Hayward, M.D. (1997) 'What can we learn about competence at the older ages from active life expectancy?', in Schaie, W., Willis, S. and Hayward, M. (eds) *Social Structural Mechanisms for Maintaining Competence in Old Age*. New York: Springer.

Crimmins, E.M., Saito, Y. and Hayward, M.D. (1993) 'Sullivan and multistate methods of estimating active life expectancy: Two methods, two answers', in Robine, J.M., Mathers, C.D., Bone, M.R. and Romieu, I. (eds) *Calculation of Health Expectancies; Harmonization, Consensus Achieved and Future Prospects*. Paris: John Libbey Eurotext.

Crimmins, E.M., Hayward, M.D. and Saito, Y. (1994) 'Changing mortality and morbidity rates and the health status and life expectancy of the older population', *Demography* 31, 159–175.

Crimmins, E.M., Hayward, M.D. and Saito, Y. (1996) 'Differentials in active life expectancy in the older population of the United States', *Journal of Gerontology: Social Sciences* 51B, S111–S120.

Crimmins, E.M., Saito, Y. and Ingegneri, D. (1997) 'Trends in disability-free life expectancy in the United States, 1970–90', *Population and Development Review* 23, 555–572.

Guilkey, D.K. and Rindfuss, R.R. (1987) 'Logistic regression multivariate life tables: A communicable approach', *Sociological Methods and Research* 16, 276–300.

Hayward, M.D. and Grady, W.R. (1990) 'Work and retirement among a cohort of older men in the United States, 1966–1983', *Demography* 27, 337–356.

Hayward, M.D. and Heron, M. (1999) 'Racial inequality in active life among older Americans', *Demography* 36, 77–91.

Hayward, M.D., Crimmins, E.M. and Saito, Y. (1998) 'Cause of death and active life expectancy in the older population of the United States', *Journal of Aging and Health* 10, 192–213.

Jagger, C. (1999) *Health Expectancy Calculation by the Sullivan Method: A Practical Guide.* Tokyo, Japan: Nihon University Population Research Institute. Research Paper Series No. 68.

Kalbfleisch, J.D. and Lawless, J.F. (1985) 'The analysis of panel data under a Markov assumption', *Journal of the American Statistical Association* 80, 863–871.

Kinsella, K. and Gist, Y.J. (1998) *International Brief: Gender and Aging.* Washington, DC: Bureau of the Census.

Laditka, S.B. and Wolf, D.A. (1998) 'New methods for analyzing active life expectancy', *Journal of Aging and Health* 10, 214–241.

Land, K.C., Guralnik, J.M. and Blazer, D.G. (1994) 'Estimating increment-decrement life tables with multiple covariates from panel data: The case of active life expectancy', *Demography* 31, 297–319.

Lee, M.A. and Rendall, M.S. (1998) 'Self-employment disadvantage in the working lives of blacks and females', University of Wisconsin. Unpublished manuscript.

Liu, X. (1995) 'Modeling transitions in health status and active life expectancy', in 8th Work-group meeting REVES, Chicago.

Liu, X., Liang, J., Muramatsu, N. and Sugisawa, H. (1995) 'Transitions in functional status and active life expectancy among older people in Japan', *Journal of Gerontology: Social Sciences* 50B, S383–S394.

Manton, K.G. and Stallard, E. (1990) 'Changes in health functioning and mortality', in Stahl, S.M. (ed.) *Legacy of Longevity.* Newbury Park, CA: Sage.

Mathers, C. (1991) *Health Expectancies in Australia 1981 and 1988.* Canberra: Australian Institute of Health and Welfare, AGPS.

Preston, S. (1982) 'Individual life cycles and population characteristics', *American Sociological Review* 47, 253–264.

Rendall, M.S. (1991) *Estimation of Variance about Working Life Expectancies for Older Americans.* Providence: Brown University, Population Studies and Training Center. Working Paper Series 91-01.

Robine, J-M., Romieu, I. and Cambois, E. (1997) 'Health expectancies and current research', *Reviews in Clinical Gerontology* 7, 73–81.

Robine, J-M., Mormiche, P. and Sermet, C. (1998) 'Examination of the causes and mechanisms of the increase in disability-free life expectancy', *Journal of Aging and Health* 10, 171–191.

Rogers, A. (1975) *Introduction to Multiregional Mathematical Demography.* New York: Wiley.

Rogers, A., Rogers, R.G. and Branch, L.G. (1989) 'A multistate analysis of active life expectancy', *Public Health Reports* 104, 222–226.

Rogers, A., Rogers, R.G. and Belanger, A. (1990) 'Longer life but worse health? Measurement and dynamics', *The Gerontologist* 30, 640–649.

Rogers, R.G., Rogers, A. and Belanger, A. (1989) 'Active life among the elderly in the United States: Multistate life-table estimates and population projections', *Milbank Quarterly* 67, 370–411.

Saito, Y., Crimmins, E.M. and Hayward, M.D. (1992) 'Stabilité des estimations de l'espérance de vie sans perte d'autonomie calculées au moyen de deux méthodes de construction de tables de survie', *Cahiers québécois de démographie* 20, 1–37.

Schoen, R. (1975) 'Constructing increment-decrement life tables', *Demography* 12, 313–324.

Schoen, R. (1988) *Modeling Multigroup Populations*. New York: Plenum.

Schoen, R. and Woodrow, K. (1980) 'Labor force status life tables for the United States, 1972', *Demography* 17, 297–322.

Sullivan, D.F. (1971) 'A single index of mortality and morbidity', *HSMHA Health Reports* 86, 347–354.

Trussell, J. and Hammerslough, C. (1983) 'A hazard-model analysis of the covariates of infant and child mortality in Sri Lanka', *Demography* 20, 1–26.

Wilkins, R. and Adams, O.B. (1983) 'Health expectancy in Canada, late 1970s: Demographic, regional, and social dimensions', *American Journal of Public Health* 73, 1073–1080.

Wilkins, R. and Adams, O.B. (1989) 'Health expectancy trends in Canada', in 1st Workgroup meeting REVES, Quebec.

Wolf, D.A. and Laditka, S.B. (1997) *Stochastic Modeling of Active Life and its Expectancy*. New York: The Maxwell Center for Demography and Economics of Aging, Syracuse University. Papers in Microsimulation Series Paper No. 4.

12

Health-adjusted Life Expectancy (HALE)

JEAN-MARIE BERTHELOT

Statistics Canada, Ottawa, Ontario, Canada

BACKGROUND

The appropriate and efficient use of limited health resources is a perennial issue among health care providers, policy-makers, and society at large. Health care expenditures constitute a significant economic and social investment for any nation, with average outlays ranging from 4% to 14% of total GDP in OECD member countries. The expectation for the return on this social capital investment is increased health, longer lives and an increase in the quality of life for its citizens.

Considering such a goal, decisions must be based on information, and ideally, evidence. Considerable gaps in knowledge exist, however, for a range of factors necessary to develop critical causal pathways to support effective health policy development. While input measures abound (e.g. number of beds and doctors per capita, average length of stay and public expenditures) and are generally of high quality, output measures are somewhat more limited, primarily to fertility and mortality outcomes, thereby limiting the scope of support for decisions.

In this chapter, we present an indicator that incorporates both mortality and a cardinal measure of morbidity into a single measure: health-adjusted life expectancy. We describe its calculation and discuss its potential policy relevance.

WHAT IS HEALTH-ADJUSTED LIFE EXPECTANCY?

Health-adjusted life expectancy (HALE) is a population health indicator that incorporates mortality and health status measures into a single statistic. HALE

Determining Health Expectancies. Edited by J-M. Robine, C. Jagger, C.D. Mathers, E.M. Crimmins and R.M. Suzman.
© 2003 John Wiley & Sons, Ltd

represents the equivalent number of years in perfect health that an individual can expect to live during his or her life if exposed at each age to the mortality and health status (morbidity) conditions that prevail today.

In 1983, Wilkins and Adams (1983) derived the first estimates of health-adjusted life expectancy for a national population (Canada). They combined the Sullivan (1971) method with the cross-sectional prevalence for six disability states, and assigned arbitrary values corresponding to perceived health-related quality of life to each of the six disability states.

As an extension of the underlying principle of health expectancy, Torrance employed a continuum of health states instead of the more limited discrete representation by using a health expectancy index based on multi-attribute health states weighted for each year of life by a utility score (Torrance, 1986; Feeny *et al*, 1994).

To be useful in estimating the HALE, health state descriptions must be quantifiable and summarised by a single number. The convention for these types of scales usually has 1.0 representing a fully healthy state; 0.0 representing death; and occasionally, numbers less than zero to indicate states worse than death, such as very painful terminal cancer. This single number is often referred to as a health state utility score.

Since the early 1990s, the Health Utilities Index (Furlong *et al*, 2001; Torrance *et al*, 1996; Feeny *et al*, 1992) and the EuroQol (Dolan, 1997; EuroQol, 1990) health status measurement systems have been used as numerical measures of health. Illustrative calculations of HALE in this paper use the provisional Health Utilities Index (HUI; Mark III) as the health status instrument (Torrance *et al*, 1992).

DATA REQUIREMENTS

HALE measures for a given population (e.g. sex, region, socioeconomic group) require two components: (1) a sequence of age-specific mortality rates and (2) a sequence of age-specific measures of average health status.

The mortality component is used to calculate the number of years lived by a given population using either single state or multistate life tables. In the case of a multistate life table, both transition rates between states and state-specific mortality are required.

Calculation of average health status requires two kinds of information. One is a carefully structured multi-attribute description of health states for a representative sample of the population, commonly referred to as the health state 'descriptive system' (Richardson and Nord, 1997). The descriptive system includes a vector of independent health attributes or dimensions, such as pain and mobility. For descriptive purposes, each attribute can be assigned or tagged with a level such as no pain, mild, moderate or severe pain. An individual's full health status therefore becomes a vector of numbers, one for each health attribute, each 'dimension' indicating a categorical level of severity, ranging from no health problem at all on that dimension, to a very severe level of health problem. Consequently, any health state descriptive system is fully described by a grid or matrix of health attributes by severity level. A mathematical function is used to synthesise the information on various levels of morbidity or functioning along a diverse set of dimensions into a single numerical score.

METHODS

Mean health state scores and age-specific mortality rates are combined to produce health-adjusted life expectancy (HALE). Conceptually, each year of life is adjusted to reflect the mean population health state score by age and sex. The HALE calculation modifies a standard LE calculation by weighting the number of life years lived in a particular age group using the mean health state score for that age group. The sum of the adjusted life years lived beyond age x can then be simply divided by the number of survivors at that age to yield HALE by age and sex.

$$LE_x = \frac{\sum_{x=a}^{\Omega} L_{(x,x+a)}}{l_x}$$

$$HALE_x = \frac{\left(\sum_{x=a}^{\Omega} L_{(x,x+a)} \times W_{(x,x+a)} \right)}{l_x}$$

where x is the age for which LE or HALE is calculated; $L_{(x,x+a)}$ is the number of life years lived for the age group $(x,x+xa)$; l_x is the number of survivors at age x; $W_{(x,x+a)}$ is the mean health status for the age group $(x,x+a)$; Ω is the last age group in the life table.

The 1994–1995 National Population Health Survey (NPHS) and the provisional HUI Mark III health status measure can be used to illustrate the calculation of general population level estimates (for males) for Canada (Table 12.1). A detailed summary of the HUI Mark III health status measure can be found in Appendix A at the end of this chapter. The mortality component is based on 1991 life tables obtained from Statistics Canada's Demography Division.

Table 12.1. Calculation of HALE for Canada, males

$W_{(x,x+a)}$ Age group	(1) $L_{(x,x+a)}$	(2) $HAL_{(x,x+a)}$	(1)*(2) $\Sigma L_{(x,x+a)}$	(3) $\Sigma L_{(x,x+a)}$	(4) $\Sigma HAL_{(x,x+a)}$	(5) l_x	LE_x $\Sigma L_{(x,x+a)}/l_x$ (3)/(5)=(6)	$HALE_x$ $\Sigma HAL_{(x,x+a)}/l_x$ (4)/(5)=(7)	LE_x- $HALE_x$ (years) (6)−(7)	$(LE_x-$ $HALE_x)/$ LE_x (%) (6)−(7)/(6)
15–24	0.929	984 768	915 061	5 968 490	5 311 175	98 930	60.3	53.7	6.6	11.0%
25–34	0.927	973 637	902 096	4 983 722	4 396 114	97 941	50.9	44.9	6.0	11.8%
35–44	0.921	959 114	883 306	4 010 085	3 494 018	96 737	41.5	36.1	5.3	12.9%
45–54	0.893	931 628	832 265	3 050 971	2 610 712	94 925	32.1	27.5	4.6	14.4%
55–64	0.870	861 611	749 207	2 119 343	1 778 447	90 755	23.4	19.6	3.8	16.1%
65–74	0.848	700 635	593 817	1 257 732	1 029 240	80 007	15.7	12.9	2.9	18.2%
75–84	0.806	420 444	338 801	557 097	435 423	57 951	9.6	7.5	2.1	21.8%
85+	0.707	136 653	96 622	136 653	96 622	25 494	5.4	3.8	1.6	29.3%

Source: HUI provisional scores from 1994–1995 National Population Health Survey (Canada) and 1991 life table data from Demography Division, Statistics Canada. Reproduced with permission. Statistics Canada information is used with the permission of the Minister of Industry, as Minister responsible for Statistic Canada. Information on the availability of the wide range of data from Statistic Canada can be obtained from Statistics Canada's Regional Offices, its World Wide Web site at http:// www.statcan.ca, and its toll-free access number 1-800-263-1136.

APPLICATION

The HALE represents the number of year-equivalents in perfect health experienced in a population. The difference between life expectancy and HALE, then, is the number of equivalent years of ill health that, on average, are expected over the course of an individual's life. HALEs can be quoted in absolute terms in the form of total year-equivalents or as a relative figure representing the percentage of remaining life expectancy in perfect health.

A time series of these percentages, assuming life expectancy itself continued to increase, would provide a clear indication of whether or not the added years of life were, on average, healthier. This is essentially the 'compression of morbidity' issue popularised by James Fries (1980, 1989). If, for example, these percentages were decreasing over time, it would likely signal that the increase in life expectancy was associated with an increasing prevalence of chronic disease morbidity, with consequent implications for health care needs.

In a recent study, Martel and Bélanger (1999) used HALE to evaluate the hypothesised compression of morbidity for Canada. They calculated changes in HALE using the last three Canadian population censuses in combination with the National Population Health Survey, the Health and Activity Limitation postcensal survey and Canadian life tables. The study supports the notion that Canadians of both sexes can expect to live more years than ever in good health. These findings apply to both younger and older populations. Over the 10-year period between 1986 and 1996 (Table 12.2), the gains made against mortality in Canada are distributed, in relative terms, about equally between healthy and non-healthy year-equivalents, achieving a form of equilibrium between gains in life expectancy and gains against morbidity.

The HALE can be broken down into components appropriate for specific analysis requirements. Disaggregated HALE and LE indicators can facilitate subgroup analysis, which, in turn, can be used to inform public policy discourse at the most general level of priority setting, to aid evaluation and targeting of public health initiatives, and to monitor populations identified at risk. Depending on data availability, health could be monitored and assessed by risk factor, specific health dimension, specific disease, socioeconomic factor, age, sex, or region. HALE, like LE, can be estimated for specific subpopulations, for example, by socioeconomic status (SES), region, health problem, or race.

Table 12.3 shows that while women are expected to live 6.3 years longer than men, they are also expected to have a higher burden of ill health. At age 15, women are expected to experience the equivalent of about two and a half more years of ill health than men; at age 65, about 1.6 years more than men. In relative terms, the burden of ill health at age 15 for women was almost 14% of their remaining life versus 11% for men and at age 65, about 23% versus 19% for men.

Table 12.2. Life expectancy (LE) and health-adjusted life expectancy (HALE) at age 15 and 65 by sex, Canada, 1986, 1991 and 1996

		Males			Females		
		LE	HALE	Difference	LE	HALE	Difference
At age 15	In years						
	1986	59.3	53.9	5.4	65.8	58.3	7.5
	1991	60.4	54.7	5.7	66.6	58.8	7.8
	1996	61.1	55.4	5.7	66.8	59.1	7.7
	As percentage						
	1986		91.0	9.0		88.6	11.4
	1991		90.6	9.4		88.3	11.7
	1996		90.6	9.4		88.4	11.6
At age 65	In years						
	1986	15.0	12.4	2.6	19.4	15.3	4.1
	1991	15.8	13.0	2.8	20.0	15.6	4.4
	1996	16.1	13.3	2.8	20.0	15.8	4.2
	As percentage						
	1986		82.7	17.3		78.9	21.1
	1991		82.0	18.0		78.0	22.0
	1996		82.4	17.6		79.1	20.9

Source: Martel and Bélanger, 1999. Reproduced with permission*

Table 12.3. Overall LE and HALE by sex, Canada

	Males		Females	
	Years	%	Years	%
Age 15:				
LE	60.3	100.0	66.6	100.0
HALE	53.7	89.0	57.4	86.2
LE − HALE	6.6	11.0	9.2	13.8
Age 65:				
LE	15.7	100.0	19.9	100.0
HALE	12.9	81.5	15.4	77.4
LE − HALE	2.9	18.5	4.5	22.6

Source: HUI provisional scores from 1994–1995 National Population Health Survey (Canada) and 1991 life table data from Demography Division, Statistics Canada. Reproduced with permission*

As for socioeconomic status, Table 12.4 presents results for several SES variables and their associated HALEs. For both males and females, large SES differences are clearly evident, with individuals in the highest education and income categories living considerably longer, and in better health, than those in

---

* Statistics Canada information is used with the permission of the Minister of Industry, as Minister responsible for Statistic Canada. Information on the availability of the wide range of data from Statistic Canada can be obtained from Statistics Canada's Regional Offices, its World Wide Web site at http://www.statcan.ca, and its toll-free access number 1-800-263-1136.

Table 12.4. HALEs at age 25 by SES and marital status, Canada

	Males		Females	
	Life expectancy	HALE	Life expectancy	HALE
Education quartile[a]				
Highest educated	47.7	42.8	53.2	46.3
2nd Quartile	47.6	41.8	52.2	44.5
3rd Quartile	45.2	39.5	52.0	44.1
Lowest educated	44.5	37.5	51.0	41.0
Income quintile				
Richest	53.5	48.8	57.6	50.5
4th Quintile	52.6	46.7	57.5	49.9
3rd Quintile	52.0	46.3	57.9	50.2
2nd Quintile	50.9	44.3	57.2	48.5
Poorest	48.2	40.9	56.3	47.0
Marital status				
Married	51.3	45.3	56.9	48.6
Single	48.9	42.7	56.2	47.7
Widowed	49.0	39.4	55.8	47.3
Divorced	49.7	44.0	53.8	46.1

[a]Highest level of education attained by age 30.
Source: Nault, Roberge and Berthelot, 1996.

the lowest categories. A steep gradient is also clearly evident for both income and education. For males, the difference between high and low categories is 5.3 year-equivalents for education and 7.9 year-equivalents for income. Similar gradients, somewhat smaller for income, are present for females.

In addition to SES variables, LE and HALE were also examined by marital status (Table 12.4). The highest LE was for the category 'married', consistent with other studies (van Poppel and Joung, 2001; Johnson *et al*, 2000). In addition, the HALE is highest for the 'married' category among both males and females.

To examine which specific functional limitations drive overall differences in LE and HALE, estimates can be decomposed by attribute contributing to the health state utility. Table 12.5 uses the attributes specific to the HUI Mark III to provide estimates of the burden of ill health for each dimension of health imbedded in the HUI Mark III 'descriptive system'. This calculation is an analogue of cause-deleted LE, for example, 'What would life expectancy be if no one died of lung cancer?' Based on this cause-deleted LE indicator, the most serious health problem would be heart disease, followed by cancer.

In this case, we refer to the 'attribute-deleted' HALE, or 'How much would HALE increase if no one suffered from ill health of type X?' While rigorous estimates are not yet available, it is likely that arthritis and dementia would

Table 12.5. Attribute-deleted HALE at age 15 by sex, Canada

	Males				Females			
	Attribute-deleted		Difference		Attribute-deleted		Difference	
Attribute	HALE A	HALE B	Years A − B	% A − B	HALE A	HALE B	Years A − B	% A − B
Overall	60.3	53.7	6.6	100.0	66.6	57.4	9.2	100.0
Sensory[a]	55.7	53.7	2.0	29.5	60.0	57.4	2.6	28.7
Pain	55.2	53.7	1.5	23.3	59.8	57.4	2.4	27.0
Emotion	55.0	53.7	1.3	19.8	59.0	57.4	1.6	15.8
Cognition	54.7	53.7	1.0	15.5	58.6	57.4	1.2	13.3
Mobility	54.0	53.7	0.3	4.8	58.1	57.4	0.7	9.0
Dexterity	53.8	53.7	0.1	1.1	57.6	57.4	0.2	2.4
Residual[b]	–	–	0.4	6.0	–	–	0.5	3.8

[a]In the HUI-3, the attribute 'sensory' is further decomposed into vision, hearing and speech.
[b]Residual is due to the multiplicative form of HUI scoring function.
Source: HUI provisional scores from 1994–1995 National Population Health Survey (Canada) and 1991 life table data from Demography Division, Statistics Canada. Reproduced with permission. (see footnote on page 240)

rank much higher on the basis of cause-deleted HALE than they do in terms of cause-deleted LE, as these diseases, while seriously debilitating, have lower fatality than other diseases. A focus on functional status rather than disease grouping per se demonstrates that pain ranks high in terms of burden of illness. As an example, at age 15 for males, the pain attribute contributed 1.5 years or 23.3% of the burden of ill health experienced by an individual over the course of his lifetime. However, the largest burden of ill health for both sexes was due to sensory limitations, the majority of which represents, in fact, vision problems, i.e. the inability to see without corrective lenses. Compared with some chronic diseases, this limitation could be considered relatively minor but very prevalent. The three top-ranking attributes, sensory, pain, and emotion, contributed close to three-quarters of the burden of ill health for each sex.

A number of limitations surrounding the use of HALEs as a national health indicator should be highlighted. First, the estimation of HALE embodies societal preferences. For example, the HUI Mark III health status measure underlying the HALE estimates is based on eliciting from individuals how they would view having to live in a specified health state. However, research suggests that considerably different results would be obtained if, instead, individuals were asked how they would view spending public money to cure the same health problems. It also appears that individuals who have suffered from a specific health problem value it differently than the bulk of the population for whom it is hypothetical. Moreover, among those for whom the health state is hypothetical, there appear to be systematic variations by socioeconomic status. These circumstances raise a fundamental issue with the HALE measure. More theoretical work is required to better understand the factors underlying individual preferences for health states.

CONCLUSION

Estimates of HALE, along with the associated family of estimates for subpopulations and components of HALE, provide a coherent and useful set of summary indicators of the health of a nation's population. In Canada, HALEs at the national population level can be calculated every two years with data from the National Population Health Survey and vital statistics. This provides a concise set of indicators that will allow monitoring, not only of trends in life expectancy, but also the extent of compression or expansion of morbidity. In addition, as with LE, morbidity estimates can provide a useful monitoring and evaluation function for both population health and clinical trials. These indicators of health status provide comparable measures, bridging the gap between public health/population health studies and experimental studies within the clinical setting.

For both researchers and policy-makers, the HALE is a unique and useful tool. Using the HALE and its subcomponents from the HUI Mark III on a regular basis, policy-makers can monitor the health of populations and subpopulations. In addition, quantitative assessment is very useful in evaluating programmes aimed at managing different aspects of the disabled population. Particular interventions can be assessed not strictly on extended survival or costs but on the equally important concept of health-related quality of life associated with morbidity. The generic nature of the HALE and HUI Mark III also means that data collected at a clinical level can be compared with similar data calculated for the entire population. Clinical data tend to focus on particular 'micro issues' relevant to a particular segment of a population that may not be readily comparable with a national population and potential public health programmes. The inclusion of HALEs in the repertoire of assessment tools for health policy goes some distance in providing evidence to support complex decision-making.

ACKNOWLEDGEMENT

The author wishes to acknowledge the contribution of Kathy White, HAMG, Statistics Canada, in preparing this manuscript for publication.

REFERENCES

Dolan, P. (1997) 'Modeling valuations for EuroQol health states', *Medical Care* 35(11), 1095–1108.

EuroQol (1990) 'A new facility for the measurement of health-related quality of life: The EuroQol Group', *Health Policy* 16(3), 199–208.

Feeny, D., Furlong, W., Barr, R.D., Torrance, G.W., Rosenbaum, P. and Weitzman, S.A. (1992) 'Comprehensive multi-attribute system for classifying the health status of survivors of childhood cancer', *Journal of Clinical Oncology* 10(6), 923–928.

Feeny, D., Torrance, G., Goldsmith, C., Furlong, W. and Boyle, M. (1994) *A Multi-attribute Approach to Population Health Status*. Hamilton, Ontario: McMaster University, Centre for Health Economics and Policy Analysis. Research Paper, 5.

Feeny, D., Furlong, W., Boyle, M. and Torrance, G.W. (1995) 'Multi-attribute health status classification systems: Health Utilities Index', *Pharmacoeconomics* 7(6), 490–502.

Fries, J. (1980) 'Aging, natural death, and the compression of morbidity', *New England Journal of Medicine* 303, 130–135.

Fries, J. (1989) 'The compression of morbidity: near or far?' *Milbank Quarterly* 67(2), 208–232.

Furlong, W., Feeny, D., Torrance, G.W., Goldsmith, C., DePauw, S., Boyle, M., Denton, M. and Zhu, Z. (1998) *Multiplicative Multi-Attribute Utility Function for the Health Utilities Index Mark III (HUI3) System: A Technical Report*. Hamilton, Ontario: McMaster University Centre for Health Economics and Policy Analysis Working Paper, 11.

Furlong, W.J., Feeny, D.H., Torrance, G.W. and Barr, R.D. (2001) 'The Health Utilities Index (HUI) system for assessing health-related quality of life in clinical studies', *Annals of Medicine* 33(5), 375–384.

Johnson, N.J., Backlund, E., Sorlie, P.D. and Loveless, C.A. (2000) 'Marital status and mortality: the National Longitudinal Mortality Study', *Annals of Epidemiology* 10(4), 224–238.

Martel, L. and Bélanger, A. (1999) 'An analysis of the change in dependence-free life expectancy in Canada between 1986 and 1996', in *Report on the Demographic Situation in Canada 1998–1999*. Ottawa: Ministry of Industry (Statistics Canada Catalogue no. 91-209-XPE).

Nault, F., Roberge, R. and Berthelot, J-M. (1996) 'Espérance de vie et espérance de vie en santé selon le sexe, l'état matrimonial et le statut socio-économique au Canada', *Cahiers Québécois de Démographie* 25(2), 286–292.

Richardson, J. and Nord, E. (1997) 'The importance of perspective in the measurement of quality-adjusted life years', *Medical Decision Making* 17(1), 33–41.

Sullivan, D. (1971) 'A single index of mortality and morbidity', *HSMHA Health Reports* 86(4), 347–354.

Torrance, G.W. (1986) 'Measurement of health state utilities for economic appraisal: A review', *Journal of Health Economics* 5, 1–30.

Torrance, G.W., Furlong, W., Feeny, D., *et al* (1992) *Provisional Health Index for the Ontario Health Survey*. Hamilton, Ontario: McMaster University Centre for Health Economics and Policy Analysis, Project No. 44400900187.

Torrance, G.W., Furlong, W., Feeny, D. and Boyle, M. (1995) 'Multi-attribute preference functions. Health Utilities Index', *Pharmacoeconomics* 7(6), 503–520.

Torrance, G.W., Feeny, D.H., Furlong, W.J., Barr, R.D., Zhang, Y. and Wang, Q. (1996) 'Multi-attribute utility function for a comprehensive health status classification system: Health Utilities Index Mark 2', *Medical Care* 34(7), 702–722.

van Poppel, F. and Joung, I. (2001) 'Long-term trends in marital status mortality differences in The Netherlands 1850–1970', *Journal of Biosocial Science* 33(20), 279–303.

von Neumann, J. and Morgenstern, O. (1953) *Theory of Games and Economic Behaviour*, 3rd edn. Princeton: Princeton University Press.

Wilkins, R. and Adams, O.B. (1983) 'Health expectancy in Canada, late 1970s: demographic, regional, and social dimensions', *American Journal of Public Health* 73(9), 1073–1080.

APPENDIX A: THE HEALTH UTILITIES INDEX

The Health Utilities Index (HUI) is a generic health status index that is able to synthesise both quantitative and qualitative aspects of health. The HUI provides a quantitative measure of a population's overall health status, as opposed to focusing on narrowly defined health indicators, risk factors or diseases. Such a measure is an analytical tool that can be used for health policy evaluation and for the assessment of health care interventions at a population and a clinical level.

The first step in the construction of a health utilities index is the specification of a set of health status attributes. These are chosen to reflect a wide range of functional capacities and to capture what most people consider the most serious health-related problems they might encounter. The method developed at McMaster University's Centre for Health Economics and Policy Analysis (CHEPA) describes an individual's overall functional health, based on eight attributes: vision, hearing, speech, mobility (ability to get around), dexterity (use of hands and fingers), cognition (memory and thinking), emotion (feelings), and pain and discomfort. An individual's health status is the vector of the observed levels of functional ability for each attribute (Figure 12.1). For

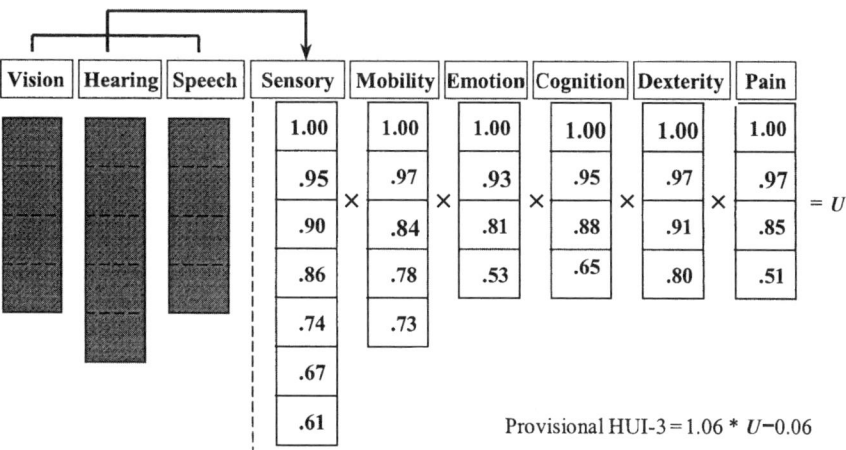

Figure 12.1. Provisional Health Utilities Index Mark III (HUI-3)

example, 'vision' ranges from perfect vision to blindness, while 'pain' ranges from no pain to completely disabling pain (Feeny *et al*, 1995).

The provisional HUI maps any one of the vectors of eight health attribute levels into a summary health utility score with 0 representing death and the score 1 representing complete health. For instance, an individual who is near-sighted, yet fully healthy on the other seven attributes, receives a score of 0.95 on this scale.

The HUI embodies the views of society concerning health status. Societal preferences are defined as an average of the preferences of individuals, insofar as they form a representative sample of the population. Preferences are evaluated using the Standard Gamble technique (Torrance *et al*, 1995), which is based on the axioms of consumer utility theory developed by von Neumann and Morgenstern (1953). For the provisional HUI Mark III, they were evaluated on the basis of the Childhood Cancer Study conducted by CHEPA at McMaster University (Feeny *et al*, 1992).

The utility scores used here are considered provisional because they are based on preference ratings using Mark II, the most recent available at the time of the analysis. Weights specific to Mark III, i.e. with sensory divided into vision, hearing and speech, have now been developed using a representative sample of the general population from the city of Hamilton, Canada (Furlong *et al*, 1998).

13

Disability-adjusted Life Years (DALYs) and Disability-adjusted Life Expectancy (DALE)

JAN J. BARENDREGT

Erasmus MC, Rotterdam, The Netherlands

INTRODUCTION

The first publication to mention the disability-adjusted life years (DALYs) was the *World Development Report 1993: Investing in Health* (World Bank, 1993). This report presented the results of the Global Burden of Disease 1990 study, an overview of the burden of morbidity and mortality by cause for the whole world subdivided into eight regions. The burden of morbidity and mortality was expressed in a new composite indicator of population health status, the DALY. In addition, recommendations for cost-effective packages of basic health care were made, based on costs per DALY gained.

Two things were thus revealed about DALYs. Firstly, DALYs were designed not just as a summary measure of population health, but for cost-effectiveness analysis as well. Secondly, while most summary measures spend years in a process to gain acceptance, DALYs were hurled onto centre stage by a major application even before peer-reviewed journal publications on the methodology were available.

Since the World Development Report a large number of publications on DALY methodology and its application have appeared, both by critical outsiders and by the designers of the DALY, Chris Murray and Alan Lopez. In the sections below we will first briefly describe the original DALY, discuss some critical comments, and then assess where the DALY methodology stands now, and discuss its health expectancy equivalent, disability-adjusted life expectancy (DALE).

Determining Health Expectancies. Edited by J-M. Robine, C. Jagger, C.D. Mathers, E.M. Crimmins and R.M. Suzman.
© 2003 John Wiley & Sons, Ltd

THE DALY METHODOLOGY

As mentioned above, DALY methodology was designed with cost-effectiveness analysis in mind. This has led to a number of design decisions that make the DALY different from health expectancies. Indeed, while the DALY has in common with health expectancies that it is a composite indicator, combining morbidity and mortality, it is not a health expectancy but a health gap indicator (Murray *et al*, 2000).

This distinction can be illustrated by the survival curve in Figure 13.1. The survival curve gives the proportion of people alive at each age, with the area under the survival curve being the life expectancy at birth. A gap measure postulates some ideal survival, for example the halved mortality curve in Figure 13.1, and then measures the difference between the actual situation and the ideal. In the figure area C gives this difference as years of life lost (YLL).

Extending this principle to morbidity we divide the area under the survival curve into years lived in full health (A) and years lived in less than full health (B). A health expectancy is then defined by:

$$HE = A + f(B)$$

or the sum of the years lived in full health and those lived in less than full health, the latter ones weighted using the function $f()$ to reflect that these years are not spent in full health. For a disability-free life expectancy (DFLE), $f(B)$ would equal 0; for a health-adjusted life expectancy (HALE), $f(B) = B.w$, with w a number between 0 and 1, reflecting the average health status of the years lived with morbidity.

A health gap indicator is defined by:

$$HG = C + g(B)$$

or the sum of YLL and the years lived in less than full health, again weighted but this time using a function $g()$. Note that the scales of the functions $f()$ and $g()$ run opposite: if the year lived in less than full health is evaluated as equal to death then $f()$ will assign it a weight of 0 and $g()$ a weight of 1, and vice versa when the year is evaluated as equal to full health. Also note that a gap measure needs a definition of ideal health (like the halved mortality survival curve in Figure 13.1), of which the current situation falls short. Such an ideal health definition cannot be but arbitrary.

The design of the DALY as a health gap indicator can be directly traced back to the intended use in cost-effectiveness analysis. A health expectancy abstracts from the structure of the population, which is undesirable in the context of cost-effectiveness analysis because both costs and effects depend on population structure. A health gap indicator can easily (but does not necessarily) include the population structure.

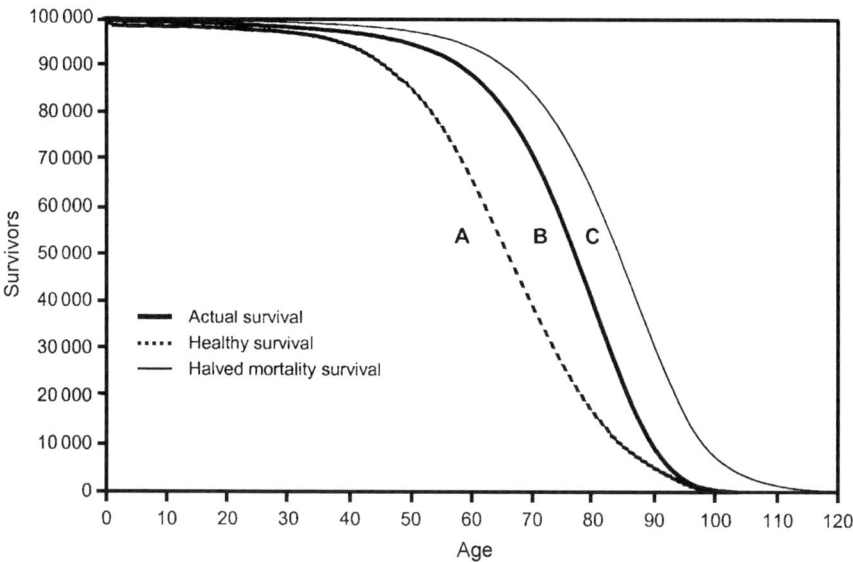

Figure 13.1. Actual survival, healthy survival, and survival with halved mortality

A central feature of DALYs is that they are disease specific from the ground up: the burden of disease is estimated on the disease-specific level, and an overall estimate is obtained by summing over diseases. This characteristic too is closely related to the cost-effectiveness and interventionist perspective. Most health care measures are disease-specific interventions, either preventive or therapeutic, and this makes it imperative to examine the effects of interventions on a disease-specific level.

The DALY methodology uses for each disease the following basic scheme. Given the disease- and age-specific mortalities the 'expected years of life lost' (YLL) due to mortality are estimated by multiplying the number of disease-specific deaths for each age by the life expectancy at that age (the so-called 'local life expectancy'), and then summing over all deaths. Years lost due to morbidity (called 'years lived with disability', or YLD) are estimated by multiplying the years lived with disease by a disability weight, a value between 0 and 1, with 0 representing full health and 1 the worst possible health state. Summing over age the thus-weighted years lived yields the years lived with disability. The sum of the years lost due to mortality and morbidity (YLL + YLD) then gives the total burden of this particular disease.

Note that the calculation of years lost due to morbidity requires considerable knowledge of disease epidemiology. The minimal knowledge would be disease prevalence by age, but in the original implementation the designers argue for the incidence perspective as being more consistent when combined with mortality (Murray, 1994). The incidence perspective also allows the inclusion of discounting to correct for time preference (see below). But of course the incidence perspective requires estimation of disease incidence and duration, the latter being determined by case fatality and recovery, thus increasing the data requirements considerably.

Add to this the objective of measuring not just the burden of disease from one or a few diseases, but the total burden of disease from all (important) diseases combined. This requires making consistent estimates of the incidence, duration and mortality of a great number of diseases, a number large enough to represent the major part of the population's health. Given these objectives and the actually available data, the researchers were forced to rely in large part on expert knowledge, while using an incidence, prevalence and mortality model to force their estimates to be at least internally consistent. It is one of the more amazing things in DALY history that critique has been directed at just about every aspect of its methodology, but has largely ignored the fundamental problem of the epidemiological data requirements.

In addition to the disease-specific perspective the original DALY implementation included the following features:

- The use of one standard life table with high life expectancy as the 'ideal health' definition. Murray argued that using the same life table world-wide, instead of different regional life tables, is necessary to compare 'like with like', to avoid valuing a death at a given age more in a high life expectancy country than in a low one (Murray, 1994).
- The use of disease-specific disability weights. This feature follows directly from the disease-specific perspective: to get from disease-specific to total morbidity a mapping for each disease to a generic morbidity indicator is needed. Expert panels evaluated 22 conditions using the person trade-off (PTO) method; remaining conditions were then assigned disability weights using these 22 conditions as indicators.
- The use of age weights. Murray cites both economic and social role arguments to justify valuing lost years of life due to mortality and morbidity differently by age. Intuitively most people will agree that the death of a newborn or a 90-year-old, while being tragic, is less so than that of a 15-year-old. The quantitative implementation of this notion is, on the other hand, not obvious.
- Discounting of future years. Although in economics it goes without saying that future costs and benefits should be discounted, it is not a generally accepted concept in the health sector that future years of life should be treated similarly. The original DALY implementation discounted future life years by 3%.

Although 'DALYs are meant to be a transparent tool' (Murray and Lopez, 1996a) this adds up to a very complex indicator indeed, with aspects from economics, demography, epidemiology and social justice. Consequently the discussion on DALYs has been wide-ranging too, and is presently anything but concluded. We will not try to give an overview of the entire discussion, but just point to a number of major controversies.

DALY CRITIQUE

As already mentioned above, all aspects of DALY methodology, as listed above, have been criticised. We will look at the critical comments in turn.

DISEASE-SPECIFIC APPROACH

The most radical critique on the disease-specific character of DALYs has come from Williams: he states that the disease-specific approach is both unnecessary and undesirable (Williams, 1999). What we need from the point of view of optimal resource allocation is, according to Williams, an intervention-specific approach. Comparing the marginal benefits of alternative interventions will guide us to the optimal resource allocation, and in the process there is no need to know the contribution of individual diseases to the total burden of disease, or the total burden itself for that matter, and trying to estimate it only diverts scarce resources.

To appreciate how radical this critique is, it is illuminating to think of the analogue in economics proper. Then Williams is saying that a system of national accounts is unnecessary and even detrimental: we only need to concentrate on formulating the policy that will deliver the highest growth of gross national product (GNP). While most economists will agree with the policy goal, very few would endorse the idea of doing away with the national accounts. Indeed, most economists will argue that a good system of national accounts is a precondition for the formulation of optimal policies. Without the data the economic policy makers of the world would be starved of information, and their macro-economic models would be useless.

In public health much the same is true. Without an understanding of the causes of morbidity and mortality, the search for the optimal policies would be blind, and an optimal outcome an unlikely event. Since intervention benefits may take a long time to emerge, many beneficial interventions would be missed because clinical trials have to end at some point. The alternative approach, modelling the disease process and using a counterfactual to assess the potential benefit of an intervention, would be impossible too because it requires precisely the kind of information gathered in a burden of disease study.

The hidden assumption in Williams' reasoning is that there are cost-effectiveness studies available for every intervention imaginable, for every (sub)population and at all times. If that were true, one could indeed simply rank interventions by outcome, and start implementing them. In practice, of course, the availability of cost-effectiveness studies is very limited, the population typically consists of middle-aged white American males without comorbidities, and by the time the results become available they are often rendered obsolete by new developments. To extrapolate from this patchy data to a real population the above-mentioned modelling and burden of disease data are necessary.

Taking Williams' critique seriously would amount to a severe setback in health policy. In practice, of course, policy makers have always relied on disease-specific burden of disease data, albeit partial data: disease-specific mortality. Naturally this leads to a concentration on diseases that cause high mortality, and relative neglect of causes of high morbidity. It is precisely the relative neglect of morbidity that has spawned the research fields that have delivered various composite health indicators such as QALYs and health expectancies. Combining total morbidity and mortality in a composite indicator is thought to be a proper way to redress the imbalanced attention to mortality. DALYs apply the same notion, but then on the disease-specific level. It is illogical to argue on the one hand that total mortality as a health indicator should be extended to include morbidity, as Williams does, and on the other hand that for disease-specific mortality the same thing is undesirable.

This is not to say that the disease-specific approach is without problems. In their basic publications Murray and Lopez already acknowledged that the disease-specific basis of the DALY introduced the problem of comorbidity (Murray, 1994). It is unclear what disability weight to use in case of comorbidity, and the sheer number of possible comorbid states makes a solution seem remote. In ageing populations, where degenerative disease is the main cause of morbidity, this problem becomes substantial.

However, the main issue with the disease-specific approach is the huge data requirement. To our knowledge, no population exists for which sufficient data is known. Getting a DALY estimate therefore implies the use of unorthodox methods, such as employing expert knowledge and disease modelling. Another possibility is to estimate only a few important diseases explicitly, and use an 'all other disability' category to get an estimate of total DALYs lost (Barendregt et al, 1998). Whichever method is used, the epidemiological data needed for the disease-specific approach are bound to remain a major bottleneck.

DISABILITY WEIGHTS

All health indicators that combine morbidity and mortality to a single number somehow have to weight the morbid state in order to do so. This weighting procedure is expressed as the functions $f(\ )$ and $g(\ )$ in the equations above. The implementation of these functions varies widely. In most health expectancy indicators it is a simple dichotomous function which assigns 1 to morbid states deemed healthy enough and 0 to the ones that are not. DALYs, like the health-adjusted life expectancy (HALE), use a continuous (or near continuous) function, but, because of the disease-specific nature of DALYs, the disability weights are disease specific as well.

These disability weights have caused no end of controversy and confusion. Some of the confusion is undoubtedly due to the fact that 'disability' weights is a bit of a misnomer. Firstly the term 'disability' has different meanings: in the American literature it includes the interaction of the morbidity with the environment, while in the definition of the International Classification of Impairments, Disabilities and Handicaps (ICIDH) it does not (in the ICIDH definition it would then be 'handicap'). Secondly, in the literature 'disability' is understood as being not able to perform specific tasks, as in the activities of daily living (ADL) questionnaire. The measuring procedure for the DALY disability weights is focused on the severity of the disease and nowhere mentions specific (dis)abilities. Therefore 'severity' weights would probably have been more appropriate.

Much of the critique on the disability weights focuses on the procedure used to obtain them. Adding to the confusion is that the results reported in the World Development Report were preliminary, and that the final results of the Global Burden of Disease 1990 study used a somewhat different method. In the preliminary version experts used six disability classes, a proportion of people with the disease getting disabled, and a distribution of those disabled over the six classes. Where the weight for each class came from is not reported (Murray and Lopez, 1994). In the final version seven disability classes were used, the proportion disabled and distribution were dropped, and the weights were obtained using a formalised method called 'person trade-off' (PTO) (Murray, 1996).

There are a number of formalised methods, in addition to PTO, to obtain health-related quality of life (HRQOL) weights: standard gamble, time trade-off, visual analogue scale, and willingness to pay. Two basic requirements of these methods are validity and reliability. Reliability in this context means that repeated measurements mostly produce the same results, and can in principle be empirically assessed. Validity is the property that the indicator actually measures what it is intended to do, but this is hard to assess because HRQOL is not directly observable (Krabbe et al, 1997).

Each of these methods tries to map the multidimensional phenomenon that is HRQOL into a single number. To help people achieve this near impossible task most methods create an artificial dilemma which has to be resolved. For example, the time trade-off method asks participants to depict themselves in a given health status during one year, and then asks how much of that year of life they are prepared to give up when the remaining part would be lived in full health.

How should the validity of such procedures be judged? Given the fact that HRQOL is not directly observable, there is no obvious gold standard. Without a gold standard two other criteria remain: plausibility ('do the results look right?') and comparability of results between methods. And here the news is mostly good. The different methods produce results that rank the severest conditions on the severe end of the scale, and vice versa. The rankings are very comparable, with differences that often can be explained (for example, the time trade-off method is confounded by time preference). And while differences between cultures exist, they are not of a degree to invalidate these procedures (and in fact, the cultural differences may very well reflect cultural differences in preferences, and not in the workings of the weighting procedures) (Üstün et al, 1999).

The adoption of a summary measure of population health, which combines mortality and morbidity, necessarily implies the use of severity weights for the morbid state, either generic or disease specific (depending on the definition of morbidity as generic or disease specific). Given that, a continuous severity function is highly preferable to a dichotomous 'healthy not-healthy' one, because the latter is very sensitive for the (highly arbitrary) choice of cut-off point, and totally insensitive to differences in health that stay within one of the two domains. For example, a paraplegic who recovers enough to walk again, but still cannot climb stairs, would not show up in a 'disability-free life expectancy' as an improvement because he is still 'disabled'.

Mapping a multidimensional phenomenon into a single number inevitably implies a loss of information. In addition to this loss of information, unwanted confounding effects may crop up. While researchers should be committed to minimising the confounding and loss of information, they also should realise that a loss-less mapping simply cannot exist. This is a sobering thought, which might help to put the, at times heated, discussion on the DALY disability weights into perspective.

AGE WEIGHTS

In the original DALY specification years lost due to mortality and morbidity were weighted according to the age at which the loss occurred. Lost years occurring at very young and very old ages are valued less than those at young adult and middle age, when people are productive and often have social responsibilities. More in particular, Murray et al used a function that valued losses between the ages of 9 and 54 at more than unity, and losses outside that range at increasingly less than unity, with a value of 0 at exact age 0.

The discussion on these age weights revolved around two questions: Should there be age weighting, and if so, should it be as proposed by Murray et al? Whether there should be age weighting at all is a personal value judgement, which for that very reason can be debated endlessly. The scarce empirical work on this notion suggests that at least for high ages people tend to attach less value to loss of health (Busschbach et al, 1993). But even if this is true, one could still argue that age weighting does not belong in a population health indicator, that every loss of life is equally important, no matter at what age it occurs. Such is the nature of value judgements.

Even when agreeing to the concept of age weighting there is still room for disagreement on the actual implementation. Williams, for example, accepts the concept as such, but proposes an alternative implementation called 'fair innings' (Williams, 1999). We have objected against the age weighting as implemented in the original DALY, mainly because it simply does not do what it proposes. As we have shown elsewhere, for mortality and chronic diseases the implementation stresses losses between the ages of 0 and 27, and downplays losses at age 28 and over (Barendregt *et al*, 1996). Contrary to the intentions as expressed by Murray *et al*, the DALY implementation stresses life lost by the very young, and not by middle-aged people. Only for morbidity with very short duration is the intended age range of 9–54 being stressed; as soon as the duration becomes longer the age range starts to shift towards the younger ages (Murray and Lopez, 1996b; Barendregt and Bonneux, 1998). If age weighting is used, then at the very least it should do the job as it was intended.

DISCOUNTING

Another highly contentious feature of the original DALY implementation is discounting. In order to understand the issues here, we will first briefly review the discounting technique and the underlying concept of 'time preference', and then discuss the implementation in the DALY.

What economists call 'time preference' is the human propensity to prefer to receive money (or other goods) as soon as possible, and postpone payments as long as possible. Economists have suggested various and often conflicting explanations for this behaviour, but few doubt its existence. Just ask a child what he prefers, one cookie now or two cookies in a month's time.

Economics is the science of making choices, given scarce resources. We want to employ our resources to maximise benefits, given our preferences. The existence of time preference may affect choices when costs and benefits do not coincide in time: we will prefer, all other things being equal, a case where benefits are upfront and costs in the future rather than the other way around.

To deal with time preference economists use the discounting procedure: costs and benefits are assigned a weight that becomes smaller the further the cost or benefit is away in time. The degree of time preference is expressed in the discount rate, with 0% standing for no time preference, 3% and 5% much used values, and 10% expressing strong time preference. The calculation of these weights is usually done by a simple exponential function, which might also be called simplistic given the complex nature of time preference (Barendregt and Bonneux, 1999).

There are two issues surrounding this discounting procedure: should it be used, and if so, what discount rate is to be employed. First the latter: economists have endlessly debated what the 'right' discount rate should be, to no avail. This is not surprising: time preference is a personal value judgement, and it differs markedly between people. The best one can do is to reach a consensus, but whatever discount rate is chosen, it will always be arbitrary (Barendregt and Bonneux, 1999). In the original DALY specification a rate of 3% was used.

Then the question whether discounting should be used. Some people argue that life years should not be discounted as a matter of principle. However, simple observation makes clear that many people trade-off current pleasures for future life years (implying that those future life years are valued less), like with smoking and overeating. It was already mentioned that the time trade-off method for assessing HRQOL is confounded by time preference, and profoundly so when a long period, say 10 instead of 1 year, is being used. Of course it is nevertheless possible to maintain that discounting should not be used for life years (it is after all a value judgement), but we think that value judgements included in indicators that are meant for policy making should broadly conform to general preferences.

Still we believe the discounting in the original DALY specification to have been misplaced, for two reasons. In our discussion of time preference two concepts are central: time and choice. Both these concepts are necessary for discounting to make sense, but we doubt they are applicable in the case of the DALY. For time to be included in the DALY it is necessary to adopt the cohort perspective: a birth cohort is followed through time as it ages, develops diseases, until it becomes extinct after something like 100 years. But this cohort perspective sits uneasily with other aspects of the DALY. First of all, it would make the DALY an indicator not of current population health, but of current birth cohort health, something rather different. And secondly, it does not make sense to multiply the future morbidity and mortality rates of this birth cohort with the current cross-sectional population numbers to obtain years of life lost (YLL) and years lived with disability (YLD): the result would be a very odd mix of present and future. Therefore the 'stationary population' perspective is the appropriate one (Shryock and Siegel, 1976). In that perspective we can look at the population cross-sectionally, hence there is no time, only age. Without time there cannot be time preference, and therefore discounting is not appropriate.

The second concept central to time preference is choice. The rationale of using discounting is that when we are faced with two or more alternatives and want to choose the one we prefer, we want to include our time preference. But in most applications of the DALY there is no choice involved. When the burden of disease is estimated, no alternatives are being considered and no choices made, we are only taking stock. In the context of cost-effectiveness analysis discounting makes sense, but most applications of the DALY, including most of the Global Burden of Disease 1990 study, were not cost-effectiveness studies. When there is no choice, there is no need to take time preference into account, hence discounting is not appropriate.

All this would not matter if discounting made no difference – but it does. When thinking in the cohort perspective the time axis is about 100 years. Discounting at 3% more than halves a burden of disease that is 25 years away, at 75 years only 10% is left. The application of discounting requires careful justification, if only because of its tremendous impact, and with the DALY the justification is still lacking.

DALY, DALE, AND OTHER DEVELOPMENTS

Despite all the controversies the DALY has clearly been a success. In the wake of the first publication in the 1993 World Development Report (World Bank, 1993) a large number of publications have been devoted to the DALY. Many articles and some books have been published by the developers of the DALY, Murray and Lopez, with more results, additions and updates.

Perhaps more significantly, there are an increasing number of studies applying the concept. There have been a number of countries carrying out a burden of disease study, and more are in progress. In addition, several cost-effectiveness studies have applied the DALY indicator.

In the field of policy making the DALY has also been successful. The WHO has adopted the concept of burden of disease as the basis for the policy recommendations it makes to the member countries and is carrying out a Global Burden of Disease 2000 study.

However, the controversial nature of the original DALY is a problem for the WHO, which is not an academic institution and depends on consensus to get its policy recommendations accepted. The typical WHO procedure to achieve consensus is by calling expert meetings, and compiling the discussions into a report with recommendations. In December 1999 a WHO expert meeting on summary measures of population health was held in Marrakech. Discussions ranged from basic concepts to valuation methods to goodness and fairness and the ethical implications of summary measures. A book with contributions from participants is currently in preparation.

With the consensus process still in progress it is not clear what the specification of the new DALY will be, but the following looks likely. The DALY will retain its disease-specific character. The built-in value judgements will be restricted to the minimum: the disease-specific disability weights. These are necessary to sum morbidity across diseases, and to combine morbidity and mortality to a single indicator. The other value judgements, age weighting and discounting, will be dropped from the basic indicator, and no new value judgements (such as for equity) will be added, but the data will be presented in such a way that users can apply these and other weights as they think fit. While the DALY can never be all things to all people, this will be a lot closer to it.

Another development has been the disability-adjusted life expectancy (DALE). As noted at the Chicago REVES conference (REVES 8, 1995), the data needed for calculating DALYs also allow calculation of its health expectancy equivalent, the DALE (Barendregt *et al*, 1998). The DALE uses a mixture of multistate and Sullivan methods: multistate models for some disease(s) of specific interest, and a Sullivan 'all other causes' disability to account for the disability not caused by the diseases of interest. This construction allows estimation of the impact on life expectancy and DALE of changes in disease epidemiology and of risk factor modification, such as smoking reduction (Barendregt and Bonneux, 1998).

The advantages of the DALE over the DALY are the ones of a health expectancy over a health gap measure: there is no need for an arbitrarily defined ideal health, it is more readily interpreted, and, at least in principle, comparable between countries and over time. In addition, leaving out the contentious value judgements such as age weighting and discounting vastly increases acceptability of the indicator. The disadvantage is that it is not fitting for cost-effectiveness analysis, where real population numbers are needed

Murray and Lopez have apparently concluded that the advantages of the DALE in some circumstances outweigh its disadvantages. The DALYs for the eight world regions of the Global Burden of Disease 1990 study have been recalculated to DALEs (Murray and Lopez, 1997). The disabilities caused by the 100 or so diseases and conditions included were added up to a total disability prevalence by age, and converted to a DALE using regional life tables and Sullivan's method.

Interestingly, one of the cherished findings of health expectancy using a dichotomous health status evaluation function is not being confirmed by DALE estimates with a near continuous function. Time and again estimates of disability-free life expectancy (DFLE) have found that women have a longer life expectancy than men, but that the DFLE is virtually the same, implying that women spend a larger part of their lives with disability. DALE estimates show that both sexes spend the same proportion (about 10% in Western countries) with disability. This supports the idea that men may spend less time with disability, but that the disability is of a more severe kind. This makes sense, because severe disability is strongly correlated with mortality. It therefore seems that, from a burden of disease perspective, the DFLE finding is an artefact of the dichotomous disability weight function.

Updated burden of disease data for 14 world regions have more recently been used as the basis for the World Health Report 2000 (World Health Organization, 2000). There DALEs for 191 member states of WHO were presented and used to assess the attainment of the countries' health systems.

Because the burden of disease data are on the level of global regions and not country-specific, these data were supplemented by non-disease- but country-specific health survey data (Mathers *et al*, 2001). The rather convoluted estimation procedure underlines once more how much the availability of epidemiological data is the bottleneck for this kind of exercise.

The World Health Report 2000 did not stop at DALEs for all WHO member states. Using additional information on the distribution of health and the financing of the health care system, among other things, the report presents for each country an index of health system performance. The report has drawn a storm of protests (Anonymous, 2001; Almeida *et al*, 2001; Houweling *et al*, 2001; Wibulpolprasert and Tangcharoensathien, 2001; Williams, 2001; Wolfson and Rowe, 2001). While most of the comments agree to some extent that estimating and comparing health systems' performance is a good thing, all point out that methodological concerns and, above all, current data availability in fact preclude making such an analysis. We can only hope that this premature exercise has not discredited the approach critically, and that it leads to increased efforts to gather the data necessary for this kind of analysis. That would be a great step forward.

CONCLUSION

In our opinion the main characteristic of both DALY and DALE as composite population health indicators is that they describe population health status based on a disease-specific approach. This characteristic is simultaneously their strength and their weakness. It is their strength because it makes it possible to link the disease-specific level to overall population health, and it is their weakness because of the data requirements this implies.

Making the link between (potential) disease-specific and risk factor interventions on the one hand, and the population health status indicator on the other, is the crux to making the indicator relevant for policy making (Barendregt *et al*, 1998). Of course one could start from the generic morbidity level, such as disability, and then attribute the morbidity to various causes, and a few attempts in this direction have been made (Nusselder, 2000). And of course, in a world of complete and perfect knowledge, both approaches would deliver the same results.

But the world is not perfect, and, as far as the availability of epidemiological data is concerned, it is not likely to become so any time soon. Therefore both approaches have their merits, with the disease-specific approach at an advantage for diseases whose epidemiology is well known.

Meanwhile, with all the sophisticated methods and refined indicators, to improve the usefulness of summary measures of population health the main way ahead remains working on better epidemiological data.

REFERENCES

Almeida, C., Braveman, P., Gold, M.R., Szwarcwald, C.L., Ribeiro, J.M., Miglionico, A., *et al* (2001) 'Methodological concerns and recommendations on policy consequences of the World Health Report 2000', *Lancet* 357(9269), 1692–1697.

Anonymous (2001) 'Why rank countries by health performance?', *Lancet* 357(9269), 1633.

Barendregt, J. and Bonneux, L. (1998) *Degenerative Disease in an Aging Population. Models and Conjectures.* Rotterdam: Erasmus University.

Barendregt, J.J. and Bonneux, L. (1999) 'The trouble with health economics', *European Journal of Public Health* 9(4), 309–312.

Barendregt, J.J., Bonneux, L. and Maas, P.J., van der (1996) 'DALYs: the age-weights on balance', *Bulletin of the World Health Organization* 74(4), 439–443.

Barendregt, J.J., Bonneux, L. and Maas, P.J. van der (1998) 'Health expectancy: from a population health indicator to a tool for policy making', *Journal of Aging and Health* 10(2), 242–258.

Busschbach, J.J., Hessing, D.J. and de Charro, F.T. (1993) 'The utility of health at different stages in life: a quantitative approach', *Social Science and Medicine* 37(2), 153–158.

Houweling, T.A., Kunst, A.E. and Mackenbach, J.P. (2001) 'World Health Report 2000: inequality index and socioeconomic inequalities in mortality', *Lancet* 357(9269), 1671–1672.

Krabbe, P.F., Essink-Bot, M.L. and Bonsel, G.J. (1997) 'The comparability and reliability of five health-state valuation methods', *Social Science and Medicine* 45(11), 1641–1652.

Mathers, C.D., Sadana, R., Salomon, J.A., Murray, C.J. and Lopez, A.D. (2001) 'Healthy life expectancy in 191 countries, 1999', *Lancet* 357(9269), 1685–1691.

Murray, C.J. (1994) 'Quantifying the burden of disease: the technical basis for disability-adjusted life years', *Bulletin of the World Health Organization* 72(3), 429–445.

Murray, C.J. (1996) 'Rethinking DALYs', in Murray, C.J. and Lopez, A.D. (eds) *The Global Burden of Disease.* Boston: Harvard School of Public Health, 1996. (Global Burden of Disease and Injury Series; vol. I.)

Murray, C.J. and Lopez, A.D. (1994) 'Quantifying disability: data, methods and results', *Bulletin of the World Health Organization* 72(3), 481–494.

Murray, C.J. and Lopez, A.D. (1996a) *Global Burden of Disease and Injury: Executive Summary.* Boston: Harvard School of Public Health, 1996. (Murray, C.J. and Lopez, A.D. (eds) Global Burden of Disease and Injury Series.)

Murray, C.J. and Lopez, A.D. (1996b) 'The incremental effect of age-weighting on YLLs, YLDs, and DALYs: a response [comment]', *Bulletin of the World Health Organization* 74(4), 445–446.

Murray, C.J.L. and Lopez, A.D. (1997) 'Regional patterns of disability-free life expectancy and disability-adjusted life expectancy: Global Burden of Disease Study', *Lancet* 349, 1347–1352.

Murray, C.J.L., Salomon, J.A. and Mathers, C.D. (2000) 'A critical examination of summary measures of population health', *Bulletin of the World Health Organization* 78, 981–994.

Nusselder, W.J. (2000) 'A method of decomposing differences in health expectancy by cause', Paper presented at the REVES 12 conference, Los Angeles, March 2000.

Shryock, H.S. and Siegel, J.S. (1976) *The Methods and Materials of Demography*, condensed edition. Orlando: Academic Press.

Üstün, T.B., Rehm, J., Chatterji, S., Saxena, S., Trotter, R., Room, R., *et al* (1999) 'Multiple-informant ranking of the disabling effects of different health conditions in 14 countries: WHO/NIH Joint Project CAR Study Group', *Lancet* 354(9173), 111–115.

Wibulpolprasert, S. and Tangcharoensathien, V. (2001) 'Health systems performance – what's next?', *Bulletin of the World Health Organization* 79(6), 489.

Williams, A. (1999) 'Calculating the global burden of disease: time for a strategic reappraisal?' *Health Economics* 8(1), 1–8.

Williams, A. (2001) 'Science or marketing at WHO? A commentary on "World Health 2000"', *Health Economics* 10(2), 93–100.

Wolfson, M. and Rowe, G. (2001) 'On measuring inequalities in health', *Bulletin of the World Health Organization* 79(6), 553–560.

World Bank (1993) *Investing in Health*. New York: Oxford University Press (World Development Report).

World Health Organization (2000) *The World Health Report 2000: Health Systems: Improving Performance*. Geneva: WHO.

14

Classification and Harmonisation

HENDRIEK BOSHUIZEN and ROM J.M. PERENBOOM*

National Institute for Public Health and the Environment, Bilthoven, The Netherlands and *TNO Prevention and Health, Leiden, The Netherlands

INTRODUCTION

When Sullivan in 1971 proposed a simple health indicator which he called 'life expectancy free of disability' (Sullivan, 1971), he combined mortality data with the prevalence rates of disability for the US population. Starting in the early 1980s, this indicator became increasingly popular. Calculations based on Sullivan's method were repeated for other countries (Colvez, 1980; Colvez and Blanchet, 1983; Wilkins and Adams, 1983; Katz *et al*, 1983; Robine and Colvez, 1986; Bebbington, 1988; Egidi, 1988). Some of those early researchers used disability data that resembled those used by Sullivan; others (Katz *et al*, 1983; Bebbington, 1988; Egidi, 1988; Crimmins *et al*, 1989; Ginneken and Water, 1990; Ginneken *et al*, 1989; Rasmussen and Brønnum-Hansen, 1990) applied the principle of combining a life table with prevalence rates to other types of data on health. The fact that the term 'disability-free life expectancy' for this indicator during the 1990s gave way to the more generic term 'health expectancy' reflects this use of the indicator for other aspects of health than disability alone.

As the number of researchers in the field increased, so did the number of versions of health expectancies. When in 1989 the International Research Network on Health Expectancy (REVES) was formed by the researchers in this field, the promotion of the international harmonisation of the data collection and calculation procedures for this health indicator was formulated as an important task for the network. Comparable calculation procedures, based on data that are collected in a comparable way, will make it possible to compare countries and thereby enhance the usefulness of this indicator for policy making.

Determining Health Expectancies. Edited by J-M. Robine, C. Jagger, C.M. Mathers, E.M. Crimmins and R.M. Suzman.
© 2003 John Wiley & Sons, Ltd

In this chapter we will describe the progress that has been made during the last 10 years with this harmonisation. As it was soon realised that the different forms of health expectancies have different uses, and therefore are not just redundant variants, classification of types of health expectancy was added to the goal of harmonisation. The process of harmonisation (and classification) relates to three different aspects:

- the harmonisation of the type of health state used,
- the harmonisation of the instruments used to measure these health states,
- the harmonisation of the calculation procedures for the integrated health measures.

We will treat these three subjects separately.

THE TYPE OF HEALTH STATUS DATA USED

Early studies (van Ginneken and van de Water, 1990; van Ginneken *et al*, 1989) showed – not unexpectedly – that when other types of health status data are used within the same population, this will result in substantially different health expectancies. A less obvious result from these studies was that this affects not only the absolute magnitude of the health expectancy calculated, but also the magnitude of the differences between groups, such as between males and females.

However, it was soon realised that different types of prevalence data differ because they measure different things. Some try to capture 'ill health' in a broad sense, like including everything that reduces quality of life, while others restrict themselves to looking at disability. Populations can be similar when looking at one aspect of health, but may differ in another aspect. A first recognition within the REVES network, underlying the first report of the REVES committee on the Conceptual Harmonisation of Statistics for the study of Disability-free Life Expectancy (Chamie, 1990), was therefore that health status has different aspects, and that health expectancies can be calculated using any one of them. Instead of 'harmonising' (forcing a common choice of one aspect of health) it was considered more fruitful to classify the aspects currently used and aim efforts toward harmonisation at a lower level: towards the use of common measurement instruments within each concept of health (Robine and Michel, 1990). An important recommendation of the REVES committee on the Conceptual Harmonisation of Statistics for the study of Disability-free Life Expectancy was to use the framework of the ICIDH (see box) as the conceptual base for such a classification (Chamie, 1990). Furthermore, the committee proposed some changes to the ICIDH framework. It proposed distinguishing between two types of disabilities: functional limitations and activity restrictions. Functional limitations are specific reductions in bodily functions, described at the level of the person, e.g. seeing, hearing, grasping or climbing stairs. Activity restrictions are reductions in daily activities such as dressing, bathing or feeding oneself. Activity restrictions thus refer to more complex activities. Functional limitations are closer to impairments, while activity restrictions are closer to handicaps.

Four basic concepts of handicaps were selected (mobility, physical independence, occupation and social integration) for which tentative questionnaire items were formulated for further discussion (Chamie, 1990).

> The International Classification of Impairments, Disabilities and Handicaps (ICIDH) is a classification for the consequences of disease, introduced by the World Health Organization in 1980. In this classification the consequences of disease are classified as impairment (any loss or abnormalities of psychological, physiological or anatomical structure of the body), disability (restriction or lack of ability to perform an activity in the manner or within the range considered normal for a human being) or handicap (disadvantage that limits or prevents the fulfilment of a role that is normal (depending on age, sex and social and cultural factors) for that individual). The ICIDH framework implies that an impairment may result in a disability, which in its turn may lead to a handicap. The reader is referred to Badley (1993) for further information on the ICIDH.

Building on this work, Mathers *et al* (1994) devised recommendations for a terminology that would bring some order into the field. Boshuizen and van de Water (Boshuizen *et al*, 1994; Boshuizen and Water, 1994, 1995) showed that the ICIDH is indeed a useful classification scheme, and could be used to bring some order into the work that had been done. However, not all work on health expectancy could be fitted into the ICIDH classification. This is largely due to health expectancies that look at health from a broader perspective and try to capture 'health' in all its dimensions, not only limited to absence of disease, impairments, disabilities and handicaps. This line of approach has yielded two types of health expectancies: the first uses self-rated (perceived) health state e.g. the Netherlands (van Ginneken *et al*, 1991; Perenboom *et al*, 1993; van de Water *et al*, 1996); Belgium (Van Oyen and Roelands, 1994); Curaçao (van Ginneken *et al*, 1994), Norway (Grotvedt and Viksand, 1994), Spain (Regidor *et al*, 1995), Italy (Egidi, 1988) and Denmark (Rasmussen and Brønnum Hansen, 1990); the other approach uses a multidimensional health index (Pettersson, 1991). It was therefore suggested that a health expectancy based on perceived health should be added to the classification scheme. Another example of a health expectancy that is difficult to fit into the ICIDH classification is that of Liu and Manton (Liu *et al*, 1990), who created a classification of disabled persons through a multivariate statistical method from data on functional limitations and activity restrictions. The empirical categorisation that resulted from this multivariate method was used to calculate health expectancies. So instead of a categorisation based on a preconceived conceptual framework such as the ICIDH, an empirical categorisation of disability was used. Empirical classifications are useful for the theoretical development of concepts on which classification systems can be based. However, as an empirical classification is data-driven, health expectancies based on these classifications are not suited as a base for comparing populations, and thus excluded from the classification scheme.

Robine *et al* (1994) proposed some further changes to the classification scheme, amongst others adding health-adjusted life expectancies (HALE) to the classification schema of health expectancies (HE), as originally proposed by Robine and Michel (1992). To date, the HALE results from a somewhat different conceptual approach from the classical health expectancy that calculates life expectancy in a particular health state. A HALE summarises the health of a population in a single number, equating a year in a particular

Table 14.1. The classification scheme for health expectancies and health-adjusted life expectancies (adapted from Robine *et al*, 1994)

Type	Concept	Health expectancy
Health state expectancy (HSE)	ICD-10: Disease	Disease-free Dementia-free
	ICIDH: Impairment Disability	Impairment-free Functional limitation-free from a list of impairments Activity restriction-free specific activity restriction-free
	Handicap	General handicap-free Independent life Active life (ADL/IADL) Mobility handicap-free Occupational handicap-free Other handicap-free
	Perceived health	In good health
Health-adjusted life expectancy (HALE)	Equivalent to years in full health	Health-adjusted

health state to a shorter time period in full health, while a classical HE provides a set of expectancies in each health state (e.g. the set of 'life expectancy with disability', and 'life expectancies without disability'). For clarity, the term health state expectancy (HSE) was introduced for the latter. As discussed more fully in Chapters 11 and 12, HALE and HSE can be viewed as the two main types of HE, rather than the HALE being one of many types of HE. Table 14.1 gives the classification scheme as proposed in 1995 (Robine *et al*, 1994), after incorporating this newer point of view.

The classification scheme in Table 14.1 makes it possible to classify different health expectancies into different categories. Such a classification shows that in the wake of Sullivan's work, at first mostly other 'disability-free life expectancies' were calculated, which we now classify as handicap-free life expectancies (see box) e.g. in the US (Colvez, 1980; Colvez and Blanchet, 1983); Canada (Wilkins and Adams, 1983); UK (Bebbington, 1988); France (Robine and Colvez, 1986); and Denmark (Rasmussen and Brønnum-Hansen,

---

Sullivan (1971) developed an indicator 'life expectancy free of disability'. In Sullivan's calculation, disability was defined as either:

- being confined to a residential institution for health care;
- having enduring limitations in the amount or kind of major activity.

Major activity is defined as housework, work, attending school, and play, for housewives, workers, school-aged children and pre-school children, respectively.

This definition agrees closely with the definition of a handicap according to the ICIDH: A handicap is a disadvantage experienced by the individual as a result of impairments and disabilities that limits or prevents the fulfilment of a role that is normal (depending on age, sex, and social and cultural factors) for that individual. So looking at Sullivan's indicator from the ICIDH conceptual framework, it would be better called 'handicap-free life expectancy'.

A similar confusion of terminology is observed in the model proposed by Nagi, where the term 'disability' is used for what the ICIDH calls 'handicap', while 'functional limitations' is used instead of what the ICIDH calls 'disabilities' (Verbrugge and Jette, 1994).

1990). Disability-free life expectancies were further calculated based on the indicator for disability proposed by the OECD, e.g. the Netherlands (van Ginneken *et al*, 1989; Perenboom *et al*, 1993; van de Water *et al*, 1996); Denmark (Rasmussen and Brønnum-Hansen, 1990); Canada (Wilkins and Adams, 1992a, 1992b)). The OECD indicator contains items on activity restrictions as well as on functional limitations, and therefore these health expectancies are not easily classified within the scheme presented in Table 14.1. Handicap-free life expectancies based on activities of daily living have mainly been calculated for the United States, under the name 'active life expectancy' (e.g. Katz *et al*, 1983; Rogers *et al*, 1990).

After the introduction of the ICIDH, surveys were developed based on the ICIDH model, and disability-free life expectancies and handicap-free life expectancies have been calculated from data resulting from those surveys. In the UK, for example, the data from the OPCS Disability Surveys were used to calculate disability-free life expectancies for 10 degrees of severity (Bebbington, 1989). In Australia, Mathers (1991) calculated both handicap-free and disability-free life expectancies from the data of the Australian Bureau of Statistics (ABS) Surveys of Disability and Handicap (1981 and 1988), and in Spain a disability-free life expectancy was calculated from data of the Survey on Disabilities, Impairments and Handicaps (Gutiérrez Fisac and Regidor Poyatos, 1991).

Although most authors calculate handicap-free or disability-free life expectancy, there is no reason not to calculate impairment-free life expectancy. This has been done most comprehensively for Ethiopia by Brown (1993), who even used the ICIDH classification codes for impairments. Others calculated impairment-free life expectancies for several global categories of impairments (Pope and Tarlov, 1991). Finally, some investigators also calculate general (chronic) disease-free life expectancy, e.g. Rasmussen and Brønnum-Hansen (1990) and Pope and Tarlov (1991). To date, however, the most commonly calculated disease-free life expectancy is the life expectancy free of dementia (e.g. Ritchie *et al*, 1993; Perenboom *et al*, 1996; Roelands *et al*, 1994; Ritchie *et al*, 1994a, 1994b; Sauvaget *et al*, 1997).

The concept of HALE was promoted strongly by its use in the Global Burden of Disease Study (Murray and Lopez, 1996). For a more comprehensive description of all types of health expectancies calculated, the reader is referred to the work of Romieu and Robine, who through the years kept track of all health expectancies calculated internationally and provided the network with reviews (Romieu *et al*, 1997; REVES, 1993; Romieu, 1991; Romieu and Robine, 1994).

Since the development of this classification, a new type of health expectancy has emerged, the 'life expectancy in good generic mental health' (Jagger *et al*, 1998). Generic mental health is mostly measured by the 12-item version of the General Health Questionnaire (GHQ-12) (Goldberg and Williams, 1988) or the

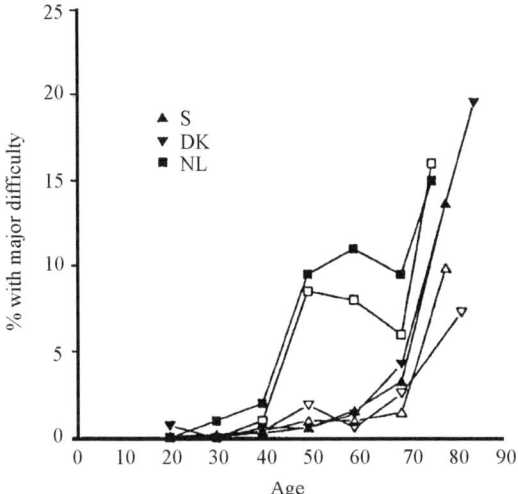

Sweden (S): Answers 'no' to the question: Are you able to read without difficulty the ordinary print in a newspaper (with or without glasses)?

Denmark (DK): Answers 'no' or 'yes, with major difficulty' to the question: Are you able to read ordinary newspaper print (with glasses, if normally worn)?

Netherlands (NL): Answers 'no' or 'yes, with major difficulty' to the question: Are your eyes good enough to be able to read the small print in a newspaper (if necessary with glasses or contact lenses)?

Figure 14.1. Percentage of women (black symbols) and men (open symbols) who have difficulties reading a newspaper, from countries using slightly different wording of this item from the OECD indicator. Reproduced with permission from Boshuizen (1993)

5-item mental health index (MHI-5), a subscale of the SF-36 (Ware *et al*, 1997). As is the case with perceived health, it is not clear where generic mental health fits into the framework of the ICIDH. For the moment we would therefore suggest regarding this as a separate category.

Although some health expectancies are classified as being of the same type, this does not make them necessarily comparable. Boshuizen *et al* (1994; Boshuizen and van de Water, 1994) took a closer look at the measurement instruments that were used to collect the data on which health expectancies are based, and concluded that within a single category of health expectancy the large majority of the health expectancies calculated are not comparable. Often small changes in the wording of questions can have a large impact on the size of the recorded prevalence rates (Boshuizen, 1993), as illustrated in Figure 14.1. Therefore a continuing effort to standardise measurement instruments is needed.

As we will show in the following section, international harmonisation of the instruments used for health status measurement is a slow, time-consuming process. Within the REVES network some progress has been made, especially in the area of dementia-free life expectancies. Members of the REVES network have calculated comparable dementia-free life expectancies, based on the DSM-III-R, for the United Kingdom (Ritchie *et al*, 1993), Belgium (Roelands *et al*, 1994), France (Ritchie *et al*, 1994b), the Netherlands (Perenboom *et al*, 1996) and Australia (Ritchie *et al*, 1994a) (see Chapter 8).

HARMONISATION OF MEASUREMENT INSTRUMENTS

Most health expectancies are based on prevalence data from national health interview surveys. In order to arrive at comparable health expectancies for different countries, the data in these surveys should be collected with common instruments.

The idea of instigating common measurement instruments in national surveys, however, is not unique to research in the field of health expectancy, but is a common goal for those involved in the monitoring of health, especially at the international level. In the 1980s, increasing contacts between statistical offices of different countries, ministries of health and public health researchers already pointed to the need for an international exchange of knowledge and instruments for health interview surveys (Bruin *et al*, 1996).

This means that from many different groups initiatives have been taken and still are being taken to harmonise data collection on health status or to develop standardised measurement instruments for health interview surveys. We will briefly discuss four initiatives, those of the Organisation for Economic Co-operation and Development (OECD), the United Nations (UN), the World Health Organization (WHO) and the European Community (EC).

INITIATIVES OF THE OECD

In the late 1970s, the OECD decided that in addition to economic indicators, it also needed indicators of well-being. One of the indicators needed was an indicator of long-term disability. As a result of a common development effort, in 1981 an indicator for long-term disability was proposed by the OECD (McWhinnie, 1981). This indicator was – with some changes – implemented in several national surveys (e.g. Canada, the Netherlands and Denmark). However, its use never became widespread, and the implemented versions use slightly different wording, which sometimes significantly influences the outcomes, as illustrated by Figure 14.1.

Health expectancies were calculated based on this indicator of disability for the Netherlands (van Ginneken and van de Water, 1990; van Ginneken *et al*, 1989, 1991; Perenboom *et al*, 1993; van de Water *et al*, 1996) Denmark (Rasmussen and Brønnum-Hansen, 1990) and Canada (Wilkins and Adams,

1992a, 1992b). The first three studies used only a subset of the items from the entire OECD instrument, while the last added more items. However, the number of items is probably less important for the resulting health expectancy than the least severe item included, and the exact wording of this least severe item.

INITIATIVES OF THE UNITED NATIONS

In 1982 the UN General Assembly adopted the World Programme of Action concerning Disabled Persons. It recommended that governments should collect data on disability, e.g. through national population censuses or health interview surveys. The Statistical Office of the UN has worked since on the design of statistical methodology and standards for data collection (Chamie, 1992). In 1994 an expert group meeting, including members of the REVES network, was organised in cooperation with Statistics Netherlands on the development of impairment, disability and handicap statistics (for short: IDH statistics), reviewing existing disability data collection methods and standards. The meeting identified a set of guidelines for use in censuses, surveys and registrations. The meeting was a first step in the preparation of a handbook on census and survey methods for the development of IDH statistics (Ooijendijk and Geurts, 1994), addressing statistical offices and research organisations and providing them with guidelines on the collection of IDH statistics in censuses and surveys, on their analysis and on the dissemination of results for policy purposes.

INITIATIVES FROM THE WORLD HEALTH ORGANIZATION

In 1977 the WHO launched its 'Health For All' programme. In 1984, the member states of the WHO European region adopted 38 targets. Target 35 states that health information systems in all member states should actively support the formulation, implementation, monitoring and evaluation of the 'Health For All' policy.

Also, due to the health monitoring initiated by the WHO 'Health For All' programme, a growing need for comparable health information was felt. At the end of the 1980s, an inventory of the coverage of indicators in health interview surveys was carried out by Statistics Netherlands, at the request of the WHO Regional Office for Europe (Evers, 1993). Included were the countries in the European Region, and Australia, Canada, Japan and the United States. The study also made an inventory of the questions used in the different countries. It showed that many questions contained the same subject matter, but that the health interview surveys could nevertheless not provide comparable information because questions on the same subject lacked uniformity. Therefore the WHO Regional Office for Europe initiated a series of Consultations to Develop

Common Methods and Instruments for Health Interview Surveys. At the first Consultation (World Health Organization, 1989) instruments were recommended for three Health for All indicators relevant to the calculation of health expectancy: Perceived health, long-term disability and temporary disability. Soon after, the Council of Europe adopted the recommended long-term disability instrument (Council of Europe, 1990), with a few additions later adopted by the second consultation (World Health Organization, 1991) as the minimum set of questions to be used in health interview surveys. At the third consultation (World Health Organization, 1993) an instrument was recommended for measuring temporary disabilities due to mental health problems. In the near future proposals are expected for standard instruments for measuring chronic physical conditions, short-term disabilities, mental health and quality of life.

In 1992 the WHO Regional Office for Europe investigated the opinions of the national bureaus for statistics on the opportunities for harmonisation, and on whether they planned to use the recommended instruments in future health interview surveys (Nossikov, 1992). This study showed that in many cases the instruments planned for use in national surveys differed to some extent from the recommended instruments. In most countries questions were asked concerning perceived health and temporary disability, but many different versions of these questions existed. Recently the comparability of European health interview surveys has been reviewed again (Hupkens *et al*, 1999). It was concluded that – with the exception of body mass index – the most frequently used measures of health still were at best only partly comparable.

This experience in trying to harmonise health interview surveys has shown that differences in existing health interview surveys in various countries, although often unnecessary, are difficult to overcome because there is considerable reluctance to change existing survey instruments (Bruin *et al*, 1996). Once a country has used a specific question in the past, it is advantageous to keep it unchanged in order to permit trend evaluation at the national level. However, for countries that start performing health interview surveys, it is easier to adopt the recommended questions.

Another important development was the publication of the World Health Report 2000 (World Health Organization, 2000), where, following the Global Burden of Disease Study (Murray and Lopez, 1996), disability-adjusted life expectancies (DALE) were calculated and compared for 191 countries. The health state data used for each country were based on a complex mixture of expert opinions, cause-specific mortality data, some epidemiological data and an obscure statistical analysis of data from household surveys. To improve on this, the WHO has initiated a comparative study in 70 countries using a new instrument based on the ICIDH, investigating seven core domains of health state. This study uses performance tests and vignettes to calibrate self-reported data between countries. It is expected to yield data that are more comparable internationally than those available to date.

INITIATIVES OF THE EUROPEAN COMMUNITY

Although public health is primarily the responsibility of the individual member states of the European Union, the European Community nevertheless is meant to contribute to a high level of health protection for its population, by actions supporting member states' policies and programmes in this field. The European Commission has recognised that relevant health information should be the basis for such actions, and that currently data are insufficiently comparable. Therefore, in 1997 a programme of community action on health monitoring was adopted. One project within this programme is the Euro-REVES II project, aiming to produce a coherent set of harmonised health expectancy indicators for the European Union. It has proposed five instruments for measuring (1) general disability; (2) general perceived health; (3) physical and sensory functional limitations; (4) problems with personal care activities; and (5) mental health. A second phase will focus on instruments for measuring (6) chronic morbidity in general; (7) more specific chronic morbidity; (8) cognitive functional limitations; (9) problems with household activities; (10) problems with activities of daily living; (11) specific aspects of perceived health (Robine *et al*, 2000).

In other projects within the Health Monitoring Programme of the European Union, the possibilities of harmonisation of data collection in health interview surveys are also addressed, by defining a set of key indicators to be monitored (ECHI, 2001), by establishing databases with information on questions used (Eijk, 1999) and by developing conversion methods for data collected by similar, but not identical instruments (Van Buuren *et al*, 2001). Within the European Community, the statistical office (EUROSTAT) collects data on a limited scale (EURO-barometer and European Community Household Panel). Although the health-related data in these surveys are limited, they might nevertheless permit some comparisons. EUROSTAT has also a taskforce on health interview surveys, whose mission includes issues of harmonisation.

THE ROLE OF THE REVES NETWORK

Members of the REVES network have been involved in most of the initiatives described above. Apart from this, within REVES in 1995 an initiative was taken by Lois Verbrugge to develop a special common measuring instrument, the global disability indicator (see Chapter 10). The idea behind this instrument was to devise a single question indicator to measure disability, similar to the question on self-rated health. It was discussed during the REVES meeting in Rome. The contribution of the Euro-REVES II project that aims at making recommendations for the EU Health Monitoring Programme has already been described above.

OTHER DEVELOPMENTS

The initiatives for harmonisation described above have resulted – until now – in only a few instances of actual data collection with recommended instruments, mostly in newly established health interview surveys, e.g. Bulgaria (Mutafova et al, 1997). In the meantime, therefore, other solutions must be sought.

Advanced statistical techniques might be useful to make the best of existing data. Imagine there are data available from three studies, of which the first measures disability with instruments A and B, the second measures it with only instrument A, while the third measures it with only B. The general principle of such techniques is now to use the relation between A and B as observed in the first study to calculate equivalent rates in all three studies. In practice, the first study will often be a survey aimed at collecting detailed information on a specific subject (where there is room for using several instruments) or a special methodological (pilot) study, while the other studies are general health surveys. As an example, such a technique (one called polytomous Rasch analysis) has been applied in order to compare severity of disability as measured by different instruments (Van Buuren and Hopman-Rock, 2001). A necessary condition for such methods is that A and B measure the same entity. In other words, the technique only works if enough overlapping information in the existing information can be found. A pilot study within the Health Monitoring Programme showed that for walking and dressing disability, this situation did not arise, and a conversion key could be made (Van Buuren et al, 2001).

Such advanced statistical methods will contribute to making the data comparable that have already been collected and will be collected in the near future with different instruments. However, these methods will always involve making assumptions. Therefore the collection of really comparable data must always be preferred.

When multiple questions are used to measure a concept such as disability, disability is usually defined as being present when it is recorded in answer to at least one question. In such cases, the questions that capture the least severe level of disability will yield the highest disability rates and thus influence the composite prevalence rate most. When working on harmonisation, therefore, these questions should get most attention.

Up to this point initiatives for harmonisation have not resulted in large-scale collection of comparable data. Some comparable data will become available from special international surveys, but the number of respondents per country in these surveys is often small relative to that of national surveys. However, new opportunities for obtaining comparable data are emerging. In recent times the standardisation of questionnaires has become more valued within the scientific community too. Those who have developed such questionnaires often actively discourage users from making changes to the wording of questions. One of the measurement instruments for health status that resulted from this autonomous development is the SF-36 (Ware *et al*, 1997). The SF-36 is an instrument developed to measure health status of the population based on the broad WHO definition of health. The instrument has eight subscales, each measuring a separate dimension of health: Physical function, Social functioning, Physical role limitations, Emotional role limitations, Mental health, Energy and vitality, Pain and General health perception. There also is a 12-item variant of the SF-36 (the SF-12). This 12-item variant (which contains one or two items from every dimension of the SF-36) has been developed to provide a shorter alternative to the SF-36 (Gandek *et al*, 1998). The SF-12 yields two summary scores, one for the mental and one for the physical component of health. The SF-36 or SF-12 have already been incorporated into a few health interview surveys (e.g. Belgium, Norway and Great Britain), and are planned to be incorporated elsewhere (e.g. the Netherlands). They have also been used in many ad hoc surveys from research institutes. The subscale for mental health has already been used for the calculation of health expectancy in Denmark (Brønnum-Hansen and Rasmussen, 1996) and the Netherlands (Perenboom and Herten, 1998, 1999). The EuroQol (Krabbe *et al*, 1999) may offer similar possibilities in the future.

HARMONISATION OF CALCULATIONS

One important methodological question is whether to use the Sullivan method, or a multistate or multiple decrement method. This topic has received much attention during REVES meetings. For a discussion the reader is referred to the excellent discussions of Crimmins *et al* (1993) and Chapter 11 of this book. In most countries, however, only the Sullivan method is feasible. Therefore we will limit our discussion to the Sullivan method.

In applying the Sullivan method there are some choices to be made. Boshuizen *et al* (1994; Boshuizen and van de Water, 1994) made an inventory of the ways in which health expectancies have been calculated, and observed two points on which calculations differ:

1. The choice of the width of the age strata
2. Whether crude age- and sex-specific prevalence data are used or random fluctuations are smoothed away using statistical models.

Mathers (1991) studied the influence of these variations. From his data it can be concluded that a stratum width of 5 years up to the age of 85 is fine enough to avoid serious bias. Smoothing did not make a substantial difference. The latter result was to be expected, as in the Sullivan method the statistical errors in each stratum are averaged out by summing the healthy years lived in each stratum. The data from Mathers (1991) even show that when smoothing is done on crudely stratified data, this could introduce substantial bias in the estimated prevalences for higher ages, due to the uncertainties involved in extrapolating outside the range of observed values. For the multistate method, however, smoothing does have an important function, as in this method, errors in incidence rates propagate themselves in the calculations at higher ages.

Recently a manual has been produced as a result of the Euro-REVES I programme, describing in detail the calculation method to be used when applying the Sullivan method (Jagger, 1997).

CONCLUSIONS: THE RESULTS OF 10 YEARS OF THE REVES NETWORK

In the past 10 years, some issues have smoothly and gradually been agreed upon. Consensus has been reached on the manner in which calculations according to the Sullivan method should best be carried out (Perenboom and Herten, 1998), and on a classification system for health expectancies (Robine *et al*, 1994). One important problem, however, still defies attempts at harmonisation: harmonisation of the basic data collection processes. This is not a problem unique to the REVES network, but is common to all those involved in health monitoring at an international level. Several attempts have been made to improve the situation, but progress is slow, due to the inertia of the process of carrying out national health surveys, where changing questions will hamper the evaluation of trends at a national level. Recommended instruments by the advocates of international harmonisation are mostly incorporated in new health interview surveys, or when a new instrument is added. Advanced statistical methods might contribute to making data collected with different instruments comparable, but will always involve making assumptions. Therefore the collection of really comparable data must always be preferred. The emerging trend towards incorporation of the SF-12 (or SF-36) in existing health interview surveys might be a very good opportunity for calculating more comparable health expectancies in the future. For other types of health expectancies, however, strong efforts to harmonise the collection of data are needed, not only for the sake of the harmonisation of health expectancy, but also because it is of general interest to other fields of health monitoring. In the dispute on the value of the DALEs calculated in the World Health Report 2000, the absence of comparable health data has been brought forcefully to the attention of policy makers. Hopefully this will accelerate the efforts for implementing standard instruments in national health surveys.

ACKNOWLEDGEMENT

The authors thank Peter Achterberg for his many very useful comments on the manuscript.

REFERENCES

Badley, E.M. (1993) 'An introduction to the concepts and classifications of the international classification of impairments, disabilities and handicaps', *Disability and Rehabilitation* 15(4), 161–178.

Bebbington, A.C. (1988) 'The expectation of life without disability in England and Wales', *Social Science and Medicine* 27(4), 321–326.

Bebbington, A.C. (1989) *Expectation of life without disability measured from the OPCS Disability surveys*, Discussion paper 651, Canterbury: PSSRU, University of Kent.

Boshuizen, H.C. (1993) 'International comparability of health expectancy calculations: aims of the project', in Robine, J-M., Mathers, C.D., Bone, M.R. and Romieu, I. (eds) *Calculation of Health Expectancies: Harmonization, Consensus Achieved and Future Perspectives*. Paris: John Libbey Eurotext.

Boshuizen, H.C. and van de Water, H.P.A. (1994) *An International Comparison of Health Expectancies*. Leiden: TNO-PG. Publ.nr. 94.046.

Boshuizen, H.C. and van de Water, H.P.A. (1995) ICIDH in the calculation of health expectancy. *Disability and Rehabilitation* 17, 358–363.

Boshuizen, H.C., van de Water, H.P.A. and Perenboom, R.J.M. (1994) 'International comparison of health expectancy: preliminary results', in Mathers, C., McCallum, J. and Robine, J-M. (eds) *Advances in Health Expectancies*. Canberra: AGPS, Australian Institute of Health and Welfare.

Brønnum-Hansen, H. and Rasmussen, N.K. (1996) 'Mental health expectancy in Denmark 1994', Paper presented at the 2nd annual meeting of Euro-REVES, London.

Brown, S.C. (1993) 'Health expectancy values in developing countries: Ethiopia as a case study', in Robine, J-M., Mathers, C.D., Bone, M.R. and Romieu, I. (eds) *Calculation of Health Expectancies: Harmonization, Consensus Achieved and Future Perspectives*. Paris: John Libbey Eurotext.

Bruin, A. de, Picavet, H.S.J. and Nossikov, A. (eds) (1996) *Health Interview Surveys. Towards International Harmonization of Methods and Instruments*. Copenhagen: WHO Regional Office for Europe.WHO Regional Publications, European Series no. 58.

Chamie, M. (1990) 'Report of the conceptual harmonization of statistics for the study of disability-free life expectancy', REVES paper no. 41. Strasbourg.

Chamie, M. (1992) 'Harmonization and use of health expectancy indices: where we stand, where we could be going', Paper 5th meeting of the international network on health expectancy (REVES 5), Ottawa.

Colvez, A. (1980) 'Evolution de l'état de santé au cours de la dernière décennie. Peut-on continuer à parler d'amélioration?' Québec: Ministère des Affaires Sociales (Document Dactylographié).

Colvez, A. and Blanchet, M. (1983) 'Potential gains in life expectancy free of disability; a tool for health planning', *International Journal of Epidemiology* 12(2), 224–229.

Council of Europe (1990) *Evaluation of the Use of the International Classification of Impairments, Disabilities and Handicaps (ICIDH) in Surveys and Health-related Statistics.* Strasbourg, France: Council of Europe.

Crimmins, E.M., Saito, Y. and Ingegneri, D. (1989) 'Changes in life expectancy and disability-free life expectancy in the United States', *Population and Development Review* 15(2), 235–267.

Crimmins, E.M., Saito, Y. and Hayward, M.D. (1993) 'Sullivan and multi-state methods of estimating active life expectancy: two methods, two answers', in Robine, J-M., Mathers, C.D., Bone, M.R. and Romieu, I. (eds) *Calculation of Health Expectancies: Harmonization, Consensus Achieved and Future Perspectives.* Paris: John Libbey Eurotext.

ECHI working group (2001) *Design for a set of European community health indicators. Final report by the ECHI project.* Bilthoven, the Netherlands: RIVM.

Egidi, V. (1988) 'Stato di salute e morbosità della popolatione', in *The Second Report on the Italian Demographic Situation.* Rome: Istituto di recerche sulla popolazione.

Eijk, B. (1999) HIS/HES database. Statistic Netherlands/KTL Finland/European commission, Voorburg.

Evers, S.M.A.A. (1993) 'Health for all indicators in health interview surveys', *Health Policy* 23, 205–218.

Gandek, B., Ware, J.E. Jr, Aaronson, N.K., *et al* (1998) 'Cross-validation of item selection and scoring for the SF-12 health survey in nine countries: results from the IQOLA project', *Journal of Clinical Epidemiology* 51(11), 1171–1178.

Goldberg, D.P. and Williams, P. (1988) *A User's Guide to the General Health Questionnaire.* Windsor, Berkshire: NFER-Nelson.

Grotvedt, L. and Viksand, G. (1994) 'Life expectancy without disease and disability in Norway', in Mathers, C., McCallum, J. and Robine, J-M. (eds) *Advances in Health Expectancies.* Canberra: AGPS, Australian Institute of Health and Welfare.

Gutiérrez Fisac, J.L. and Regidor Poyatos, E. (1991) 'Esperanza de vida libre de incapacidad: un indicator global del estado de salud', *Medicina Clinica* 96, 453–455.

Hupkens, C.L.H., van den Berg, J. and van der Zee, J. (1999) 'National Health interview surveys in Europe: an overview', *Health Policy* 47, 145–168.

Jagger, C. (1997) *Health Expectancy Calculation by the Sullivan Method: a Practical Guide.* Montpellier, France: Euro-REVES.

Jagger, C., Ritchie, K., Brønnum-Hansen, H., Deeg, D., Gispert, R., Grimley-Evans, J., Hibbett, M., Lawlor, B., the Medical Research Council Cognitive Function and Ageing Study Group, Perenboom, R., Polge, C. and Van Oyen, H. (1998) 'Mental health expectancy – the European perspective: a synopsis of results presented at the Conference of the European Network for the Calculation of Health Expectancies (Euro-REVES)', *Acta Psychiatrica Scandinavica* 98, 85–91.

Katz, S., Branch, L.G., Branson, M.H., Papsidero, J.A., Beck, J.C. and Greer, D.S. (1983) 'Active life expectancy', *New England Journal of Medicine* 309(2), 1218–1224.

Krabbe, P.F., Stouthard, M.E.A., Essink-Bot, M.L. and Bonse, G.J. (1999) 'The effect of adding a cognitive dimension to the EuroQol Multiattribute health-status classification system', *Journal of Clinical Epidemiology* 52(4), 293–301.

Liu, K., Manton, K.G. and Liu, B.M. (1990) 'Morbidity, disability and long-term care of the elderly: implications for insurance financing', *Milbank Quarterly* 68(3), 445–492.

Mathers, C. (1991) *Health Expectancies in Australia 1981 and 1988.* Canberra: Australian Institute of Health, AGPS.

Mathers, C.D., Robine, J-M. and Wilkins, R. (1994) 'Health expectancy indicators: recommendations for terminology', in Mathers, C., McCallum, J. and Robine, J-M.

(eds) *Advances in Health Expectancies*. Canberra: AGPS, Australian Institute of Health and Welfare.

McWhinnie, J.R. (1981) 'Disability assessment in population surveys: results of the O.E.C.D. common development effort', *Revue d'Epidemiologie et de Santé Publique*, 29, 413–419.

Murray, C.J.L. and Lopez, A.D. (1996) *The Global Burden of Disease: a comprehensive assessment of mortality and disability from diseases, injuries and risk factors in 1990 and projected to 2020*. Harvard: Harvard School of Public Health.

Mutafova, M., van de Water, H.P.A., Perenboom, R.J.M., Boshuizen, H.C. and Maleshkov, C.H. (1997) 'Health expectancy calculations: a novel approach to studying population health in Bulgaria', *Bulletin of the World Health Organization* 75(2), 147–153.

Nossikov, A. (1992) 'Measurement of health for all indicators in health interview surveys planned for 1993/1994 and some notes on prospects for survey harmonization'. Paper prepared for the third consultation to develop common methods and instruments for health interview surveys, 22–24 September 1992 (document ICP/HST/124).

Ooijendijk, W.T.M. and Geurts, J. (1994) *Draft Handbook: Development of IDH Statistics*. Voorburg, the Netherlands: CBS.

Perenboom, R.J.M. and van Herten, L.M. (1998) *Levensverwachting in goede geestelijke gezondheid: inventarisatie van potentiele instrumenten en gegevens* (Mental health expectancy: an inventory of potential instruments and data). Leiden, the Netherlands: TNO Prevention and Health.

Perenboom, R.J.M. and van Herten, L.M. (1999) 'Mental health expectancy in the Netherlands, a new approach, based on the MHI-5 of the SF-36', Paper presented at the 11th meeting of REVES, London.

Perenboom, R.J.M., Boshuizen, H.C. and van de Water, H.P.A. (1993) 'Trends in health expectancies in the Netherlands, 1981–1990', in Robine, J-M., Mathers, C.D., Bone, M.R. and Romieu, I. (eds) *Calculation of Health Expectancies: Harmonization, Consensus Achieved and Future Perspectives*. Paris: John Libbey Eurotext.

Perenboom, R.J.M., Boshuizen, H.C., Breteler, M.M.B., Ott, A. and van de Water, H.P.A. (1996) 'Dementia-free life expectancy (DemFLE) in the Netherlands', *Social Science and Medicine* 43, 1703–1707.

Pettersson, H.A. (1991) 'Swedish population health index', Paper presented at the fourth international workshop on healthy life expectancy (REVES), Noordwijkerhout.

Pope, A.M. and Tarlov, A.R. (eds) (1991) *Disability in America. Towards a National Agenda for Prevention. Report of the Committee on a National Agenda for the Prevention of Disabilities*. Washington, DC: National Academy Press.

Rasmussen, N.K. and Brønnum-Hansen, H. (1990) 'The expectation of life without disability in Denmark', Presentation to the XII Scientific meeting of the international Epidemiological Association. Los Angeles, California, USA.

Regidor, E., Rodriguez, C. and Gutiérrez-Fisac, J.L. (1995) *Indicatores de Salud: Tercera evaluacion en Espana del programa regional europeo Salud Para Todos*. Madrid: Ministerio de Sanidad y Consumo.

REVES (1993) Statistical Yearbook series 'Health Expectancy', Montpellier: REVES.

Ritchie, K., Jagger, C., Brayne, C. and Letenneur, L. (1993) 'Dementia-free life expectancy: preliminary calculations for France and the United Kingdom', in Robine, J-M., Mathers, C.D., Bone, M.R. and Romieu, I. (eds) *Calculation of Health Expectancies: Harmonization, Consensus Achieved and Future Perspectives*. Paris: John Libbey Eurotext.

Ritchie, K., Mathers, C. and Jorm, A. (1994a) 'Dementia-free life expectancy in Australia', *Australian Journal of Public Health* 18, 149–152.

Ritchie, K., Robine, J-M., Letenneur, L. and Dartigues, J.F. (1994b) 'Dementia-free life expectancy in France', *American Journal of Public Health* 84, 232–236.

Robine, J-M. and Colvez, A. (1986) 'Espérance de vie sans incapacité et ses composantes: de nouveaux indicateurs pour mesurer la santé et les besoins de la population', *Population* 1, 27–46.

Robine, J-M. and Michel, J-P. (1990) 'Recommendations for international guidelines for comparisons of healthy life expectancy: Working paper for the REVES meeting in Geneva', in 2nd Workgroup meeting REVES, Geneva (REVES paper 27).

Robine, J-M. and Michel, J.-P. (1992). 'Les Espérances de santé: vers une harmonisation internationale des indicateurs de santé', in 5th Workgroup meeting REVES, Ottawa.

Robine, J-M., Romieu, I., Cambois, E., van de Water, H.P.A. and Boshuizen, H.C. (1994) *Contribution of the Network on Health Expectancy and the Disability Process to the World Health Organization (WHO)*. Montpellier, France: REVES.

Robine, J-M., Jagger, C. and Egidi, V. (eds) (2000) *Selection of a coherent set of health indicators. A first step towards a user's guide to health expectancies for the European Union*. Montpellier, France: Euro-REVES.

Roelands, M., van Oyen, H. and Baro, F. (1994) 'Dementia free life expectancy in Belgium', *European Journal of Public Health* 4, 33–37.

Rogers, A., Rogers, R.G. and Belanger, A. (1990) 'Longer life but worse health? Measurement and dynamics', *The Gerontologist* 30(5), 640–649.

Romieu, I. (1991) 'Report on the Bibliography series', in 4th Workgroup meeting REVES, Noordwijkerhout. Reves paper 65.

Romieu, I. and Robine, J-M. (1994) 'World atlas on health expectancy calculations', in Mathers, C., McCallum, J. and Robine, J-M. (eds) *Advances in Health Expectancies*. Canberra: AGPS, Australian Institute of Health and Welfare.

Romieu, I., Robine, J-M. and Jee, M. (1997) *Health Expectancies in OECD Countries*. Montpellier, France: REVES. Reves paper 317.

Sauvaget, C., Tsuji, I., Minami, Y., *et al* (1997) 'Dementia-free life expectancy among elderly Japanese', *Gerontology* 43, 168–175.

Sullivan, D.F. (1971) 'A single index of mortality and morbidity', *HSMHA Health Reports* 86(4), 347–354.

Van Buuren, S. and Hopman-Rock, M. (2001) 'Revision of the ICIDH Severity of Disabilities Scale by data linking and item response theory', *Statistics in Medicine* 20(7), 1061–1076.

Van Buuren, S., Eyres, S., Tennant, A. and Hopman-Rock (2001) *Response conversion: A new technology for comparing existing health information*, Report 2001.097. Leiden, the Netherlands: TNO Prevention and Health.

van Ginneken, J.K.S. van. and van de Water, H.P.A. (1990) 'A comparison of four methods to determine life expectancy free of disability in the Netherlands', in 2nd Workgroup meeting REVES, Geneva. Reves paper no. 37.

van Ginneken, J.K.S., Dissevelt, A.G. and Bonte, J.T.P. (1989) Summary of results of calculation of life expectancy free of disability in the Netherlands in 1981–85', in Robine, J-M., Blanchet, M. and Dowd, J.E. (eds) *Health Expectancy*. London: HMSO.

van Ginneken, J.K.S., Disseveld, A.G., van de Water, H.P.A. and van Sonsbeek, J.L.A. (1991) 'Results of two methods to determine health expectancy in the Netherlands 1981–1985', *Social Science and Medicine* 32, 1129–1136.

van Ginneken, J.K., van Leusden, H.M. and van de Hel, M. (1994) 'Healthy life expectancy in Curaçao, Netherlands Antilles, in 1992', in Mathers, C., McCallum, J.

and Robine, J-M. (eds) *Advances in Health Expectancies.* Canberra: AGPS, Australian Institute of Health and Welfare.

Van Oyen, H. and Roelands, M. (1994) 'Estimates of health expectancy in Belgium', in Mathers, C., McCallum, J. and Robine, J-M. (eds) *Advances in Health Expectancies.* Canberra: AGPS, Australian Institute of Health and Welfare.

van de Water, H.P.A., Boshuizen, H.C. and Perenboom, R.J.M. (1996) 'Health expectancy in the Netherlands', *European Journal of Public Health* 6, 21–28.

Verbrugge, L.M. and Jette, A.M. (1994) 'The disablement process', *Social Science and Medicine* 38(1), 1–14.

Ware, J.E., Snow, K.K., Kosinski, M., *et al* (1997) *SF-36 Health Survey: Manual and Interpretation Guide*, 2 edn. Boston: The Health Institute, New England Medical Center.

Wilkins, R. and Adams, O.B. (1983) 'Health expectancy in Canada, late 1970s: Demographic, regional, and social dimensions', *American Journal of Public Health* 73(9), 1073–1080.

Wilkins, R. and Adams, O.B. (1992a) 'Health expectancy in Canada, 1986', in Robine, J-M., Blanchet, M. and Dowd, J.E. (eds) *Health Expectancy*, London: HMSO.

Wilkins, R. and Adams, O.B. (1992b) 'Health expectancy trends in Canada, 1951–1986', in Robine, J-M., Blanchet, M. and Dowd, J.E (eds) *Health Expectancy*, London: HMSO.

World Health Organization, Regional Office for Europe (1989) *Consultation to develop common methods and instruments for health interview surveys.* Voorburg: Statistics Netherlands.

World Health Organization, Regional Office for Europe (1991) *Second consultation to develop common methods and instruments for health interview surveys.* Voorburg: Statistics Netherlands.

World Health Organization, Regional Office for Europe (1993) *Third consultation to develop common methods and instruments for health interview surveys.* Voorburg: Statistics Netherlands.

World Health Organization (2000) *The World Health Report 2000 Health Systems: Improving Performance.* Geneva: WHO.

PART IV

Health Expectancies in the Different Regions of the World

Introduction

COLIN D. MATHERS

WHO, Geneva, Switzerland

In the last two decades, considerable international effort has been put into the development of summary measures of population health that integrate information on mortality and non-fatal health outcomes, and international policy interest in such indicators is increasing. The following section contains chapters which review estimates of health expectancies for populations in the various regions of the world.

The concept of combining population health state prevalence data with mortality data in a life table to generate estimates of expected years of life in various health states was first proposed in the 1960s (Sanders, 1964; Sullivan, 1966, 1971) and disability-free life expectancy (DFLE) was calculated for a number of countries during the 1980s. REVES has focused much of its efforts on the harmonization of calculation methods and identification of the conditions necessary for comparison of health expectancy estimates, both across populations and over time (Bone, 1992; Mathers and Robine, 1993).

Since the late 1980s, there has been a dramatic increase in the number of health expectancy calculations carried out, almost all using the Sullivan method (Robine *et al*, 1999). In 1993, OECD included disability-free life expectancy among the health indicators reported in its health database (OECD, 1993) and by 1999 the number of OECD countries for which some estimates of disability-free life expectancy were available had grown to 12 (OECD, 1999). In the *World Health Report 2000*, the World Health Organization (WHO) reported for the first time on the average levels of population health for its 191 member countries using a health expectancy measure (WHO, 2000). New estimates of healthy life expectancy for the year 2000 were published in the *World Health Report 2001* using improved methods and incorporating cross-population comparable survey data from 63 surveys in 55 countries (see Chapter 17). Other chapters in this section review health expectancy estimates for Asian countries (Chapter 15), North American

Determining Health Expectancies. Edited by J-M. Robine, C. Jagger, C.D. Mathers, E.M. Crimmins and R.M. Suzman.
© 2003 John Wiley & Sons, Ltd

countries (Chapter 19), Latin American countries (Chapter 16), Australia and New Zealand (Chapter 20) and European countries (Chapter 18).

Without being able to measure and summarize population health, it is impossible to know if health policies are working – if levels of health are improving and inequalities are being reduced. Health policy is not aimed only at reducing mortality. Substantial resources are devoted to reducing the incidence of conditions that cause ill health but not death and to reducing their impact on people's lives. So it is important to capture both fatal and non-fatal health outcomes in any summary measure of population health. For this reason, there is great interest in the calculation and comparison of health expectancies across countries.

As a summary measure of the average level of health in a population, health expectancies have two advantages over other summary measures. The first is that it is relatively easy to explain the concept of an equivalent 'healthy' life expectancy to a non-technical audience. The second is that health expectancies are measured in units (expected years of life) that are meaningful to and within the common experience of non-technical audiences (unlike other indicators such as mortality rates or incidence rates).

It is clear from the chapters following that two main challenges exist that prevent the meaningful comparison of household interview data across populations. The first is that existing nationally representative surveys use different questions and response scales to assess health status. The second concerns limitations in the cross-population comparability of self-report data. As Boshuizen and Perenboom show in Chapter 14, there is very little consistency in definitions of health states and survey instruments used across the world to measure prevalence of health states for the calculation of health expectancies. They document the substantial efforts that REVES and international agencies have devoted to the harmonization of health measurement and the standardization of questionnaire instruments and methods.

In the 1990s, a number of cross-national surveys became available that used a common instrument and consistent sampling methods. The best known of these is the European Community Household Panel survey conducted in 13 countries in the mid-1990s. It became apparent from these surveys that standardized instruments did not solve the problems of comparability across countries (Sadana *et al*, 2002). These problems relate much more fundamentally to unmeasured differences in expectations and norms for health. Recent analyses of surveys containing both self-report and objective measurements of health status have documented systematic biases in self-report data according to age, sex, socioeconomic disadvantage, and other measures of social disadvantage within populations (Moesgard-Iberg *et al*, 2002; Thomas and Frankenberg, 2002). These issues have been discussed further by Buratta and Egidi (Chapter 9).

During the last two years, WHO has embarked on large-scale efforts to improve the methodological and empirical basis for the measurement of population health, and has initiated a data collection strategy consisting of household and/or postal or telephone surveys in representative samples of the general populations using a standardized instrument together with new statistical methods for correcting biases in self-reported health (Üstün et al, 2001). Reporting bias between different groups of people (in different cultures or demographic groups) is controlled with new techniques for comparability (Murray et al, 2002). The self-reports of individuals of their own health are calibrated against well-known performance tests (i.e. self-report vision is measured against standard Snellen's visual acuity test) or against short descriptions in vignettes that mark known anchor points of difficulty (e.g. people with different levels of mobility such as a paraplegic person or an athlete who runs 4 km each day).

The reviews in the following chapters of health expectancy calculations that have been carried out in various regions of the world highlight the methodological challenges regarding comparability of health status data across populations and cultures. REVES, OECD, WHO and other international organizations have all identified this as the key issue to be addressed if health expectancies are to become useful summary measures of variations and trends in population health. Promising new strategies for improving the comparability of self-report health status data are being developed.

REFERENCES

Bone, M.R. (1992) 'International efforts to measure health expectancy', *Journal of Epidemiology and Community Health* 46, 555–558.

Mathers, C.D. and Robine, J.M. (1993) 'Health expectancy indicators: a review of the work of REVES to date', in Robine, J-M., Mathers, C.D., Bone; M.R. and Romieu, I. (eds) *Calculation of Health Expectancies; Harmonization, Consensus Achieved and Future Perspectives (Calcul des espérances de vie en santé : harmonisation, acquis et perspectives)*. Paris: John Libbey Eurotext.

Moesgaard-Iburg, K., Murray, C.J.L., Tandon, A. and Salomon, J. (2002) 'Comparability of measurement of health domains: self-reported, physician-assessed and observed measures of health status', in Murray, C.J.L., Salomon, J.A., Mathers, C.D. and Lopez, A.D. (eds) *Summary Measures of Population Health: Concepts, Ethics, Measurement and Applications*. Geneva: World Health Organization.

Murray, C.J.L., Tandon, A., Salomon, J. and Mathers, C.D. (2002) 'New approaches to enhance cross-population comparability of survey results', in Murray, C.J.L., Salomon, J.A., Mathers, C.D. and Lopez, A.D. (eds) *Summary Measures of Population Health: Concepts, Ethics, Measurement and Applications*. Geneva: World Health Organization.

OECD (1993) *OECD Health Systems: Facts and Trends 1960–1991*. Paris: OECD.

OECD (1999) *Eco-santé. OECD Health Database 1999*. Paris: OECD.

Robine, J.M., Romieu, I. and Cambois, E. (1999) 'Health expectancy indicators', *Bulletin of the World Health Organization* 77(2), 181–185.

Sadana, R., Mathers, C.D., Lopez, A., Murray, C.J.L. and Moesgaard-Iberg, K. (2002) 'Comparative analysis of more than 50 household surveys of health status' results', in Murray, C.J.L., Salomon, J.A., Mathers, C.D. and Lopez, A.D. (eds) *Summary Measures of Population Health: Concepts, Ethics, Measurement and Applications.* Geneva: World Health Organization.

Sanders, B.S. (1964) 'Measuring community health levels', *American Journal of Public Health*, 54, 1063–1070.

Sullivan, D.F. (1966) 'Conceptual problems in developing an index of health', *Vital and Health Statistics Series* 2, no. 17.

Sullivan, D.F. (1971) 'A single index of mortality and morbidity', *HSMHA Health Reports*, 86, 347–354.

Thomas, D. and Frankenberg, E. (2002) 'The measurement and interpretation of health in social surveys', in Murray, C.J.L., Salomon, J.A., Mathers, C.D. and Lopez, A.D. (eds) *Summary Measures of Population Health: Concepts, Ethics, Measurement and Applications.* Geneva: World Health Organization.

Üstün, T.B., Chatterji, S., Villanueva, M., Bendib, L., Sadana, R., Valentine, N., Mathers, C., Ortiz, J., Tandon, A., Salomon, J., Yang, C., Xie Wan, J. and Murray, C.J.L. (2001) *WHO Multi-country Household Survey Study on Health and Responsiveness, 2000–2001.* Geneva: World Health Organization (GPE discussion paper No. 37).

World Health Organization (2000) *World Health Report 2000.* Geneva: World Health Organization.

15

Health Expectancy in Asian Countries

YASUHIKO SAITO, XIAOCHUN QIAO* and SUTTHICHAI JITAPUNKUL[†]
Nihon University,Tokyo, Japan, *The People's University of China, Beijing, China
and [†]Chulongkorn University, Bangkok,Thailand

INTRODUCTION

On 12 October 1999, the world population exceeded 6 billion people (UNFPA, 1999). About 60% of the world's population live in Asia (United Nations, 1999), and the two most populous countries, namely China and India, are in this region. Six countries in Asia have more than 100 million people, contributing to nearly half of the world's population (World Bank, 1999). The level of economic development varies tremendously in the region as indicated by gross national product (GNP) per capita, from a high of $38 160 in Japan to $220 in Nepal in 1997 (World Bank, 1999). An indicator of health, expected life at birth, also varies widely among countries in the region: Japan has the world's highest life expectancy at 80 years while Nepal's is only 57 years in 1997 (World Bank, 1999).

The level of population aging is another indicator of the diversity of this region. However, the issue of population aging is and will be a very important topic to study for each individual country and the Asian region as a whole. This is because the number of those aged 65 and over is projected to increase from 186 million in 1995 to 477 million in 2025 and the proportion will almost double from 5.4% to 10.1% over the same period (United Nations, 1999). In 2025, the proportion of those 65 and over is projected to be more than 20% in Japan, Hong Kong and Singapore, 10% in South Korea, Taiwan, China, Sri Lanka and Thailand, and over 7% in Malaysia, India, Indonesia, Myanmar (Burma), Philippines and Vietnam. In other words, the numbers of those 65 and over will be increasing at a very high rate. At the same time, they will be living longer. Life expectancy for Asia was estimated as 64.5 years for both

Determining Health Expectancies. Edited by J-M. Robine, C. Jagger, C.D. Mathers, E.M. Crimmins and R.M. Suzman.

sexes combined during the 1990–1995 period and projected to reach 73.2 years during the 2020–2025 period (United Nations, 1999). However, it is not clear whether higher life expectancy will be accompanied by better health. Without accurate and reliable information on the health status of the elderly, it will be difficult to formulate policies to improve their health.

In Asia, the concept of health expectancy is not yet widely known, although it has been computed in several countries. In this chapter, we review studies on health expectancy conducted in several Asian countries. Health expectancy was first calculated in 1974 in Japan by the Council of National Living among Asian countries. Since then several other studies have also been conducted in Japan and in other countries. Since Japan has the largest number of studies of health expectancy, we begin by reviewing the Japanese studies, followed by those conducted in other Asian countries.

JAPAN

As mentioned above, the Council of National Living probably published what is the first calculation of health expectancy in an Asian country in 1974. Although it is not clear exactly how 'average healthy life expectancy' was calculated, weights for different health states were employed. Average life expectancy free from disease was estimated as well as the length of life with diseases. In addition, a weighted health expectancy is calculated by using weights by health states relative to perfect health. For a hospitalized period the weight is 1/6 and for a period of work loss without hospitalization it is 1/2. However, there are no firm reasons to regard that a year of hospitalized life is the same as 2 months of perfect life and work loss without hospitalization as 6 months. This is probably the reason the authors suggested caution in interpretation of their results as 'individual figures do not go beyond the level of referential data, which, however, suggest the general tendency'. The result is shown in Table 15.1. Functional loss includes injury and disease, mental disorder, mental retardation and physical handicap. While life expectancy and average healthy life expectancy at birth increase from 70.88 and 68.08 in 1966 to 71.93 and 68.78 in 1970, respectively, the percentage of average healthy life expectancy to life expectancy decreased slightly at birth. This indicates that overall health status in Japan slightly decreased between 1966 and 1970 even though the length of life increased.

Other studies on health expectancy in Japan have used three methods of calculating health expectancy: the Sullivan method, the double-decrement life table method, and population-based multistate life table method. We introduce these studies by the method used.

Table 15.1. Average healthy life expectancy at birth and age 65 in Japan: 1966 and 1970

Age	Year	Life expectancy	Average years with function loss	Average healthy life expectancy	Percent of average healthy life expectancy
0	1966	70.88	2.80	68.08	96.0
	1970	71.93	3.15	68.78	95.6
65	1966	13.81	1.18	12.63	91.5
	1970	13.97	1.35	12.62	90.3

Source: The Council of National Living, 1974, *Social Indicators of Japan*, Table 2, p. 104.

SULLIVAN METHOD

Nanjo and Shigematsu (1987) presented bed disability-free life expectancy using the Sullivan method. They used data from national health surveys and measured health status by the number of days in bed because of health reasons. The result is shown in Table 15.2. For both males and females at birth and age 65, life expectancy and bed disability-free life expectancy increased consistently from 1975 to 1985. The proportion of bed disability-free life expectancy to life expectancy also increased between 1975 and 1985, but the change is minimal at birth (0.4 percentage points for both sexes) and very small at age 65 (1.4 percentage points for males and 1.5 percentage points for females).

Table 15.2. Bed disability-free life expectancy at birth and age 65 by sex in Japan: 1975–1985

Age	Year	Life expectancy	Length of life with bed disability	Bed disability-free life expectancy	Percent of bed disability-free life expectancy
Males					
0	1975	71.7	2.4	69.3	96.6
	1980	73.4	2.5	70.9	96.6
	1985	74.8	2.3	72.6	97.0
65	1975	13.7	1.4	12.3	89.5
	1980	14.6	1.4	13.2	90.4
	1985	15.5	1.4	14.1	90.9
Females					
0	1975	76.9	2.9	74.0	96.2
	1980	78.8	2.9	75.9	96.4
	1985	80.5	2.7	77.7	96.6
65	1975	16.6	1.8	14.7	89.0
	1980	17.7	1.8	15.8	89.6
	1985	18.9	1.8	17.1	90.5

Source: Zenji Nanjo and Takao Shigematsu, 1987, 'Kenkou seimeihyo sakusei ni tsuite' (Calculation of health expectancy), Paper presented at a regional meeting of Population Association of Japan, Fukuoka, Japan.

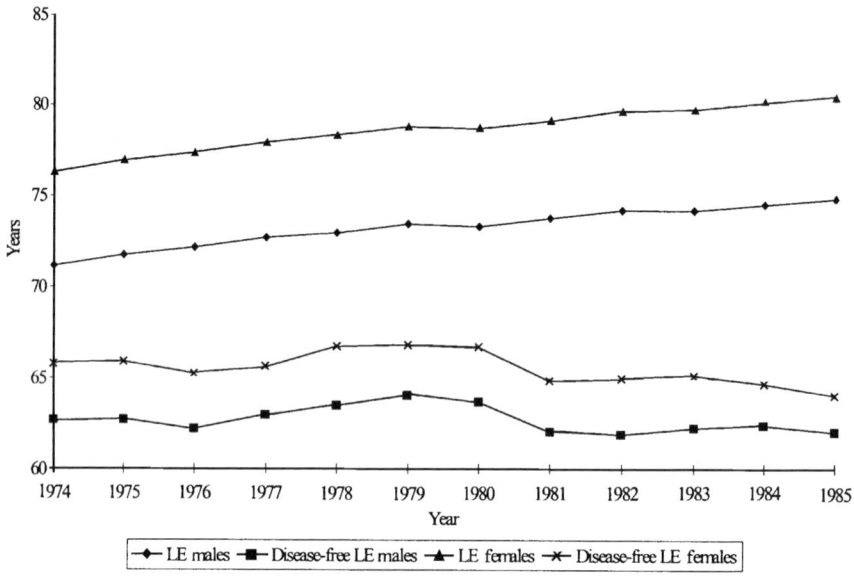

Figure 15.1. Life expectancy and disease-free life expectancy by sex in Japan: 1974–1985

Gunji and Hayashi (1991) computed both disease-free life expectancy and bed disability-free life expectancy by sex in Japan for the period 1974 to 1985. The trends in life expectancy and disease-free life expectancy are shown in Figure 15.1. While life expectancy increased from 71.2 years in 1974 to 74.8 years in 1985 for males and from 76.3 to 80.5 for females over the same period, disease-free life expectancy decreased from 62.7 to 62.0 for males and from 65.8 to 64.1 for females. As a result, the proportion of disease-free life expectancy to life expectancy decreased from 88.1% in 1974 to 82.9% in 1985 for males and from 86.2% to 79.6% for females (Figure 15.2). The health status of the Japanese as a whole had worsened during the period if the prevalence of disease was used as the indicator of health. The trend in the proportion of bed disability-free life expectancy to life expectancy at birth is also shown in Figure 15.2. This is consistent with results of Nanjo and Shigematsu.

Bed disability-free life expectancy and disability-free life expectancy for 1990 were computed by Inoue *et al* (1997) as shown in Table 15.3. The definition of bed disability-free life expectancy in their study is comparable to the 1987 Nanjo and Shigematsu study. The figures and trends of bed disability-free life expectancy are very consistent for both sexes, both at birth and age 65 with the exception of females at age 65. Increases in life expectancy were accompanied by increases in bed disability-free life expectancy and in the proportion of bed disability-free life expectancy. However, the health status of females measured

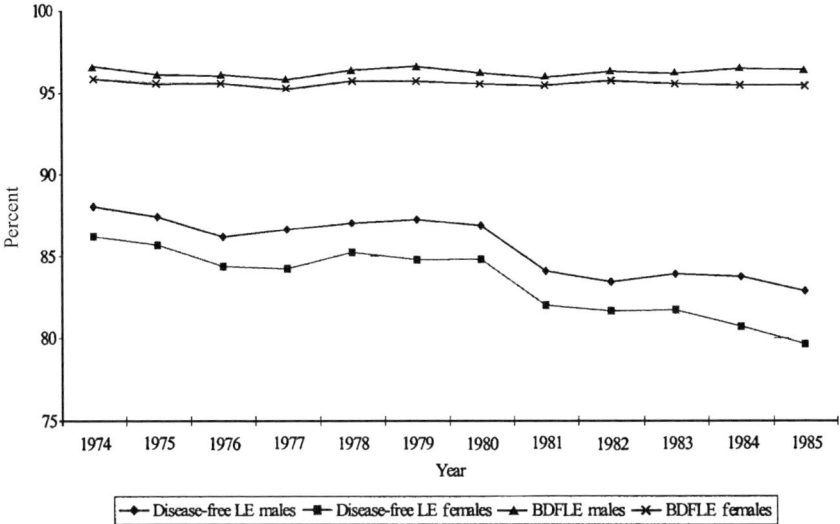

Figure 15.2. Proportion of disease-free and bed disability-free life expectancy (BDFLE) to life expectancy by sex in Japan: 1974–1985

by the proportion of bed disability-free life expectancy to life expectancy at age 65 slightly worsened from 90.5% in 1985 to 86.2% in 1990.

Disability-free life expectancy at birth by sex in 1990 computed by Inoue and colleagues appears to be very different from the disability-free life expectancy at birth for 1985 computed by Gunji and Hayashi even after accounting for the different time period. Disability-free life expectancy computed by Inoue and colleagues was 72.5 and 76.4 in 1990 for males and females, respectively,

Table 15.3. Bed disability-free and disability-free life expectancy by sex in Japan: 1990

Age	Life expectancy	Bed disability-free life expectancy	Percent of bed disability-free life expectancy	Disability-free life expectancy	Percent of disability-free life expectancy
Males					
0	75.9	74.2	97.8	72.5	95.5
65	16.2	14.8	91.6	13.8	85.3
Females					
0	81.9	78.7	96.1	76.4	93.3
65	20.0	17.2	86.2	15.9	79.5

Source: Toshitaka Inoue, Takao Shigematsu and Zenji Nanjo (1997) 'Nihon no 1990nen kenkou seimeihyo–sekai saichoju no shitsu no kenkou' (Health life tables in Japan, 1990, men: A quality of the longest life expectancy in the world), *Minzoku Eisei*, 63(4), 231, Table 2.

whereas the figure computed by Gunji and Hayashi was 62.0 and 64.1 in 1985. Over the same period life expectancy increased from 74.8 years to 75.9 years for males and from 80.5 years to 81.9 years for females. Increases in disability-free life expectancy were more than 10 years while increases in life expectancy were only about one year. Inoue and colleagues explain that these different results could be due to different estimations of prevalence rates, even though both studies used similar definitions of disability.

Kamimura (1996) calculated health expectancy using 'activities of daily living' (ADL) as a measure of health. He used six items of ADLs included in the 'Kokumin Seikatsu Kiso Chosa' (national survey on everyday life) conducted in 1992. Those who do not receive any assistance from others on any of the six ADLs – washing face and brushing teeth, dressing, eating, toileting, bathing, and walking – are defined as active or independent. A limitation of this study is that data on mortality, morbidity, or health are from different points in time.

A study by Hashimoto (1998) employed a similar measure of health, that is, dependence defined as those who need assistance to perform daily activities. He computed independent life expectancy at age 65 by sex for Japan and by prefecture based on the estimated age-specific prevalence of dependence. Independence is the reverse of dependence and computed by subtracting prevalence of dependence from unity. In order to estimate the prevalence of dependence, he divided those aged 65 and over into four categories according to place of residence: community dwelling, hospital, and two kinds of institutions for the elderly. The reason for this is the availability of data. For community dwelling populations Hashimoto employed six ADL items including washing face and brushing teeth, dressing, eating, toileting, bathing, and walking, from 'Kokumin Seikatsu Kiso Chosa' conducted in 1995. A serious drawback of this study is the use of published data which are not tabulated by age, leading to assumptions regarding the distribution of those classified as inactive by age.

In Japan, there are 47 prefectures in total; selected results are shown in Table 15.4. In 1995, males had 16.5 years and females had 20.9 years of life expectancy at age 65. Independent life expectancy was 14.9 years (90.6% of life expectancy) and 18.3 years (87.3% of life expectancy) for males and females, respectively. Okinawa prefecture has the longest life expectancy and independent life expectancy for both sexes. However, in terms of ranking, the proportion of independent life expectancy to life expectancy, it is 40th for males and last for females. In contrast, while Osaka prefecture has one of the lowest levels of life expectancy for males and females, its rank for independent life expectancy is better – 26th for males and 22nd for females. Yamanashi prefecture seems to have a very balanced life expectancy and independent life expectancy.

Ikuta *et al* (1999) estimated life expectancy and health expectancy for a specific occupational category – dentists – for the period 1991–1997 for

Table 15.4. Independent life expectancy at age 65 by sex for Japan and by prefecture: 1995

	Life expectancy				Independent life expectancy		Proportion of independent life expectancy	
	Males		Females		Males	Females	Males	Females
Prefecture	Years	Ranking	Years	Ranking	Years	Years	Ranking	Ranking
Japan	16.48		20.94		14.93	18.29		
Okinawa	18.22	1	24.82	1	16.26	20.44	40	47
Aomori	15.80	47	20.86	43	14.05	17.62	43	43
Osaka	15.87	46	20.41	47	14.34	17.79	26	22
Yamanashi	16.94	11	24.78	10	15.69	19.57	1	2
Chiba	16.77	18	21.30	28	15.51	19.15	2	1
Tokyo	16.78	17	21.33	24	15.35	18.74	5	15

Source: Shuji Hashimoto (1998) 'Hoken iryo fukushi ni kansuru chiiki shihyou no sougouteki kaihatsu to ouyou ni kansuru kenkyu'. Research Report.

Saitama prefecture. They defined bed disability as those who were hospitalized for 10 days or more and bed-ridden for 30 days or more at home and computed bed disability-free life expectancy. Their definition of bed disability-free life expectancy is different from the one used in the previous studies because it does not include bed days less than 10. The study found that dentists at age 65 on average had 17.9 years of life expectancy and 17.4 years of bed disability-free life expectancy or 97.6% of life expectancy.

DOUBLE-DECREMENT LIFE TABLE METHOD

Kai *et al* (1991) computed active life expectancy using modified ADL measures and the double-decrement life table method for Saku City in Nagano prefecture. A longitudinal survey conducted there in 1988 and 1989 was used to estimate active life expectancy. Health states were defined as active if six ADL items were performed independently and inactive for the rest. The six ADL items were bathing, dressing, toileting, standing, eating and continence. Computed results are shown in Table 15.5. Because of the limitation of the method, active life expectancies refer only to those who were active at the first wave of the survey and do not take into account people returning to the active state from the inactive state between two surveys. Although the number of people returning to the active state in the study by Kai *et al* is small during the one-year period, other studies have reported a significant number of transitions (Branch *et al*, 1984; Manton, 1988; Rogers *et al*, 1990; Crimmins and Saito, 1993). The number of people returning to the active state depends on the

Table 15.5. Active life expectancy for Saku City in Nagano prefecture by sex: 1988–1989

	Active life expectancy		Percent of active life expectancy to life expectancy	
Age	Males	Females	Males	Females
60	15.1	15.3	61	53
65	11.6	11.7	56	48
70	8.4	8.3	51	42
75	6.3	5.8	51	38
80	4.3	4.0	50	34
85	2.3	2.8	42	36
90	2.4	2.1	78	48

Source: Kai *et al* (1991) 'Quality of life: A possible health index for the elderly', *Asia-Pacific Journal of Public Health* 5(3), 224, Tables 2 and 3.

number and kind of items in the ADL measures, severity to be measured, and length of an interval.

Honma *et al* (1998) also computed active life expectancy. Their calculation is for a regional population and employed a follow-up survey of 36 months from September 1992 to August 1995.

Sauvaget *et al* (1997) computed dementia-free life expectancy for those aged 65 and over without mental disorder living in Sendai City, Miyagi prefecture, using the double-decrement life table method. They utilized the Sendai Longitudinal Study of Aging conducted in 1988 and 1991 (Table 15.6). The use of the double-decrement life table method is less problematic in computing dementia-free life expectancy compared to active life expectancy because the possibility of demented people returning to normal mental state is slight. Dementia-free life expectancy at age 65 between 1988 and 1991 in Sendai City was 15.8 years for males and 17.8 year for females. Females could expect to live, on average, 2 years longer without dementia. However, they are also expected to live almost 3 years longer with the state of dementia. At age 90, females are expected to live a half of their remaining life with dementia. Sauvaget and colleagues indicate that Japanese elderly, especially females, are likely to spend more years with dementia compared to elderly living in other developed countries.

POPULATION-BASED MULTISTATE LIFE TABLE METHOD

Tsuji *et al* (1995) computed active life expectancy using the population-based multistate life table method for those aged 65 and over living in Sendai City (Table 15.7). They used the same data as for the study by Sauvaget and colleagues mentioned above. The definition of dependent or inactive is the state

Table 15.6. Dementia-free life expectancy by sex for Sendai City: 1988–1991

Age	Males			Females		
	Life expectancy	Dementia-free life expectancy	Percent of dementia-free life expectancy	Life expectancy	Dementia-free life expectancy	Percent of dementia-free life expectancy
65	17.7	15.8	89.3	22.6	17.8	78.8
70	13.6	11.9	87.5	18.2	13.6	74.7
75	10.1	8.6	85.1	14.3	10.0	69.9
80	7.2	5.8	80.6	10.8	7.0	64.8
85	4.9	3.8	77.6	7.9	4.6	58.2
90	3.2	2.4	75.0	5.7	2.8	49.1

Source: Sauvaget *et al* (1997) 'Dementia-free life expectancy among elderly Japanese', *Gerontology* 43, 173, Table 2. Reproduced with permission

of needing assistance to perform at least one of the following ADLs: bathing, dressing, toileting and eating. Four series of age-specific transition rates for the period of 1988–1991 were estimated, i.e., active to inactive, inactive to active, active to death, and inactive to death. Based on these transition schedules, active and inactive life expectancies were computed. One advantage of utilizing the multistate life table method to compute health expectancy is that it takes into account differential mortality. Transition rates from active and inactive to death are the same as mortality rates by health status. Their estimated life expectancy was similar to that computed for Sendai City in 1990 for both males and females. Males have 16.1 remaining years of life at age 65, on average, of which

Table 15.7. Active life expectancy by sex for Sendai City, Japan: 1988–1991

Age	Males			Females		
	Life expectancy	Active life expectancy	Percent of active life expectancy	Life expectancy	Active life expectancy	Percent of active life expectancy
65	16.1	14.7	91.3	20.4	17.7	86.8
70	12.6	11.2	88.9	16.4	13.6	82.9
75	9.0	7.9	87.8	12.5	9.8	78.4
80	6.4	5.2	81.3	9.0	6.6	73.3
85	4.7	3.3	70.2	6.2	4.1	66.1
90	3.5	3.1	88.6	3.7	2.7	73.0

Source: Tsuji *et al* (1995) 'Active life expectancy among elderly Japanese', *Journal of Gerontology: Medical Sciences* 50A(3), M174, Table 3. ©The Gerontological Society of America. Reproduced by permission of the publisher

Table 15.8. Active life expectancy for Japanese elderly: 1987–1990

Age	Life expectancy	Active life expectancy	Percent of active life expectancy
60	23.04	18.67	81.03
63	20.43	16.15	79.05
66	17.88	13.65	76.34
69	15.49	11.31	73.01
72	13.26	9.14	68.93
75	11.18	7.18	64.22
78	9.40	5.54	58.94
81	7.96	4.25	53.39
84	6.54	3.11	47.55
87	5.20	2.08	40.00
90	4.41	1.38	31.29
93	3.80	0.92	24.21
96	3.26	0.61	18.71

Source: Liu *et al* (1995) 'Transitions in functional status and active life expectancy among older people in Japan', *Journal of Gerontology: Social Sciences* 50B(6), S391, Table 6. ©The Gerontological Society of America. Reproduced by permission of the publisher

14.7 years or 91.3% of remaining years are expected to be active. Females are expected to live longer (20.4 years) and active life (17.7 years) but the proportion of active life to life expectancy is 4.5 percentage points smaller than that of males.

Liu *et al* (1995) also employed the multistate life table method to compute health expectancy for the Japanese elderly aged 60 and over (Table 15.8). Data are from the first and second waves of a longitudinal study that is still ongoing, as the fifth wave of the survey was conducted in 1999. Their measures of health are bathing oneself, climbing two or three flights of stairs, and walking about 200–300 meters or a few blocks. Those who have any degree of difficulty in performing at least one of the three activities were classified as 'functionally disabled'. As the surveys are three years apart, conducted in 1987 and 1990, Liu *et al* computed life expectancy and active life expectancy every three years of age starting at age 60. Their estimated life expectancy (23.04 years) for both sexes is slightly higher than that for the Japanese population (22.23 years) in 1989. Active life expectancy was 18.7 years at age 60, 7.2 years at age 75, and 1.4 years at age 90. At age 75 and 90, the percentage of active life expectancy computed is 64.2% and 31.3%, respectively, and is much lower than the percentage of active life expectancy for females at each age computed by Tsuji and colleagues. There are many possible reasons for the differences between the two studies. One main difference is the definition of the 'active' state; another is that activities used for the definition of functionally disabled in the study of Liu and colleagues require more energy and strength and are more difficult to perform than the ADL items.

Table 15.9. Disability-free life expectancy by sex for China: 1987

	Males			Females		
Age	Life expectancy	Disability-free life expectancy	Percent of disability-free life expectancy	Life expectancy	Disability-free life expectancy	Percent of disability-free life expectancy
0	66.6	61.6	92.5	69.5	63.7	91.7
15	55.6	50.8	91.4	58.6	52.7	89.9
25	46.2	41.6	90.0	49.2	43.5	88.4
45	27.9	23.7	84.9	30.8	25.5	82.8
65	12.5	8.9	71.2	14.6	9.9	67.8
75	7.4	4.2	56.8	8.7	4.7	54.0

Source: Grab *et al* (1991) 'Estimate of disability-free life expectancy in China', paper presented at the 4th meeting of REVES, Noordwijkerhout, Netherlands.

CHINA

Grab *et al* (1991) calculated disability-free life expectancy in China. They applied the Sullivan method and utilized the National Sampling Survey of Handicapped conducted in 1987 to estimate disability prevalence. There were five types of disabilities, i.e., visual disability, hearing and speech disability, mental disability, physical disability, and psychotic disability. They defined disability as those with at least one of these five types of disabilities and computed disability-free life expectancy. Three different tabulations are available: by sex, by sex and type of disability, and by sex and region. Disability-free life expectancy by sex is shown in Table 15.9. As observed in other developed countries, life expectancy and disability-free life expectancy are longer for females but the proportion of disability-free life expectancy to life expectancy is smaller at all ages for females.

One limitation of this study is the use of life tables for 1982 constructed by Calot and Caselli (1988). Data for disability and mortality are five years apart. Therefore, the calculated disability-free life expectancy may not represent conditions in China in 1987. Another possible source of bias is that the survey did not include those living in institutions. Although the proportion of those who are institutionalized might be negligible, they are included in the calculation of the life table.

Qiao *et al* (1993) calculated health expectancy by the Sullivan method for Xichang prefecture in Sichuan province, China. The Xichang Health Quality Survey conducted between December 1989 and January 1990 was used to compute prevalence rates of four health states. Measures used to define these health states were ADLs including bathing, dressing, going to the toilet,

Table 15.10. Health expectancy by age and sex for Xichang, China: 1990

Age	Life expectancy	ADL/IADL no trouble	ADL/IADL trouble	IADL unable	ADL unable
Males					
15	54.0	49.0	3.2	1.0	0.8
25	44.6	39.5	3.3	0.9	0.8
35	35.4	30.4	3.3	0.9	0.8
45	26.6	21.5	3.4	0.8	0.9
55	18.3	13.1	3.5	0.8	0.9
65	10.9	6.1	3.1	0.8	0.9
75	6.8	2.6	2.3	0.7	1.1
Females					
15	56.1	48.1	5.1	1.8	1.1
25	46.9	38.8	5.2	1.8	1.1
35	37.8	29.6	5.3	1.8	1.1
45	28.7	20.5	5.3	1.8	1.1
55	20.1	12.1	5.1	1.6	1.2
65	12.1	5.3	4.1	1.5	1.1
75	6.5	1.9	2.0	1.4	1.2

Source: Z.-K. Qiao *et al* (1993) 'Health expectancy of adults in Xichang, China, 1990: autonomy in various activities of daily living', in J.-M. Robine, C.D. Mathers, M.R. Bone and I. Romieu (eds) *Calculation of Health Expectancy: Harmonization, Consensus Achieved and Future Perspective.* John Libbey Eurotext, p. 364. Reproduced with permission

transferring, continence, feeding, and grooming, and instrumental activities of daily living (IADLs) including food preparation, housekeeping, shopping, and handling money. The four health states are: unable to do at least one ADL (ADL unable); able to do all ADLs but unable to do at least one IADL (IADL unable); able to do both ADLs and IADLs but having difficulty performing at least one ADL or IADL (ADL/IADL trouble); and no difficulty performing ADLs and IADLs (ADL/IADL no trouble). Abridged life tables based on the 1990 census of China were also constructed.

Results are shown in Table 15.10. At age 15, males have 54.0 years of remaining life with 49.0 years without any difficulties performing any ADLs and IADLs. The proportion of ADL/IADL no trouble at age 15 is 90.7% and reduces to 56.0% at age 65. However, at age 65, 84.4% of remaining life is spent able to do ADLs and IADLs. Life expectancy for females at age 15 is 56.1 years, which is 2.1 years longer than for males. But, female health expectancy without ADL/IADL difficulty is smaller than that for males. In general, males have lower life expectancy at each age but have a longer healthy life and proportion of healthy life.

Health expectancy by region was also computed. In addition, the study computed health expectancy by sex using weights for each health state on the assumption that expectancy adjusted by the health states is better than one without any adjustments. However, the rationale for the weights employed is unclear.

Wang (1993) published a book in Chinese entitled *Living Long is not Equal to Living Healthy*. In her study, she used the Sullivan method to calculate health expectancies by age, sex, and place of residence (urban/rural). Using data from the Survey on China's Support Systems for the Elderly conducted in 1992, she computed active life expectancy based on four ADLs. These ADLs are dressing, eating, bathing and toileting. At age 60, life expectancy was 16.30 years for males living in urban areas and 15.77 years for their counterparts living in rural areas. Estimated active life expectancies for them are not very different, 14.90 years for urban dwellers and 14.76 years for those living in rural areas. The proportion of active life expectancy for those living in rural areas is slightly higher than for the elderly living in urban areas. The same pattern is observed in the female population. Life expectancy is 19.26 and 18.36, and active life expectancy is 16.78 and 16.79 for urban area and rural areas, respectively.

Qiao (1997) also calculated four types of health expectancies for China using the Sullivan method. Several data sources were used: data on health from the 1987 National Sampling Survey of Handicapped, 1987 Sampling Survey of the Elderly Aged 60 and Over, and 1992 Survey on China's Support Systems for the Elderly. Life tables were estimated from the 1990 National Population Census, and 1% Population Sampling Survey conducted in 1987 and 1995.

The 1987 National Sampling Survey of Handicapped used by Grab and colleagues was also used to estimate the prevalence of disability defined as those with visual, hearing and speech, mental, physical, or psychotic disability. Based on the estimated prevalence rates, disability-free life expectancy was computed by sex. At birth, life expectancy for males was 67.3 years and 62.3 years were expected to be disability-free. For females, the estimates were 70.6 years and 64.5 years, respectively. Both life expectancy and disability-free life expectancy are longer for females but the proportion of disability-free life expectancy is longer for males. At age 65, life expectancy is 12.6 and disability-free life expectancy is 9.0 for males, and 15.0 and 10.2 for females.

Perceived health compared with persons of similar age and independence were measured in the Sampling Survey of the Elderly Aged 60 and Over conducted in 1987. For the measure of independence, respondents were asked if they could take care of themselves in daily living. Response categories were 'no problem', 'some problems', 'very difficult', and 'unable'. The Survey on China's Support Systems for the Elderly in 1992 included several indicators of health. Perceived health was measured 'healthy', 'fair', and 'not healthy'. Four ADL measures, i.e., dressing, eating, bathing and toileting, were used to define independence. In addition, a question on presence of chronic disease was asked.

Although the measures used in these two surveys are not exactly the same, Qiao (1997) computed active life expectancy and perceived healthy life expectancy at two dates as shown in Table 15.11. Life expectancy for males at age 65 increased from 12.6 years in 1987 to 13.0 years in 1992, and for females from 15.0 years to 15.6 years over the same period. Qiao also computed disease-free life expectancy for 1992. Three types of health expectancy for 1992, including active life expectancy, perceived healthy life expectancy, and disease-free life expectancy, are shown in Table 15.12 by 5-year age group and sex.

Table 15.11. Life expectancy, perceived healthy life expectancy, and active life expectancy by sex for China: 1987 and 1992

Year	Age	Life expectancy	Active life expectancy	Percent of active life expectancy	Perceived healthy life expectancy	Percent of perceived healthy life expectancy
Males
1987	65	12.60	9.62	76.4	9.35	74.8
	80	5.52	2.85	51.6	4.26	77.1
1992	65	13.04	11.89	91.2	10.24	78.6
	80	5.78	4.62	80.0	4.38	75.9
Females
1987	65	15.02	11.46	76.3	10.70	70.6
	80	6.51	3.70	56.8	4.85	74.5
1992	65	15.58	13.74	88.2	11.66	74.8
	80	7.07	5.13	72.6	5.15	72.8

Source: X.-C. Qiao (1997) 'Health expectancy of China', Paper presented at 10th REVES meeting, Tokyo.

Table 15.12. Various health expectancies by sex for China: 1992

Age	Life expectancy	Active life expectancy	Perceived healthy life expectancy	Disease-free life expectancy
Males
65	13.0	11.9	10.2	4.2
70	10.1	9.0	7.8	3.2
75	7.7	6.6	5.9	2.4
80	5.8	4.6	4.4	1.9
85	4.3	3.2	3.2	1.5
Females
65	15.6	13.7	11.7	4.4
70	12.2	10.3	9.0	3.4
75	9.4	7.6	6.8	2.7
80	7.1	5.1	5.1	2.1
85	5.4	3.5	3.9	1.7

Source: X.-C. Qiao (1997) 'Health Expectancy of China', Paper presented at 10th REVES meeting, Tokyo.

Table 15.13. Total, disability-free, and disease-free life expectancy by sex in Taiwan: 1986 and 1991

	Males			Females		
Age	Total life expectancy	Disability-free life expectancy	Disease-free life expectancy	Total life expectancy	Disability-free life expectancy	Disease-free life expectancy
1986						
15	56.2	42.4	36.4	60.5	49.6	43.2
25	46.9	34.7	28.9	50.9	41.5	35.6
45	28.7	21.0	16.3	31.8	25.0	19.7
65	12.9	7.6	2.6	14.5	9.1	3.1
75	6.5	4.0	2.7	7.4	4.2	2.6
1991						
15	58.3	44.5	37.6	63.5	52.6	44.7
25	49.0	37.3	30.6	53.8	45.1	37.1
45	31.0	23.6	16.9	34.7	28.2	20.0
65	15.5	11.7	2.8	17.5	12.9	2.7
75	9.7	6.9	2.6	10.8	7.4	2.6

Source: Tu and Chen (1994) 'Recent changes in healthy life expectancy and their implications for medical costs in Taiwan', in C.D. Mathers, J. McCallum and J.-M. Robine (eds), *Advances in Health Expectancies.* Canberra, Australia, p. 375, Table 1. Reproduced with permission

TAIWAN

Studies on health expectancy in Taiwan have been carried out by Tu and Chen (1994a, 1994b). They applied the multiple-decrement life table method, which is a direct extension of the double-decrement life table method and allows more than two kinds of exits from a disability-free state. Tu and Chen used the Taiwan-Fukien Demographic Fact Book (Republic of China, Department of Health, 1987–1990) for mortality data and the Supplement of Elderly Living Conditions to the Monthly Survey of Human Resources, conducted in 1986 and 1991 by the Directorate-General of Budget, Accounting, and Statistics for health data. Disability was defined for the working-age group as a state of incapacity to perform major self-care and job-related functions, and for those aged 65 and over as a state of being functionally dependent. They added a morbid state defined as a state with diseases in their model. Results from this study (Tu and Chen, 1994b) are shown in Table 15.13. It should be pointed out that the model begins with those who are disability free as the method implies. Therefore, all the results should have been for those who were in the disability-free state at the beginning as only those who are healthy can move to a disability state. Also the mortality schedule for those without disability should have been used for the study because the mortality schedule for the general population would be higher than that for those without disability or disease.

Studies of health expectancy are often limited by data availability. However, in Taiwan a longitudinal study was initiated in 1989 called 'Survey of Health and Living Status of the Elderly' and the follow-up interviews were conducted in 1993 and 1996. Tu *et al* (1997) studied changes in morbidity and chronic disability in an elderly population in Taiwan using the first and second wave of the longitudinal study. As yet, they have not computed health expectancy using the data.

HEALTH EXPECTANCY FOR EIGHT ASIAN COUNTRIES

So far, we have introduced studies on health expectancy by country. However, Lamb (1999) calculated active life expectancy based on the Sullivan method for eight Asian countries. A number of data sets are used to estimate the prevalence of disability in this study. These data sets were collected by the World Health Organization's 'Health and Social Aspects of Aging' project in 1984 in WPRO (Western Pacific Regional Office) countries – Malaysia, Philippines and South Korea; and in 1989 in SEARO (South East Asian Regional Office) countries – Burma, Indonesia, North Korea, Sri Lanka and Thailand. Non-institutionalized persons aged 60 years and over were interviewed in these countries. Measures of health included in the survey were ADL activities on whether one can eat, dress and undress oneself, take care of one's appearance, walk, get in and out of bed or the place where one sleeps, and take a bath or shower. Response categories to the question on these activities are without help, with some help, or unable to do (or totally dependent for the last two items). Respondents were classified as disabled if they needed help in completing, or were unable to do at least one of the six activities. Country-specific abridged life tables by sex from the Center for International Research, Bureau of the Census, US Department of Commerce are employed for the study. These life tables are assumed to reflect the mortality experience of the populations for the approximate times of the surveys. A caveat should be mentioned here. The data for health are from the non-institutionalized population but the country-specific life tables Lamb used are probably nationally representative. Although institutionalized populations are negligible in these countries, this is a possible source of bias in the calculation of health expectancy.

Results are shown for WPRO countries in Table 15.14 and for SEARO countries in Table 15.15. For all countries included, females generally have a longer life expectancy and active life expectancy. However, Filipino males have a longer life expectancy after age 70 and males at older ages in Indonesia, Sri Lanka, Thailand, and Philippines have a longer active life expectancy. With the

Table 15.14. Active life expectancy for WPRO countries: 1984

	Males			Females		
Age	Total life expectancy	Active life expectancy	Percent of active life expectancy	Total life expectancy	Active life expectancy	Percent of active life expectancy
Malaysia						
60	14.18	13.28	93.6	16.54	15.53	93.9
65	11.30	10.49	92.9	13.20	12.13	91.9
70	8.89	8.12	91.4	10.27	9.12	88.8
75	6.74	6.08	90.2	7.86	6.64	84.5
80	4.66	3.78	81.2	5.43	4.17	76.9
Philippines						
60	16.75	14.84	88.6	17.40	15.03	86.4
65	13.61	11.62	85.4	13.69	11.56	84.5
70	10.36	8.33	80.4	10.04	8.05	80.1
75	8.08	5.85	72.4	7.30	5.46	74.8
80	6.07	3.82	62.9	5.47	3.11	56.9
South Korea						
60	13.63	10.56	77.5	18.65	14.23	76.3
65	10.65	8.01	75.2	14.84	10.66	71.9
70	8.29	6.03	72.7	11.40	7.41	65.0
75	6.27	4.29	68.3	8.68	5.12	59.0
80	4.88	2.70	55.2	6.30	3.43	54.5

Source: Vicki L. Lamb (1999) 'Active life expectancy of the elderly in selected Asian countries', NUPRI Research Paper Series No. 69. Tokyo, Japan: Nihon University Population Research Institute, p. 13, Table 1. Reproduced with permission

exception of Burma, the proportion of active life expectancy to total life expectancy is higher for males at almost all ages. Also as a general pattern, females tend to lose their ability to perform ADL activities more rapidly as age advances. These patterns suggest that males are more likely to be affected by acute or mortal diseases and females by chronic conditions.

Among individual countries studied by Lamb, Sri Lanka has the longest life expectancy for both males and females. However, the proportion of active life expectancy is the lowest for females and the second lowest for males. In contrast, countries like Indonesia and Malaysia have relatively lower life expectancy but their proportion of active life expectancy is very high. Longer life expectancy does not seem to mean healthier life. The relationship between length of total life expectancy and the proportion of active life expectancy in Thailand has a peculiar pattern. Life expectancy for both males and females is ranked very high, and their proportion of active life expectancy is also ranked very high among those eight countries.

Table 15.15. Active life expectancy for SEARO countries: 1989

	Males			Females		
Age	Total life expectancy	Active life expectancy	Percent of active life expectancy	Total life expectancy	Active life expectancy	Percent of active life expectancy
Burma (Myanmar)						
60	14.56	11.86	81.5	16.30	13.40	82.2
65	11.66	8.80	75.5	13.08	10.19	77.9
70	9.11	5.97	65.5	10.22	7.29	71.3
75	6.97	4.19	60.1	7.78	4.76	61.2
80	5.31	2.66	50.0	5.84	2.76	47.3
Indonesia						
60	14.40	13.66	94.9	15.89	14.49	91.2
65	11.62	10.86	93.5	12.87	11.34	88.1
70	9.20	8.43	91.6	10.30	8.61	83.6
75	7.15	6.53	91.3	8.14	6.16	75.6
80	5.56	5.70	84.5	6.45	4.17	64.7
North Korea						
60	14.79	13.30	90.0	18.94	16.15	85.3
65	11.91	10.67	89.6	15.42	12.67	82.2
70	9.49	8.21	86.5	12.30	9.55	77.7
75	7.50	6.16	82.1	9.58	6.84	71.4
80	5.86	4.60	78.4	7.18	4.65	64.8
Sri Lanka						
60	18.12	14.14	78.0	20.13	14.68	72.9
65	14.60	10.76	73.7	16.17	10.94	67.6
70	11.52	7.66	66.5	12.66	7.86	62.1
75	8.83	5.14	58.3	9.50	5.14	54.1
80	6.18	2.78	45.0	6.51	2.77	42.6
Thailand						
60	16.01	15.22	95.1	19.06	17.42	91.4
65	12.95	12.10	93.4	15.58	13.89	89.2
70	10.04	9.13	91.0	12.39	10.56	85.2
75	7.77	7.13	91.8	9.63	7.55	78.4
80	5.47	4.89	89.4	6.49	4.32	66.6

Source: Vicki L. Lamb (1999) 'Active life expectancy of the elderly in selected Asian countries', NUPRI Research Paper Series No. 69. Tokyo, Japan: Nihon University Population Research Institute, p. 14, Table 2. Reproduced with permission

Table 15.16. Life expectancy and disability-free life expectancy by sex for South Korea: 1989

	Males			Females		
Age	Life expectancy	Disability-free life expectancy	Percent of disability-free life expectancy	Life expectancy	Disability-free life expectancy	Percent of disability-free life expectancy
0	66.73	60.48	90.6	74.88	63.80	85.2
60	15.07	10.97	72.8	19.93	12.78	64.1
65	11.94	8.37	70.1	15.96	9.79	61.3
70	9.16	6.24	68.1	12.33	7.24	58.7
75	6.85	4.66	68.0	9.20	5.13	55.8
80	5.06	3.12	61.7	6.61	3.66	55.4

Source: Lee (1997) 'A study on disability-free life expectancy of the Elderly in Korea', Paper presented at 10th meeting of REVES, Tokyo, Japan.

SOUTH KOREA

Lee (1997) estimated disability-free life expectancy by the Sullivan method for 1989 in South Korea. He employed 1989 life tables for mortality data and the National Health Survey in 1989 for health data. Those who were not able to perform usual activities were defined as disabled. Table 15.16 shows life expectancy, disability-free life expectancy, and the proportion of disability-free life expectancy by sex at selected ages. At birth, males and females were expected to live, on the average, 66.7 years and 74.9 years, respectively. There is an 8-year difference in life expectancy between sexes. Disability-free life expectancy is 60.5 years for males and 63.8 years for females. At age 60, males can expect to spend 11.0 years in disability-free state and females have 12.8 years of disability-free life expectancy. The proportions of these years to total life expectancies are 72.8% and 64.1%.

It is interesting to compare these figures in 1989 with Lamb's study for 1984 although their measures for health are not exactly comparable. While life expectancy increased 1.4 years for males and 1.3 years for females at age 60, disability-free life expectancy only increased 0.4 years for males and decreased 1.4 years for females. This change may be attributable to the differences in definition of health. The proportion of disability-free life expectancy also decreased from 1984 to 1989, especially for females.

In 1998, the National Health and Welfare Survey for the Elderly Persons was conducted in South Korea. This survey included questions on ADLs, IADLs and diseases. The preliminary work on health expectancy was carried out by participants at the NUPRI Training Workshop on Health

Table 15.17. Healthy life expectancy by sex for Thailand: 1986 and 1995

Age	Males			Females		
	Life expectancy	Healthy life expectancy	Percent of healthy life expectancy	Life expectancy	Healthy life expectancy	Percent of healthy life expectancy
1986						
60	15.52	9.46	60.9	18.56	10.38	55.9
65	12.53	7.33	58.5	15.15	8.18	54.0
70	9.69	5.43	56.1	12.03	6.23	51.8
75	7.49	4.07	54.3	9.33	4.43	47.5
80	5.20	2.68	51.5	6.17	2.89	46.3
1995						
60	20.29	13.45	66.3	23.89	13.61	57.0
65	17.14	10.78	62.9	20.20	11.20	55.4
70	14.18	8.02	56.6	16.89	8.96	53.0
75	11.87	6.34	53.4	14.60	7.49	51.3
80	10.90	5.87	53.8	13.60	6.95	51.1

Source: Jitapunkul and Chayovan (2000) 'Healthy life expectancy of Thai elderly: Did it improve during the soap-bubble economic period?' *Journal of Medical Association of Thailand* 83(8), 861–864.

Expectancy for Developing Countries held in Tokyo, Japan, in July 1999. Their results will show the trend in health status of the elderly over the last 10 years.

THAILAND

In Thailand, studies on health expectancy were conducted by Jitapunkul and his colleagues using the Sullivan method. Jitapunkul and Chayovan (2000) computed healthy life expectancy for Thai elderly for 1986 and 1995. The two surveys used were the Socio-Economic Consequences of the Ageing of the Population (SECAPT) conducted in 1986 and the Survey of the Welfare of Elderly in Thailand (SWET) conducted in 1995. Although the wording was slightly different, both surveys included a question on perceived health. The exact wording of the question in SECAPT is 'During the past week, how did you feel about your health in general?' and in SWET is 'How do you feel about your health in general?' Response categories for the former are 'very good', 'fair', 'as usual', and 'bad'; and for the latter are 'very healthy', 'rather healthy', 'moderate', 'rather weak', and 'weak'. In the study, they defined 'good health' as those who answered 'very good', 'fair', or 'as usual' in SECAPT; and 'very healthy', 'rather healthy', or 'moderate' in SWET. The life tables of the corresponding years are used to compute healthy life expectancies. Results from their study are shown in Table 15.17. Total life expectancy, healthy life expectancy, and the proportion of healthy life expectancy increased for both sexes between 1986 and 1995. The absolute increase in the percentage of healthy life expectancy to total life expectancy is larger for males than for females. Males are more likely to feel they are healthy. At age 60 in 1995, they feel they are healthy for 66% of their remaining life, while females expect to live 60% of their remaining life feeling healthy.

Jitapunkul *et al* (1999) also computed several types of health expectancy for Thailand. Using the National Health Examination Survey II conducted by the Ministry of Public Health in 1997, Jitapunkul and his colleagues computed active life expectancy, disability-free life expectancy without short-term disability, and disability-free life expectancy with short-term disability. Need for assistance with ADL items including eating, grooming, transferring, toileting, dressing and bathing is the criterion for active life expectancy. Those who have long-term conditions or health problems for six months or longer are classified as disabled. Short-term disability is defined as a state of being restricted on daily activities due to health problems during the two weeks preceding the survey date. Abridged life tables for 1996 are used to compute these health expectancies. Active life expectancy and disability-free life expectancy with and without short-term disability are shown in Table 15.18. Females have a longer life expectancy and active life expectancy but a smaller

Table 15.18. Active life expectancy, disability-free life expectancy by sex for Thailand: 1996

Age	Total life expectancy	Active life expectancy	Percent of active life expectancy	Disability-free life expectancy with short-term disability	Disability-free life expectancy without short-term disability
Males					
60	20.29	18.65	91.9	16.39	15.44
65	17.14	15.51	90.5	13.53	12.77
70	14.18	12.63	89.1	10.93	10.29
75	11.87	10.37	87.4	8.96	8.38
80	10.90	8.96	82.2	7.89	7.27
Females					
60	23.89	21.30	89.2	18.18	16.66
65	20.20	17.59	87.1	14.77	13.55
70	16.89	14.34	84.9	11.84	10.92
75	14.60	12.03	82.4	9.84	9.08
80	13.60	10.76	79.1	8.71	8.20

Source: Sutthichai Jitapunkul, Chaiyos Kunanusont, Wiput Phoolcharoen and Paibul Suriyawongpaisal (1999) *Health Problems of the Elderly in Thailand.* Bangkok: National Health Foundation and Ministry of Public Health.

proportion of active life expectancy at each age. Males average 20.3 years of remaining life at age 60 and of these they expect to spend 1.6 years (20.29 – 18.65) as inactive, 2.3 years (18.65 – 16.39) with long-term disability, and 1 year (16.39–15.44) with short-term disability in 1996. Corresponding figures for females are 2.6 years, 3.1 years, and 1.5 years, respectively.

Although the ADL items are not exactly the same, it is interesting to compare the results from Lamb's study previously presented (see Table 15.15) and the study by Jitapunkul and his colleagues. Active life expectancy increased from 15.2 years in 1989 to 18.6 years in 1996 for males aged 60 and from 17.4 years to 21.3 years for females aged 60 over the same period, while life expectancy increased from 16.0 years to 20.3 years for males and from 19.1 years to 23.9 years for females. However, the proportion of active life expectancy decreased for both sexes between 1989 and 1996.

Disability-free life expectancies with short-term disability were also computed for the Thai elderly by region (Jitapunkul *et al*, 1999). As shown in Table 15.19, those 60 years and over living in Bangkok had the longest life expectancy for both sexes in 1996; however, they spent proportionally more time in the disabled

Table 15.19. Disability-free life expectancy with short-term disability by sex and region in Thailand: 1996

	Males			Females		
Region	Life expectancy	Disability-free life expectancy with short-term disability	Percent of disability-free life expectancy with short-term disability	Life expectancy	Disability-free life expectancy with short-term disability	Percent of disability-free life expectancy with short-term disability
At age 60						
Bangkok	25.41	17.80	70.05	27.99	16.11	57.56
Central	20.50	15.58	76.00	23.26	15.78	67.84
South	20.83	17.44	83.72	24.59	19.18	78.00
North east	18.00	15.42	85.67	22.17	18.90	85.25
North	22.01	18.13	82.37	26.45	22.61	85.48
At age 80						
Bangkok	14.60	8.25	56.51	17.75	7.24	40.79
Central	10.76	7.68	71.37	11.66	6.12	54.49
South	10.93	8.43	77.13	15.25	10.42	68.33
North east	9.53	7.15	75.03	11.97	8.98	75.02
North	12.50	9.30	74.40	17.52	13.69	78.14

Source: Sutthichai Jitapunkul, Chaiyos Kunanusont, Wiput Phoolcharoen and Paibul Suriyawongpaisal (1999) *Health Problems of the Elderly in Thailand.* Bangkok, National Health Foundation and Ministry of Public Health.

state compared to those in the other regions. The average health status of elderly people in the northern regions was better than in the other regions. A very interesting finding from this study is that a region with a higher gross domestic product (GDP) per capita has a lower proportion of disability-free life expectancy with short-term disability to life expectancy. This finding suggests a possible relationship between the prevalence of disability among the Thai elderly and urbanization and development. This relationship was associated with an effect of urban environment such as a change in life style or an increase in the prevalence of chronic diseases, in particular hypertension and stroke. Jitapunkul and colleagues suggest that with urbanization occurring very rapidly, morbidity-disability may be on the rise in Thailand.

SINGAPORE

At a Training Workshop on Health Expectancy at the Nihon University Population Research Institute, two participants from Singapore presented their calculation of life expectancy without chronic illness based on the Sullivan method. They used abridged life tables for 1995 and the National Survey of Senior Citizens conducted in 1995. Their results are shown in Table 15.20. Males are expected to live 23.3 years more at age 55 with 16.6 years without chronic illness. The corresponding figures for females are 27.6 and 18.6 years, respectively. As observed in many other studies, females have a longer life expectancy and life expectancy without chronic illness but a smaller proportion

Table 15.20. Life expectancy without chronic illness by sex for Singapore: 1995

	Males			Females		
Age	Life expectancy	Chronic illness-free life expectancy	Percent of chronic illness-free life expectancy	Life expectancy	Chronic illness-free life expectancy	Percent of chronic illness-free life expectancy
55	23.3	16.6	71.2	27.6	18.6	67.4
60	19.4	13.3	68.6	23.3	15.3	65.7
65	16.0	10.6	66.3	19.4	12.5	64.4
70	13.1	8.9	67.9	15.9	10.3	64.8
75	10.8	7.4	68.5	13.1	8.5	64.9
80	9.2	6.0	65.2	10.8	6.9	63.9
85	8.3	5.3	63.9	9.1	5.8	63.7

Source: Results presented at NUPRI Training Workshop on Health Expectancy for Developing Countries, Tokyo, Japan. July 1999.

Table 15.21. Summary table of studies on health expectancy in Asian countries

Author	Year of study	Population	Type of health expectancy	Measure	Year computed	Method	Age available	Break-down
Japan								
The Council of National Living	1974	National	Average healthy life expectancy	Functional loss	1966 and 1970	NA	0, 15, 25, 45, 65	Sex
Nanjo and Shigematsu	1987	National	Bed disability-free	Number of days in bed	1975, 1980 and 1985	Sullivan	0–75 by 10	Sex
Gunji and Hayashi	1991	National	Disease-free	Have disease or injury	1974–1985	Sullivan	0	Sex
			Bed disability-free	Number of days in bed	1974–1985	Sullivan	0	Sex
Inoue *et al*	1997	National	Bed disability-free	Number of days in bed	1990	Sullivan	0–50 by 10, 55–80 by 5	Sex
Kamimura	1996	National	Active life	Help on ADL	1992	Sullivan	0–50 by 10, 60–90 by 5	Sex
Hashimoto	1998	National	Active life	Help on ADL	1995	Sullivan	65–85 by 10	Sex, region
Ikuta *et al*	1999	Dentists	Bed disability-free	Number of days in bed	1991–1997 pooled	Sullivan	25–85 by 5	None
Kai *et al*	1991	Regional	Active life	ADL	1988–1989	Double-decrement	60–90 by 5	Sex
Honma *et al*	1998	Regional	Active life	ADL	1992–1996	Double-decrement	70–90 by 5	Sex
Sauvaget *et al*	1997	Regional	Dementia-free	Dementia	1988–1991	Double-decrement	65–90 by 5	Sex
Tsuji *et al*	1995	Regional	Active life	Help on ADL	1988–1991	Multistate	65–90	Sex
Liu *et al*	1995	National	Active life	Functionally disabled	1987–1990	Multistate	60–96 by 3	None

China								
Grab et al	1991	National	Disability-free	5 types of disability	1987	Sullivan	0, 15, 25, 45, 65, 75	Sex
Z.-K. Qiao et al	1993	Regional	Active life	ADL/IADL	1989–1990	Sullivan	15–75 by 10	Sex, place of residence
Wang	1993	National	Active life	ADL	1992	Sullivan	60	Sex, place of residence
X.-C. Qiao	1997	National	Disability-free	5 types of disability	1987	Sullivan	0, 65, 80	Sex
			Perceived health	Perceived health	1987 and 1992	Sullivan	65, 80	Sex
			Active life	ADL	1987 and 1992	Sullivan	65, 80	Sex
			Disease-free	Have disease or injury	1992	Sullivan	65, 80	Sex
Taiwan								
Tu and Chen	1994	National	Disability-free	Independence	1986–1991	Double-decrement	15, 25, 45, 65, 75	Sex
			Disease-free	Have disease	1986–1991	Double-decrement	15, 25, 45, 65, 75	Sex
Korea								
Lamb	1999	National	Active life	ADL	1984	Sullivan	60–80 by 5	Sex
Lee	1997	National	Disability-free	Usual activities	1989	Sullivan	0, 60–80 by 5	Sex
Thailand								
Jitapunkul and Chayovan	2000	National	Perceived health	Perceived health	1986, 1995	Sullivan	60–80 by 5	Sex
Lamb	1999	National	Active life	ADL	1989	Sullivan	60–80 by 5	Sex
Jitapunkul et al	1998	National	Disability-free active life	Help on ADL	1996	Sullivan	60–80 by 5	Sex
Singapore								
NUPRI training workshop	1999	National	Disease-free	Chronic disease	1995	Sullivan	55–85 by 5	Sex
Malaysia								
Lamb	1999	National	Active life	ADL	1984	Sullivan	60–80 by 5	Sex

(continued)

Table 15.21. (*continued*)

Author	Year of study	Population	Type of health expectancy	Measure	Year computed	Method	Age available	Break-down
Philippines Lamb	1999	National	Active life	ADL	1984	Sullivan	60–80 by 5	Sex
Burma Lamb	1999	National	Active life	ADL	1989	Sullivan	60–80 by 5	Sex
Indonesia Lamb	1999	National	Active life	ADL	1989	Sullivan	60–80 by 5	Sex
North Korea Lamb	1999	National	Active life	ADL	1989	Sullivan	60–80 by 5	Sex
Sri Lanka Lamb	1999	National	Active life	ADL	1989	Sullivan	60–80 by 5	Sex

of life expectancy without chronic illness. However, the differences in the proportion between sexes are small at all ages. For both sexes, the proportion of life expectancy without chronic illness does not decline even at older age groups.

CONCLUSION

We summarize the characteristics of the major studies on health expectancy in Asian countries in Table 15.21. The Sullivan method is the most prevalent method for computing health expectancy in Asian countries due to data availability. In order to apply other methods such as the multistate life table method and the double-decrement life table method, longitudinal surveys are required, which are relatively rare in Asia. The information obtained from the Sullivan method and multistate life table method is different (Crimmins *et al*, 1993). Many studies of health expectancy introduced here are for older age groups although health expectancy is not limited to the elderly. This is partly because quality of life measured by health status is more relevant to the elderly. In addition, in many studies ADLs are used as the measure of health. While these are probably a good measure of health status for older people they may not be appropriate for younger populations. This limits some estimates of health expectancy to the older population.

Studies on health expectancy in Asian countries are relatively few at this moment, because research priorities differ across countries and the concept of health expectancy is relatively new in the region. However, we expect studies using health expectancy to increase in the future with the increase in the older population in each country. Also researchers interested in the concept of health expectancy are increasing. Participants at the NUPRI Training Workshop mentioned above are computing health expectancy for the Philippines using the 1996 Philippine Elderly Survey. Participants from Malaysia are also computing health expectancy using their health survey. Health expectancy is a very useful measure to monitor health status of populations and should be linked to policy making and this is on our research agenda in the new millennium.

REFERENCES

Branch, L.G.S., Katz, K., Kniepmann K. and Papsidero, J.A. (1984). 'A prospective study of functional status among community elders', *American Journal of Public Health* 74(3), 266–268.

Calot, G. and Caselli, G. (1988) 'La mortalité en Chine d'après le recensement de 1982', document prepared for the Seminar on Mortality Transition in South and East Asia, Beijing.

Council of National Living (1974) *Social Indicators of Japan.* Tokyo: The Council of National Living, Research Committee.

Crimmins, E.M. and Saito, Y. (1993) 'Getting better and getting worse: Transitions in functional status among older Americans', *Journal of Aging and Health* 5(1), 3–36.

Crimmins, E.M., Saito, Y. and Hayward, M.D. (1993) 'Sullivan and multi-state methods of estimating active life expectancy: two methods, two answers', in Robine, J-M., Mathers, C.D., Bone, M.R. and Romieu, I. (eds) *Calculation of Health Expectancies: Harmonization, Consensus Achieved and Future Perspectives.* Paris: John Libbey Eurotext.

Grab, B., Dowd, J.E. and Michel, J.-P. (1991) 'Estimate of disability-free life expectancy in China', Paper presented at the 4th meeting of REVES, Noordwijkerhout, Netherlands.

Gunji, T and Hayashi, R. (1991) 'Shitsu o kouryo shita kenkou shihyou to sono katsuyou', Paper presented at Population Association of Japan.

Hashimoto, S. (1998) 'Hoken iryo fukushi ni kansuru chiiki shihyou no sougouteki kaihatsu to ouyou ni kansuru kenkyu'. Research report.

Honma, Y., Naruse Y. and Kagamimori, S. (1998) 'Koureisha no nichijou seikatsu jiritsudo to seimei yogo, katsudouteki yomyou tono kanren ni tsuite' (Active life expectancy, life expectancy and ADL in Japanese elderly), *Nihon Koushuu Eisei Zasshi* (Japanese Journal of Public Health) 45(10), 1018–1029.

Ikuta, A., Yokoyama, E., Shinbo, H., Miyake, T., Terui, T., Nozaki, S., Nasu, K. and Saito, Y. (1999) 'Shika ishi ni okeru katsudouteki heikin yomyou no kenkyu: 1991–1997 nen' (Health expectancy research for dentists: 1991–1997). Paper presented at Japan Society for Occupational Health meetings, May, Tokyo.

Inoue, T., Shigematsu T. and Nanjo, Z. (1997) 'Nihon no 1990nen kenkou seimeihyo – sekai saichoju no shitsu no kenkou' (Health life tables in Japan, 1990: A quality of the longest life expectancy in the world), *Minzoku Eisei* (Japanese Journal of Public Health), 63(4), 226–240.

Jitapunkul, S. and Chayovan, N. (2000) 'Healthy life expectancy of Thai elderly: Did it improve during the soap-bubble economic period?' *Journal of Medical Association of Thailand* 83(8), 861–864.

Jitapunkul, S., Kunanusont, C., Phoolcharoen, W. and Suriyawongpaisal, P. (1999) *Health Problems of the Elderly in Thailand.* Bangkok: National Health Foundation and Ministry of Public Health [in Thai].

Kai, I., Ohi, G., Kobayashi, Y., Ishizaki, T., Hisata, M. and Kiuchi M. (1991) 'Quality of Life: A Possible Health Index for the Elderly', *Asia-Pacific Journal of Public Health* 5(3), 221–227.

Kamimura, K. (1996) 'Kenkou yomei no sokutei ni kansuru kenkyuu houkokusho'. Research report.

Lamb, V.L. (1999) 'Active life expectancy of the elderly in selected Asian countries', NUPRI Research Paper Series No. 69. Tokyo, Japan: Nihon University Population Research Institute.

Lee, S.-K. (1997) 'A study on disability-free life expectancy of the elderly in Korea', Paper presented at 10th meeting of REVES, Tokyo, Japan.

Liu, X., Liang, J., Muramatsu, N. and Sugisawa H. (1995) 'Transitions in functional status and active life expectancy among older people in Japan', *Journal of Gerontology: Social Sciences* 50B(6), S383–S394.

Manton, K.G. (1988) 'A longitudinal study of functional change and mortality in the United States', *Journal of Gerontology: Social Sciences* 43(5), S153–S161.

Nanjo, Z. and Shigematsu, T. (1987) 'Kenkou seimeihyo sakusei ni tsuite' (Calculation of health expectancy). Paper presented at a regional meeting of Population Association of Japan, Fukuoka, Japan.

Qiao, X.-C. (1997) 'Health Expectancy of China', Paper presented at 10th REVES meeting, Tokyo, Japan.

Qiao, Z.-K., Wilkins, R., Yang, M., Lan, Y., Chen, X., Xu, Y. and Ng, E. (1993) 'Health expectancy of adults in Xichang, China, 1990: autonomy in various activities of daily living', in Robine, J-M., Mathers, C.D., Bone, M.R. and Romieu, I. (eds) *Calculation of Health Expectancies: Harmonization, Consensus Achieved and Future Perspectives*. Paris: John Libbey Eurotext.

Rogers, A., Rogers, R.G. and Belanger, A. (1990) 'Longer life but worse health? Measurement and dynamics', *The Gerontologist* 30(5), 640–649.

Sauvaget, C., Tsuji, I., Minami, Y., Fukao, A., Hisamichi, S., Asano, H. and Sato, M. (1997) 'Dementia-free life expectancy among elderly Japanese', *Gerontology*, 43, 168–175.

Tsuji, I., Minami, Y., Fukao, A., Hisamichi, S., Asano, H. and Sato, M. (1995) 'Active life expectancy among elderly Japanese', *Journal of Gerontology: Medical Sciences* 50A(3), M173–M176.

Tu, E.J.-C. and Chen, K.-J. (1994a) 'Changes in active life expectancy in Taiwan: Compression or expansion?' *Social Science and Medicine* 39, 1657–1665.

Tu, E.J.-C. and Chen, K.-J. (1994b) 'Recent changes in healthy life expectancy and their implications for medical costs in Taiwan', in Mathers, C., McCallum, J. and Robine, J-M. (eds) *Advances in Health Expectancies*. Canberra: AGPS, Australian Institute of Health and Welfare.

Tu, E.J.-C., Chen, K.-J. and Chang, M.-C. (1997) 'Changes in morbidity and chronic disability in an elderly population: Taiwan, 1989–1993', Paper presented at 10th REVES meeting, Tokyo, Japan.

UNFPA (1999) *The State of World Population, 1999*. New York: United Nations.

United Nations (1999) *World Population Prospects: The 1998 Revision*. New York: United Nations.

Wang, M. (1993) *Living Long is not Equal to Living Healthy: Quality of Life and Medical Security*. Beijing: China Economic Press.

World Bank (1999) *1999 World Development Indicators*. Washington, DC: World Bank.

16

Ageing and Health Expectancies in Urban Latin America

ROBERTO HAM-CHANDE

El Colegio de la Frontera Norte, Tijuana, Mexico

The Americas are that large part of the world that geographically separates the Pacific and Atlantic oceans. Socioeconomically the Americas are divided in two. One part is North America, essentially Canada and the United States,[1] the only two countries of the Americas that are fully developed. Both have the cultural characteristic of being predominantly English speaking. On the other side there is Latin America, a vast subcontinent of 20.3 million square kilometres, comprising many geographical regions and experiencing all of the known climates and environments.

Politically Latin America is composed of 45 nations and other territories. Statistics from the year 2000 report more than 519 million inhabitants (UN, 2000), divided into hundreds of ethnicities, at the same time concentrated in a few huge metropolises, living in multitudes of medium-size cities and scattered in hundreds of thousands of rural settlements. The population is socially and economically polarized into a diversity that has been moulded during the second half of the last millennium. The turning point was the arrival of the European settlers, whose origins are principally from the Iberian peninsula, Spain and Portugal, with the subsequent colonization and racial mixing. These antecedents provide the cultural and ethnic background for the Latin adjective of this part of the Americas. Actually ethnicity in Latin America is more multifaceted and rounded out with the demographic flows that have come from other parts of Europe, Africa and Asia.

No other great multinational region in the world has such a social and cultural cohesion through a common language for most of its inhabitants, as is the case of the Spanish language in Latin America. Brazil is an exception to this

---

[1] Some atlases and statistics consider Greenland and Iceland as part of the Americas.

Determining Health Expectancies. Edited by J-M. Robine, C. Jagger, C.D. Mathers, E.M. Crimmins and R.M. Suzman.
© 2003 John Wiley & Sons, Ltd

linguistic uniformity with the speaking of Portuguese. However, these two languages are similar, facilitating the extended knowledge of Spanish among the educated Brazilian population seeking economic and social links with their Latin American neighbourhood.

From a geographical perspective, in Latin America we distinguish three large regions.

Central America is composed of Mexico with its 99 million inhabitants and the long and narrow isthmus, approximately 1700 km in length, that connects the two massive subcontinents of North America and South America. This string of countries is composed of seven republics (Guatemala, Belize, Honduras, El Salvador, Nicaragua, Costa Rica and Panama), home to 36 million people.

South America is the largest geographical region of Latin America, with 13 nations and possessions (Brazil, Colombia, Argentina, Peru, Venezuela, Chile, Ecuador, Bolivia, Paraguay, Uruguay, Suriname, Guyana and French Guiana). It is also the home for the greatest part of the Latin America population, with 320 million inhabitants.

The Caribbean is composed of 24 islands or archipelagos, each one constituting a nation or a political entity, and with a total of 38 million inhabitants. (The nations in this region with more than 1 million people are Cuba, Dominican Republic, Haiti, Puerto Rico, Jamaica, Trinidad-Tobago.)

In the Caribbean there are other classifications and criteria, depending on the characteristics that are emphasized; for instance there are 11 English speaking entities and a Dutch possession, therefore non-Latin, but there are also places where French is the language, thus non-Hispanic. In some instances Puerto Rico is regarded as part of the United States. However, there remains no doubt of its Latin population and culture, including the generalized use of the Spanish language. The concept of the Caribbean is also conceived not only by its islands but as the Caribbean Sea basin, hence also including Florida, the Yucatan peninsula, Central America, and the northern coasts of South America.

POPULATION DYNAMICS

Overall demographic dynamics for Latin America are shown in Table 16.1. Data include population sizes, life expectancies for males and females, total fertility rates and population distribution by age groups. The numbers from 1950 to 1990 and the projections from 2000 to 2050 come from the Population Division of the Organization of the United Nations (UN, 2000).[2] During the second half of the 20th century the population size of Latin America multiplied by 3.2, growing from 167.0 to 519.1 million. It is expected that during the first

---

[2] The resulting projections are from the medium hypotheses on fertility and mortality.

Table 16.1. Demographic indicators for Latin America, 1950–2050

Year	Pop	LE-m	LE-f	TFR	%(0–14)	%(15–64)	%(65+)
1950	166 994	49.7	53.1	5.9	40.0	56.3	3.7
1960	218 225	54.9	58.9	6.0	42.2	53.8	3.9
1970	284 796	58.6	63.3	5.0	42.4	53.4	4.2
1980	361 398	61.9	68.1	3.9	39.6	55.9	4.5
1990	440 472	64.8	71.5	3.0	36.0	59.3	4.7
2000	519 143	67.2	73.6	2.5	31.5	63.1	5.4
2010	595 037	69.4	75.7	2.3	27.8	65.9	6.4
2020	665 093	71.3	77.5	2.2	24.9	66.9	8.3
2030	725 536	73.0	79.1	2.1	22.6	66.4	11.0
2040	773 554	74.3	80.3	2.1	21.0	65.0	14.0
2050	808 910	75.2	81.1	2.1	20.0	63.2	16.8

Pop = Population in thousands; LE-m = life expectancy at birth for males; LE-f = life expectancy at birth for females; TFR = total fertility rate; %(0–14) = % population aged 0–14 years; %(15–64) = % population aged 15–64 years; %(65+) = % population aged 65 years and over.
Source: United Nations (2000) *World Population Prospects – 1998.* Reproduced with permission

half of the 21st century demographic growth will slow down. Projections estimate a population size of 808.9 million by 2050, implying a multiplication factor of 1.6. The rapid pace of population increase experienced in the decades before 1970 is explained mainly by the high total fertility rates, combined with declines achieved in mortality levels reflected in constant gains in life expectancies. Total fertility rate was over 6.0 between 1960 and 1970, and then started a decline that will take the region to replacement level after 2030. It is also clear that the part of the projection that assumes the total fertility rate will level off at 2.1 after 2030 is a psychological barrier rejecting decreasing population size and theoretical extinction. Nevertheless it is probable that in the next decades Latin America will reach rates of fertility below the population growth.

Subsequent deceleration of population growth after 1970 is a product of a sharp lowering in birth rates accompanied by steady mortality improvements. In 1950 life expectancies were around 50 years for males and 53 years for females; by 2000 they were 67 years and 74 years, respectively, and are expected to reach 75 years and 81 years by the middle of the current century. Clearly, not only is the intensity of population growth decreasing but age structures are also changing.

From the beginning of the 20th century until 1970 the proportion of children and adolescents (0–14) in the population grew, to later decrease. In contrast, the proportion of the young and adult population (15–64) decreased until 1970, when it began to rise. The aged population (65+) has been continuously increasing with a sharp acceleration after 1990. Statistics depicting the second half of the 20th century are a reflection of past facts and events. Estimations for the first half of this century indeed have all the uncertainties that come with any projection; nevertheless, there is an evident trend leading to an intense demographic ageing. The percentage of the population aged 65+ went from 3.7 in 1950 to just 4.7 in 1990. After that numbers climb to 5.4 in 2000 and to an estimated 16.8 by 2050.

Certainly Latin America will profit from some or much of the progress that science and medical technology are now promising through breakthroughs in health maintenance and therapy. It now appears that with just a part of the improvements in medical care and health prevention that are foreseen, most probably life expectancies will be higher than those assumed in the projection. The question is 'In what measure will it be possible to benefit from such research and improvements?' For Latin America that answer will mainly come from social and economic performance that will allow the purchase and application of new developments in the medical fields.

However, in the prospective views over the 21st century the ageing process always appears not only unavoidable but accelerated, no matter which reasonable set of projection hypotheses is adopted. The expected figures show a continuing decline in percentage terms for the youngest population group (0–14), strong increases in the aged population (65+), and also the growing participation of the adult population (15–64) until a maximum is reached at some point during the decade of the 2030s. The consensus is that the demographic structure in Latin America shows an ageing process, characterized by a population in the intermediate ages (15–64) that will have a greater percentage and absolute participation during the following three or four decades.

AGEING IN LATIN AMERICA AND THE WORLD

The ageing index $100*P(65+)/P(0-14)$ provides a measure of the degree of demographic ageing by relating the numbers constituting the elderly part of the population $P(65+)$ to those of the youngest section $P(0-14)$.[3] Figure 16.1 shows a comparison of this index for the world and by major regions, including Latin America.

Europe has been and will be the most aged region. It is expected not only that it will continue in that position but that the gap with the rest of the world will be widening. North America (Canada and United States) follows as the second oldest region with Oceania third. Asia and Latin America are at a level close to the global averages. Finally, Africa is the continent furthest behind in the ageing process.

The figure refers to average behaviour within very large continents, regardless of their great internal variability in socioeconomic and demographic

---

[3]   As was defined by T. Kuroda.

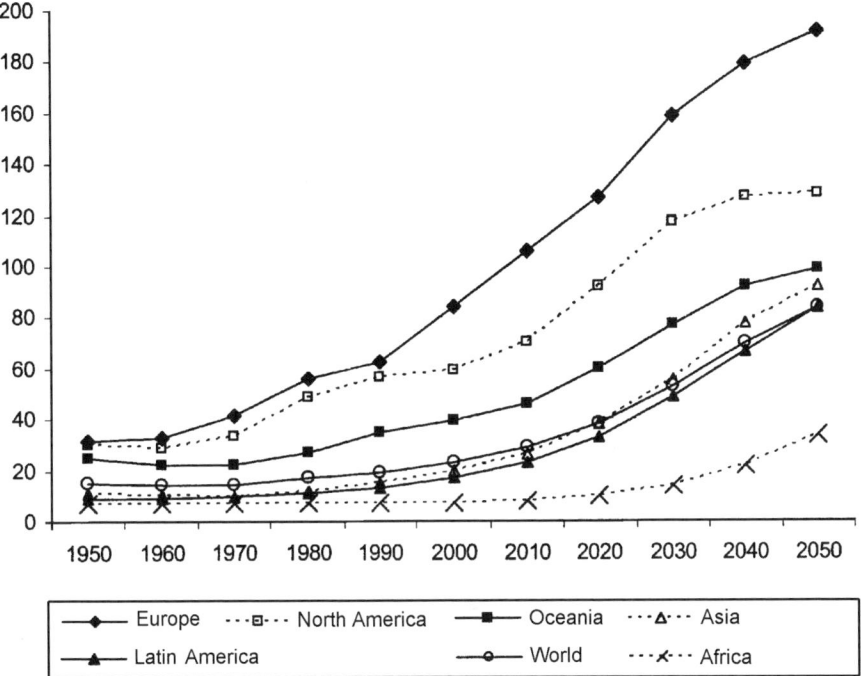

Figure 16.1. Ageing indexes in major regions of the world, 1950–2050. Ageing index $= 100*P(65+)/P(0$–$14)$. Source of data: UN, *World Population Prospects – 1998*. United Nations, 2000

conditions. For instance, the ageing process in Japan is very different from the rest of the Asian trends, which are dominated by the large population sizes of China and India. A similar situation occurs in Latin America that cannot be ignored.

AGEING DIVERSITY IN LATIN AMERICA

The figures in Figure 16.1 are a general demographic description based on averages for the whole Latin America region. However, as has been stated earlier, the countries (and indeed regions within countries) are very diverse in terms of geography, socioeconomic development, health problems and indeed in their stage of the epidemiological and demographic transitions. With such great variability within regions, averages over large areas or whole countries have little meaning for practical purposes and perspectives from smaller units are required.

Table 16.2. Population and demographic transition indicators in major countries of Latin America, 2000

Country	Population (thousands)	% Popu- lation	Σ % popu- lation	Period E(0) > 65	Period TFR < 4.0	%(65+) in 2000	Demo- graphic transition
Brazil	170 115	32.8	32.8	1990–95	1980–85	5.1	Intermediate
Mexico	98 881	19.0	51.8	1975–80	1985–90	4.7	Intermediate
Colombia	42 321	8.2	60.0	1980–85	1980–85	4.7	Intermediate
Argentina	37 032	7.1	67.1	1960–65	b. 1950	9.7	Early
Peru	25 662	4.9	72.1	1990–95	1985–90	4.8	Intermediate
Venezuela	24 170	4.7	76.7	1970–75	1980–85	4.4	Intermediate
Chile	15 211	2.9	79.7	1975-80	1970–75	7.2	Early
Ecuador	12 646	2.4	82.1	1985–90	1985–90	4.7	Intermediate
Guatemala	11 385	2.2	84.3	2000–05	2005–10	3.6	Late
Cuba	11 201	2.2	86.4	1960–65	1955–60	9.6	Early
Dominican Republic	8 495	1.6	88.1	1980–85	1980–85	4.5	Intermediate
Bolivia	8 329	1.6	89.7	2005–10	2000–05	4.0	Late

Period E(0) > 65: period for which life expectancy at birth started to be over 65 years.
Period TFR < 4: period for which total fertility rate started to be lower than 4.
% (65+) in 2000: Percentage of population over 65 years old.
Data from: United Nations (2000) *World Population Prospects – 1998*.

A large part of the geographical area and population size is concentrated in a few nations. Table 16.2 displays demographic indicators on the times and degrees of the demographic transition of the 12 major countries of Latin America, ordered by population size. The figures show that two countries, Brazil and Mexico, hold slightly over half the total population in Latin America; that in the first six is concentrated more than three-quarters, and that the listed dozen contain 90%. Thus by studying these 12 countries one can gain an almost complete appreciation of the overall demographic situation of Latin America.

Table 16.2 shows the periods in which decreases in mortality have resulted in life expectancies over 65 years and when total fertility rates became lower than 4.0. It also displays the percentage of the population aged 65+ in the year 2000. These indicators are used to classify countries as early, intermediate or late in regard to each one's demographic transition experience. Countries achieving life expectancies above 65 before 1980, a total fertility rate smaller than 4.0 before 1970 and percentages of population (65+) above 7.0% in the year 2000 are considered to have had an *early* demographic transition and to be at a relatively high degree of demographic ageing. Countries that reached the year 2000 without achieving life expectancies over 65, whose total fertility rate is still over 4.0 and with percentages of population (65+) lower than 4.0%, are those in a *late* demographic transition with only an incipient ageing process. All others are at an *intermediate* stage, in both their demographic transition and their degree of ageing.

This exercise was performed not just for these 12 nations, but for all the Latin American countries, and revealed that 12.4% of the population is in countries with an early demographic transition, 66.5% in countries at an intermediate stage and 21.1% in countries in a late process.

It should be added that the diversity in the demographic transition is correlated with the great polarization of the epidemiological transition. Shifts toward chronic diseases and degenerative conditions are occurring together with a decline in infectious and parasitic illnesses. This is a reflection of the socioeconomic heterogeneity whose more pernicious manifestation is the social and economic inequality in Latin America. The most direct and revealing indicators deal with the income distribution, showing an unfair situation where wealth is concentrated among the few, there is a middle-income class, but many people live below the poverty line.

AGEING INDEX IN LATIN AMERICA

Using the ageing index, Figure 16.2 shows the diversity of the ageing process in Latin America in 2000 and how it is expected to be in 2050. The selected countries are those that in 2000 have more than a million inhabitants. They are ranked from the demographically youngest to the oldest. Those with the youngest structures are in Central America (Nicaragua, Guatemala and Honduras) with indexes around 8. Most of Latin America nations have intermediate ageing indexes between 12 and 18. The most aged countries are the southern ones (Chile, Argentina and Uruguay) together with some in the Caribbean (Trinidad-Tobago, Puerto Rico and Cuba). This group of the oldest nations has indexes between 25 and 50.

The same figure clarifies the intensity of the ageing process that is expected in the following decades. The ageing index for Latin America is 17.2 and this number will be 83.7 in 2050. Around these averages there is great variability in the degree of ageing between countries with some important changes. The youngest nations in the year 2050 will be as old as the most aged nations of today. The largest part of Latin America will be in nations with indexes between 80 and 100. The four countries with higher ageing levels will all be in the Caribbean (Jamaica, Trinidad-Tobago, Puerto Rico and Cuba). Cuba will be by far the oldest, with an ageing index of 170.

DIFFERENTIALS IN LIFE EXPECTANCIES

Life expectancies are a summary of mortality levels in a population and also a reflection of the general health conditions. As such they are interrelated with the degree of development, thus following their heterogeneity. As

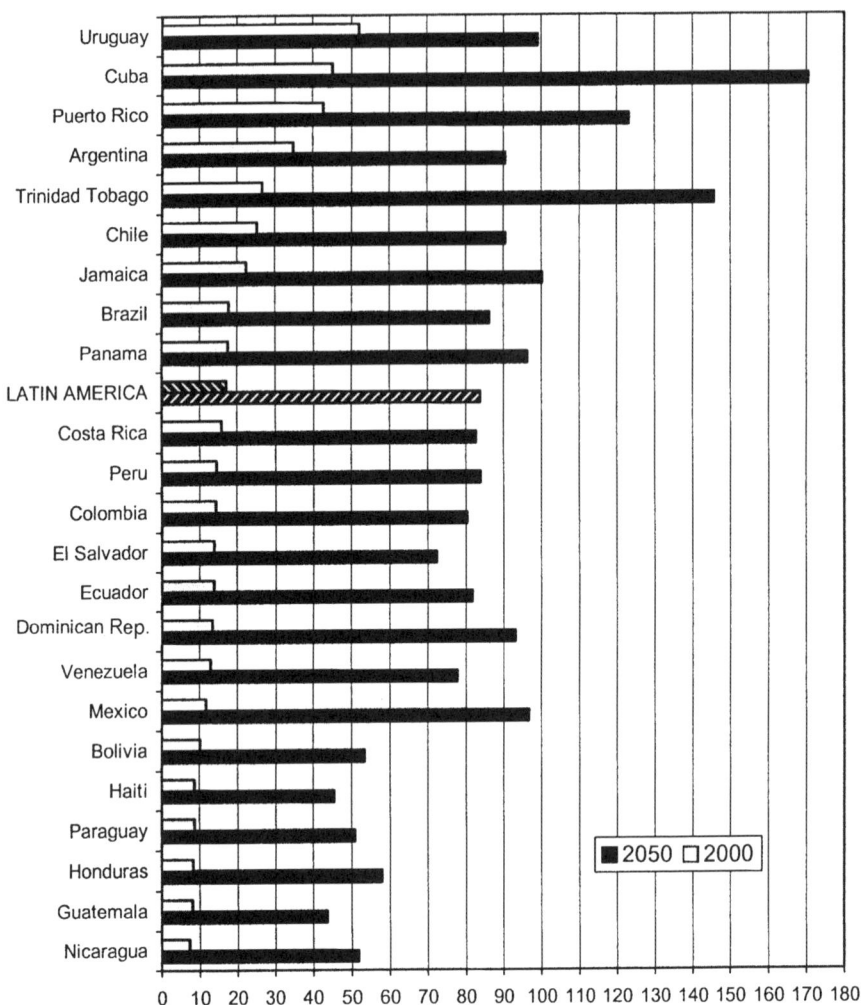

Figure 16.2. Ageing indexes for Latin America, 2000 and 2050. Ageing index $= 100^{*}P(65+)/P(0\text{–}14)$. Source of data: UN, *World Population Prospects – 1998*. United Nations, 2000

statistical indicators life expectancies have the advantages of availability, a concrete and straightforward meaning, comparability, and easy understanding. These characteristics help in the study of past population dynamics and its perspectives for the future. Table 16.3 presents life expectancies at birth, at age 65 and at age 80, in three pairs of the most populated Latin American countries that are examples of the early, intermediate and late status in their demographic transition. The figures are

Table 16.3. Life expectancies at birth, at 65 and 80 years old, by sex, in selected Latin American countries of early, intermediate and late demographic transition, 1950–1955, 1995–2000 and 2045–2050

Period	E(0)			E(65)			E(80)		
	1950–1955	1995–2000	2045–2050	1950–1955	1995–2000	2045–2050	1950–1955	1995–2000	2045–2050
Males									
(a) Argentina	60.4	69.7	76.9	12.1	16.1	17.5	5.5	5.9	8.2
Chile	52.9	71.1	77.5	11.8	16.3	17.8	5.4	6.9	8.5
(b) Brazil	49.3	65.5	74.5	12.2	17.3	17.1	5.4	7.2	8.2
Mexico	49.2	68.9	76.5	12.7	17.3	18.3	5.8	7.4	8.8
(c) Guatemala	41.9	64.7	74.5	11.4	15.4	17.6	4.9	7.3	8.4
Bolivia	38.5	59.8	74.5	9.9	15.2	17.3	4.1	5.9	8.4
Females									
(a) Argentina	65.1	76.8	84.0	14.5	20.4	22.2	6.5	8.0	10.5
Chile	56.8	78.1	84.0	13.7	20.2	22.0	6.4	8.6	10.6
(b) Brazil	52.8	70.1	82.5	12.7	19.7	21.5	5.5	8.0	10.5
Mexico	52.4	75.0	82.7	13.4	20.1	21.9	6.1	8.5	10.7
(c) Guatemala	42.3	69.8	80.5	11.8	18.3	21.1	5.5	8.3	10.2
Bolivia	42.5	63.2	79.0	10.7	16.8	20.4	4.3	6.5	10.0

Demographic transition: (a) early; (b) intermediate; (c) late.
E(0) = Life expectancy at birth; E(65) = life expectancy at age 65; E(80) = life expectancy at age 80.
Data from: CELADE, 2001. *Boletín Demográfico No. 67.* Santiago, Chile.

the estimates for the five-year periods 1950–1955, 1995–2000 and those projected for 2045–2050 (CELADE, 2001).

In these countries life expectancies are increasing at all ages, a common experience for all Latin American nations and practically all over the world.[4] Figures for 1950–1955 show that there have been huge differences in life expectancies among Latin American nations, obviously related to development levels and the pace of demographic transition. As expected, among the examples Guatemala and Bolivia have the lowest figures, Mexico and Brazil are intermediate and Argentina and Chile have the highest life expectancies. Life expectancies in 1995–2000 not only show increases but also that gaps are closing between countries. In the estimates for 2045–2050 it is anticipated that differences in life expectancies from country to country will be substantially shortened.

---

[4] Exceptions are the nations in Africa beset by the AIDS epidemic and Russia with its recent socioeconomic problems, alcoholism and violence.

In 1950–1955 the difference between life expectancies at birth in Argentina and Bolivia was 22 years; in 1995–2000 it decreased to 10 years and in the United Nations population projection for 2045–2050 it is expected to drop even further and be merely around 2 years. The larger relative gains in Bolivia in comparison to Argentina during the second half of the 20th century were due to the possibility of reducing high infantile mortality rates. In the coming decades the reductions in adult and elderly mortality will be more and more important for the increments in life expectancies. These potential diminutions have lower limits and are more difficult to achieve. In addition, life expectancies at ages 65 and 80 refer to selected survivors, which makes them similar in mortality rates, thus showing smaller differences between countries and in time.

BUILDING INFORMATION AND KNOWLEDGE

The increments in life expectancies in Latin America are another expression of the demographic ageing process that is occurring in the region. Although this process is common for the entire world, Latin America has characteristics that make it particularly important: ageing is taking place at a great speed within a context of incomplete development, in such a way that to unsolved social and economic problems now are added the needs of an elderly population that is rapidly increasing. Besides the financial crisis of social security, the most pressing requirements come from health care and maintenance. The challenges include building knowledge and information on demographic ageing, its interrelations with social and economic variables, and their impact on health systems. Necessary tasks include the collection of appropriate and pertinent information and statistics.

To address this, the Pan American Health Office is coordinating a multi-centre project on Health and Well-Being of the Elderly, known as SABE by its acronym in Spanish.[5] The emphasis of the project is on health issues, under the specific objective of carrying out a survey to provide a database on the topic. This project has necessitated the construction of concepts, the elaboration of theoretical frameworks and the creation of methodological instruments suitable for Latin America. This research project takes into consideration that in the region demographic ageing and its relationships with health and well-being are not a set of uniform phenomena. Rather their characteristics are as variable as the social, economic and demographic conditions. With the aim of covering the social and economic heterogeneity of Latin America, the study was organized to include seven Latin American countries: Argentina, Barbados, Brazil, Chile, Cuba, Mexico and Uruguay.

---

[5] The name of the project in Spanish is *Salud y Bienestar en el Envejecimiento*.

In a first stage, a central objective of the SABE project was to evaluate the current health conditions of the elderly in major urban areas and to provide comparative studies between participant countries. Of special interest is the characterization of patterns of morbidity, assessments of physical, mental and functional deficiencies, as well as the access and use of health services available to the elderly. In this analysis it is also of relevance to determine the differences that exist between cohorts, social classes and the variations by gender, as well as the relationships between all these variables.

The cities included in the first stage were: Buenos Aires (Argentina), Bridgetown (Barbados), São Paulo (Brazil), Santiago (Chile), Havana (Cuba), Mexico City (Mexico) and Montevideo (Uruguay). The target population for the SABE survey was composed of usual residents of the selected geographical areas that at the moment of the interview were aged 60 years and over.[6] Information was captured by a home interview, using exactly the same structured questionnaire in all the seven survey sites.

SIGNIFICANT CHRONIC ILLNESSES

Among the several topics included in the SABE survey the prevalence of diagnosed chronic illnesses is of utmost relevance. Table 16.4 shows those conditions with the highest prevalence, for each of the surveyed cities,[7] separately by sex and age groups (60–74) and (75+).

Of the chronic illnesses impacting on the elderly population, hypertension and arthritis stand out because of their high prevalence rates, particularly among women. Buenos Aires, Santiago and São Paulo are the cities showing the worst rates of hypertension for men while Mexico City has the lowest rates. For women hypertension rates are high everywhere. Second in importance is arthritis, a heavy burden for women. Diabetes rates are also particularly high in Mexico City for both sexes as well as for women in Bridgetown. Heart disease rates are highest in Buenos Aires and São Paulo. Although at lower rates, lung diseases are also reported in significant numbers.

SOCIOECONOMIC DETERMINANTS

Latin American countries and their regions and cities show diverse demographic and health profiles resulting from their historical backgrounds and socioeconomic conditions. Part of this diversity is reflected in the different mortality levels and morbidity outcomes. A significant and sensitive indicator

---

[6] An exemption was Mexico City, where women 50 and over were included.

[7] At the time when this chapter was being written the database for Havana, Cuba, was not ready.

Table 16.4. Prevalence (%) of diagnosed chronic disease in population (60–74) and (75+), by sex. Selected major cities in Latin America, 2000

	Hypertension		Diabetes		Arthritis		Heart disease		Lung disease	
	60–74	75+	60–74	75+	60–74	75+	60–74	75+	60–74	75+
Men										
Bridgetown	36.5	39.9	18.2	19.4	29.8	36.3	10.5	14.3	2.2	4.8
Buenos Aires	47.1	46.7	14.7	11.7	36.2	37.4	21.7	18.6	10.4	9.8
Mexico City	35.4	32.2	21.9	24.1	15.4	17.7	8.0	17.0	7.2	11.7
Montevideo	39.3	33.4	12.8	11.5	29.6	38.2	21.0	26.7	10.9	10.9
Santiago	42.9	51.6	12.3	12.9	13.3	15.3	30.6	30.6	11.4	18.5
São Paulo	50.2	46.3	17.5	15.4	19.5	23.4	20.0	24.5	13.9	15.4
Women										
Bridgetown	56.9	50.9	25.1	23.9	55.2	59.7	8.9	16.6	4.8	5.0
Buenos Aires	50.2	52.4	11.3	11.4	61.4	65.0	18.0	21.9	4.9	10.0
Mexico City	49.1	48.0	20.6	21.3	28.9	36.7	9.8	10.7	9.5	15.4
Montevideo	49.7	49.0	15.0	13.1	56.3	59.4	20.5	32.9	7.8	9.6
Santiago	54.5	58.3	12.3	12.9	39.1	44.2	33.6	37.9	10.0	16.0
São Paulo	55.3	60.6	19.3	17.8	38.6	43.1	17.4	24.6	10.8	11.6

Data from: *Survey on Health and Well-being of the Elderly in Latin America* – SABE. Pan American Health Organization (PAHO), 2000.

of the socioeconomic level of a person or a society is the degree of education. Table 16.5 shows the percentages of the population 60 years and over that never went to school, those that only had primary studies and those that attended at least high school or more. The information is provided for the studied cities, by sex and divided in two large groups of age.

These results describe the educational levels of the now elderly population that should have had an elementary education before 1950. Bridgetown has the smallest percentages of the elderly population who never went to school and the highest percentage of those having only primary instruction. The proportion of people that had at least high-school education and above is relatively high. These relatively good indicators can be explained by the fact that Barbados is a small island that holds unusual social and economic opportunities for its small size population.

Buenos Aires and Montevideo also have a small percentage of the elderly population who did not go to school. Most of the elderly had elementary school and a substantial part went to high school and beyond. These two cities are neighbouring, although separated by the great mouth of the De la Plata river, and are ethnically very similar in their Italian and Spanish ancestry, with cultural and urban traces of the great development that they had during the first half of the 20th century. Those past conditions allowed good educational

Table 16.5. Schooling in population aged 60 and over, by sex and age group, in selected cities of Latin America, 2000

		Women			Men		
		No schooling	Primary	High school +	No schooling	Primary	High school +
Bridgetown	60–74	0.4	73.4	26.1	0.0	70.9	29.1
	75+	1.5	83.5	14.9	2.2	81.1	16.7
Buenos Aires	60–74	4.8	65.6	29.6	2.1	60.6	37.3
	75+	2.5	79.9	16.8	1.3	62.3	36.4
Mexico	60–74	19.9	59.8	20.3	15.7	59.9	24.2
	75+	27.5	57.8	14.1	16.6	67.8	15.0
Montevideo	60–74	3.8	68.1	28.1	1.6	65.2	33.2
	75+	8.2	70.9	20.9	5.5	71.0	23.5
Santiago	60–74	11.3	62.2	26.5	7.2	62.2	30.6
	75+	17.1	58.9	23.1	9.0	56.6	34.4
São Paulo	60–74	19.8	67.9	11.7	14.8	65.2	19.8
	75+	34.3	58.2	6.4	29.0	59.9	9.5

Source of data: *SABE survey*. Pan American Health Organization (PAHO), 2000.

opportunities for the people that would be the elderly population at the beginning of this century.

Santiago has lower educational levels than Buenos Aires and Montevideo, as a result of later development. On the other hand, Mexico City and São Paulo are the two largest cities in Latin America, growing mainly because of large inflows of population from rural areas. The low levels of education in these two big cities reflect the lower socioeconomic conditions that Mexico and Brazil had during the first decades of the 20th century. Following another well-known tendency, educational levels are higher for men in comparison to women. Nevertheless, the gap is smaller in those cities with higher levels of education.

Differences in educational levels are indicative of the socioeconomic differences between the elderly population in the cities that were surveyed by SABE. In turn these differences should have implications for the health of the aged population, clearly exemplified in Table 16.6. The numbers are the proportions of the population 60 years and over, under the three levels of education considered, that report disability in at least one of the basic activities of daily living (ADLs) asked about in the SABE survey. Data is presented for each city and for each sex.

The numbers clearly show how the lack of schooling impacts in higher prevalences of disability. The percentage of people having difficulty with ADLs is substantially higher in those that never went to school. These figures also show the higher disability levels for women. The differences found among cities require further examination in order to elucidate the reasons; these might

Table 16.6. Proportion of population aged 60 and with at least one deteriorated basic ADL or IADL, by sex and schooling, in selected cities in Latin America, 2000

	Men			Women		
	No schooling	Primary	High school+	No schooling	Primary	High school+
Bridgetown	16.7	7.6	4.4	22.2	11.3	7.8
Buenos Aires	9.2	8.3	3.0	14.0	12.2	5.6
Mexico	16.5	7.8	3.7	11.3	10.6	8.0
Montevideo	24.0	4.4	3.4	15.9	9.5	3.7
Santiago	17.6	9.7	9.3	28.1	19.0	14.6
São Paulo	15.5	13.2	3.1	18.4	12.6	9.3

Source of data: *SABE survey*. Pan American Health Organization (PAHO), 2000.

include not only other social and economic factors but also the reliability of the data collected.

LIFE AND HEALTH EXPECTANCIES

Just as life expectancy is a summary of mortality acting over the whole age range, a way of summarizing the health status associated with ageing is through estimating life expectancies with and without disabilities. In Table 16.7 using SABE data, life expectancies are shown for women 65 years and over, along with life expectancies without disability, as measured by the ability to perform all ADLs and instrumental ADLs (IADLs) without any difficulty.[8]

Although life expectancies at age 65, 75 and 85 are very similar among the six selected major urban areas in Latin America for females, the proportion of life free of disability – as measured by the ability to perform all ADLs and IADLs without any difficulty – varies significantly. At age 65, when life expectancy varies by a maximum of 0.7 years, the proportion of life free of disability varies from 89.9% (Montevideo, Uruguay) to 79.3% (Santiago, Chile), a gap of more than 10%. At age 75, when life expectancy varies by a maximum of 0.8 year, the proportion of life free of disability varies from 84.7% (Montevideo) to 69.1% (Santiago), a gap of more than 15.0%. At age 85, life expectancy still varies by a maximum of 0.7 year, the proportion of life free of disability varies from 74.0% (Montevideo again) to 48.9% (Santiago), a gap of more than 25.0%. In terms of disability-free life expectancy (DFLE) for females at age 65 years, the six areas rank in the following order: Montevideo (17.1 years), Bridgetown (16.7), Buenos Aires and São Paulo (15.8), Mexico (15.7) and Santiago (14.7).

---

[8] Estimates use the Sullivan method.

Table 16.7. Life expectancies and life expectancies without disability in women at ages 65, 75 and 85 in six selected major urban areas in Latin America, 2000

	Age 65			Age 75			Age 85		
	LE years	DFLE years	DFLE/ LE %	LE years	DFLE years	DFLE/ LE %	LE years	DFLE years	DFLE/ LE %
Buenos Aires	18.3	15.8	86.2	10.7	8.4	78.4	5.8	3.6	61.4
Bridgetown	18.8	16.7	88.6	11.5	9.6	83.3	6.4	4.6	73.1
São Paulo	18.3	15.8	85.9	10.7	8.4	78.5	5.8	3.7	63.1
Santiago	18.6	14.7	79.3	11.2	7.8	69.1	6.4	3.1	48.9
Mexico City	18.4	15.7	85.0	11.3	8.6	76.6	6.5	3.8	59.0
Montevideo	19.0	17.1	89.9	11.5	9.8	84.7	6.5	4.8	74.0

Data from: CELADE (2001). *Boletín Demográfico 67.* Santiago, Chile and PAHO (2000). *Survey on Health and Well-being of the Elderly in Latin America* – SABE.

Thus, these calculations of disability-free life expectancy raise the important issue of the quality of life in the major urban areas in Latin America, and its determinants. Why in urban areas where life expectancies are so similar can their proportion free of disability be so dissimilar? Further analysis of the SABE survey and possible future extensions must tackle this issue, being a basis for the design and construction of new sources of information that should be nationwide and longitudinal, as part of the search to identify and manage determinants of health and demographic ageing in Latin America.

REFERENCES

CELADE (2001) *Boletín Demográfico No. 67.* Santiago, Chile: Centro Latinoamericano de Demografía.

PAHO (2000) *Survey on Health and Well-being of the Elderly in Latin America – SABE.* Washington, DC: Pan American Health Organization.

United Nations (2000) *World Population Prospects – 1998.* New York: United Nations Population Division.

17

Global Patterns of Health Expectancy in the Year 2000

COLIN D. MATHERS, CHRISTOPHER J.L. MURRAY, ALAN D. LOPEZ, JOSHUA A. SALOMON and RITU SADANA
World Health Organization, Geneva, Switzerland

INTRODUCTION

In its World Health Report 2000, the World Health Organization (WHO) for the first time reported on the average levels of population health for its 191 member countries using a summary measure that combines information on mortality and disability (WHO, 2000). The primary summary measure of population health used was disability-adjusted life expectancy, or DALE, which measures the equivalent number of years of life expected to be lived in full health (Mathers *et al*, 2001b). In the following year, updated estimates for the year 2000 were published in the World Health Report 2001 (WHO, 2001) using improved methods and incorporating cross-population comparable survey data from 63 surveys in 55 countries. To better reflect the inclusion of all states of health in the summary measure of population health, the name of the indicator was changed from disability-adjusted life expectancy (DALE) to health-adjusted or healthy life expectancy (HALE).[1]

The World Health Report 2000 also carried out an assessment of the performance of health systems of member countries in achieving three main (intrinsic) goals for health systems: health, responsiveness and fairness in financing (WHO, 2000). WHO's work on operationalizing the measurement of goal attainment is focused on measuring these three goals as well as relating

---

[1] Note that the term healthy life expectancy, as used in this chapter and by WHO in its publications, refers to HALE and not to a health expectancy calculated directly from self-reports of perceived health, using a single global health question.

Determining Health Expectancies. Edited by J-M. Robine, C. Jagger, C.D. Mathers, E.M. Crimmins and R.M. Suzman.

goal attainment to resource use in order to evaluate the performance and efficiency of health systems (WHO, 2000; Murray and Frenk, 2000).

There are two main classes of summary measures: health gaps and health expectancies. The disability-adjusted life year (DALY) is the best-known health gap measure and quantifies the gap between a population's actual health and some defined goal (Murray and Lopez, 1996). HALE belongs to the family of health expectancies, summarizing the total life expectancy into equivalent years of 'full health' by taking into account the distribution of health states (disability) in the population. WHO has chosen to use HALE as a summary measure of level of population health because it is relatively easy to explain the concept of an equivalent 'healthy' life expectancy and because it is measured in units (years of life) that are meaningful to non-technical audiences (unlike other indicators such as mortality rates or incidence rates).

HALE is also preferable as a summary measure of population to indicators such as disability-free life expectancy (DFLE) which incorporate a dichotomous weighting scheme. Because time spent in any health state categorized as disabled is assigned arbitrarily a weight of zero (equivalent to death), DFLE is not sensitive to differences in the severity distribution of disability in populations. In contrast, HALE adds up expectation of life for different health states with adjustment for severity distribution.

Health expectancy estimates based on self-reported health status information are not comparable across countries due to differences in survey instruments and cultural differences in reporting of health (Robine *et al*, 1996). Analyses of over 50 national health surveys for the calculation of healthy life expectancy in the World Health Report 2000 identified severe limitations in the comparability of self-report health status data from different populations, even when identical survey instruments and methods were used (Sadana *et al*, 2002). We have demonstrated how these comparability problems relate not only to differences in survey design and methods, but more fundamentally to unmeasured differences in expectations and norms for health. For example, the cut points of scales for a given domain such as mobility may have very different meanings across different cultures, across socioeconomic groups within a society, across age groups or between men and women (Sadana *et al*, 2002; Murray *et al*, 2002). In order to improve the methodological and empirical basis for the measurement of population health, WHO has initiated a data collection strategy with member states consisting of household and/or postal or telephone surveys in representative samples of the general populations using a standardized instrument together with new statistical methods for correcting biases in self-reported health (Üstün *et al*, 2001).

In constructing estimates of HALE for 191 countries for the year 2000, we have sought to address some of the methodological challenges regarding comparability of health status data across populations and cultures. This chapter briefly describes methods and data sources used to prepare the HALE estimates for the 191 member countries of WHO, and then examines the implications of the results for our understanding of global patterns of female–male differences in healthy life expectancy at age 60, and their proximate disease and injury causes.

METHODS

Calculation of HALE requires three inputs. First, life expectancy at each age is calculated in the standard way. Second, estimates of the prevalence of various states of health at each age are required. Finally, a method of valuing this time compared to full health must be developed. Data and methods for each of these components are briefly described below. Because comparable health status prevalence data are not yet available for all countries, a three-stage strategy was used to estimate severity-weighted health state prevalences for countries:

- firstly, data from the Global Burden of Disease 2000 study (GBD 2000) (Murray *et al*, 2001) were used to estimate severity-adjusted disability prevalences by age and sex for all 191 countries;
- secondly, data on health state prevalences and health state valuations from the WHO survey program were used to make independent estimates of severity-adjusted disability prevalences by age and sex for 55 countries;
- finally, for the survey countries, 'posterior' prevalences were calculated as weighted averages of the GBD 2000-based prevalences and the survey prevalences. The relationship between the GBD 2000-based prevalences and the survey prevalences among the survey countries was then used to adjust the GBD 2000-based prevalences for the non-survey countries.

LIFE TABLES AND CAUSE OF DEATH DISTRIBUTIONS FOR COUNTRIES

New life tables and detailed cause of death distributions were developed for all 191 WHO member states for the year 2000, starting with a systematic review of all available evidence from surveys, censuses, sample registration systems, population laboratories and national vital registration systems on levels and trends of child and adult mortality (Lopez *et al*, 2002). In countries with a substantial HIV epidemic, separate estimates were made of the numbers and distributions of deaths due to HIV/AIDS and these deaths incorporated into the life table estimates (Salomon and Murray, 2001). Complete or incomplete vital registration data together with sample registration systems cover 76% of global mortality. Survey data and indirect demographic techniques provide information on levels of child and adult mortality for the remaining 24% of estimated global mortality. Cause of death patterns were carefully analyzed to take into account incomplete coverage of vital registration in countries and the likely differences in cause of death patterns that would be expected in the low coverage areas of countries with incomplete data (Salomon and Murray, 2000). In addition, information from sample registration systems, population laboratories and epidemiological analyses of specific conditions were used to improve estimates of the cause of death patterns.

GBD 2000 ESTIMATES OF SEVERITY-WEIGHTED DISABILITY FOR COUNTRIES

WHO is currently updating and revising estimates of the Global Burden of Disease for the year 2000. The burden of disease methodology provides a way to link information at the population level on disease causes and occurrence to information on both short-term and long-term health outcomes, including impairments, disability and death (Murray and Lopez, 1996). These revisions draw on a wide range of data sources, and various methods have been developed to reconcile often fragmented and partial estimates of epidemiological parameters that are available from different studies (Murray *et al*, 2001). These data, together with the new and revised estimates of deaths by cause, age and sex for all member states, were used to develop internally consistent estimates of incidence, prevalence, duration and YLD (years lived with disability), for over 130 major causes, for 17 sub-regions of the 6 WHO regions of the world. As well as the usual incidence-based YLD, prevalence rates and prevalence-based YLD rates were also calculated by cause, age and sex, giving direct estimates of the severity-weighted prevalence of health states attributable to each cause (Mathers *et al*, 2001a). These estimates are used here to summarize the broad patterns of causes of disability in different regions of the world.

The regional YLD rates from the Global Burden of Disease 2000 project were also used to estimate country-specific YLD rates by age and sex for the calculation of HALE. Where feasible, country-specific prevalence estimates were made for a number of causes (including childhood immunizable diseases, malnutrition, HIV/AIDS, cancers and diabetes). For other causes, regional disability estimates were used, together with country-specific cause of death information, to develop country-specific estimates of severity-weighted prevalence of health states of less than good health (Mathers *et al*, 2001a).

Summation of prevalence YLD over all causes would result in over-estimation of disability prevalence because of comorbidity between conditions. We corrected for independent comorbidity between major cause groups as follows:

$$D_{s,x} = 1 - \prod_g (1 - \mathrm{PYLD}_{s,x,g})$$

where $PYLD_{s,x,g}$ is the prevalence YLD per 1000 population for sex s, age x and cause g and $D_{s,x}$ gives the overall severity-weighted prevalence of disability by age and sex.

HEALTH SURVEY DATA

In order to gather population health data in a truly comparable manner across all member states, WHO launched a survey in 1999 through a series of carefully designed steps (Üstün *et al*, 2001). The health module was based on selected domains of the International Classification of Functioning, Disability and Health (ICF). It was developed after a rigorous scientific review of various existing assessment instruments, international consultations with experts and with representatives of national and international statistical agencies, and pilot studies in 10 countries.

Comparability is fundamental to the use of survey results for calculating summary measures of population health but has been under-emphasized in instrument development. The WHO survey program has as its first objective the assessment of health in different domains for nationally representative adult population samples in a way that is comparable across populations. To do this, the survey includes case vignettes and some measured tests on selected domains that are intended to calibrate the description that respondents provide of their own health. WHO has developed statistical methods for correcting biases in self-reported health using these data, based on the hierarchical ordered probit (HOPIT) model (Murray *et al*, 2002). The calibrated responses for 63 surveys in 55 countries were used to estimate the true prevalence of different states of health by age and sex for the HALE estimates reported here (Mathers *et al*, 2001a).

Just over one-half (34) of the surveys were household interview surveys, two were telephone surveys, and the remainder postal surveys. Thirty-five of the surveys were carried out in 31 European countries, 22 surveys in 19 developing countries, and the remainder in Canada, USA, Australia and New Zealand.

VALUING HEALTH STATES

In order to use time as a common currency for years of life lived in various states of health and for time lost due to premature mortality, we must numerically value time lived in non-fatal health states. The health state valuations (or *disability weights*) used in HALE calculations represent societal preferences for different health states. They range from 0 representing a state of good or ideal health (preferred to all other states) to 1 representing states equivalent to being dead. These weights do not represent the lived experience of any disability or health state, or imply any societal value of the person in a

Table 17.1. Core domains of health used in WHO Health Status Survey Module for measurement and valuation of health states

1. Mobility	4. Pain and discomfort
2. Self-care	5. Affect (anxiety/depression)
3. Usual activities	6. Cognition

disability or health state. Rather they quantify societal preferences for health states in relation to the societal 'ideal' of good health.

An additional objective of the WHO survey program is to measure the value that individuals assign to descriptions of health states derived from decrements in major domains of body functions and activities. The WHO survey program uses a two-tiered data collection strategy involving the general population surveys described above, combined with more detailed surveys among respondents with high levels of educational attainment in the same sites.

In the household surveys, individuals provide descriptions for a series of hypothetical health states along six core domains of health, listed in Table 17.1, followed by valuations of these states using a simple thermometer-type (visual analog) scale. The more detailed surveys include more abstract and cognitively demanding valuation tasks (standard gamble, time trade-off and person trade-off) that have limited reliability in general population surveys but have been applied widely in industrialized countries among convenience samples of educated respondents.

Statistical methods have been used to estimate the relationships between valuations elicited using visual analog scale and those elicited with other valuation techniques in order to measure the underlying health state severities that inform responses on each of the different measurement methods. A valuation function based on estimation of the relationships between levels on the core domains of health for a particular health state and the valuation of that health state has then been used together with the calibrated prevalences of health states to estimate the overall severity-weighted prevalence of health states for the 61 surveys in 55 countries (Mathers *et al*, 2001a).

POSTERIOR HEALTH STATE PREVALENCES FOR THE CALCULATION OF HALE

The prevalence estimates for all 191 countries based on the GBD-based prior estimates (described above) and the prevalence estimates for the countries with health surveys were combined using Bayesian methods to obtain posterior health state prevalences for all member states. Bayesian statistical analysis techniques use evidence (the health surveys) together with prior probability distributions (the GBD-based prevalence estimates) to calculate new posterior probability distributions. For the HALE estimates reported here, both the evidence (survey mean severity-weighted prevalences by age and sex) and the prior means were assumed to be normally distributed, allowing the posterior mean severity-weighted prevalence to be calculated as the weighted sum of the survey mean and the prior mean, where the weights are inversely proportional to the standard errors of the uncertainties for each (Mathers *et al*, 2001a).

Evidence from the surveys was also used to update the prior estimates for non-survey countries. Least squares ordinary regression was used to model the relationship between the posterior prevalences and the prior prevalences for the survey countries. The fitted model was then used to estimate posterior severity-weighted prevalences for all non-survey countries, in order (1) to ensure that the use of the survey data did not introduce a prevalence differential between survey and non-survey countries, and (2) to take the survey evidence into account in making the best possible prevalence estimates for non-survey countries.

CALCULATION OF HALE

HALE was calculated using Sullivan's method based on abridged country life tables and the posterior estimates of severity-weighted prevalence of disability (Mathers *et al*, 2001a). The abridged life tables used five-year age intervals, up to an open-ended interval of 100+ years. The first interval was subdivided into 0 years and 1–4 years. Posterior prevalences were calculated for the GBD age groups (0–4, 5–14, 15–29, 30–44, 45–59, 60–69, 70–79, 80+) and were assumed to be constant for the five-year age groups within each GBD age group. More detailed calculations showed that error in the final estimate of HALE introduced by this approximation was less than 0.1 years.

UNCERTAINTY ANALYSIS

Uncertainty distributions for the HALE estimates for each country were also calculated to take into account uncertainty in the life table quantities and in the posterior prevalence estimates. Uncertainty intervals were estimated for life expectancies and other life table parameters for WHO member countries as described by Salomon *et al* (2001). To capture the uncertainty due to sampling, indirect estimation techniques and projections, a total of between 600 and 1000 life tables were developed for each member state in order to quantify the uncertainty distribution of key life table parameters. In countries with a substantial HIV epidemic, recent estimates of the level and uncertainty range of the magnitude of HIV/AIDS deaths by age and sex were incorporated into the life table uncertainty analysis.

The degree of uncertainty in country-level weighted disability prevalences was also estimated for each country. This was mainly determined by levels of uncertainty in

(a) GBD prior prevalence estimates (including uncertainty in epidemiological estimates for prevalence, incidence and/or severity of disability associated with specific conditions, and in health state preferences),
(b) uncertainty in the survey-based prevalence estimates (including measurement uncertainty arising from sample size limitations, from potential systematic biases in sampling frames, and from uncertainty in the statistical adjustments for cross-population comparability),
(c) uncertainty arising from the estimation of posterior prevalence.

Uncertainty in the posterior estimates derived from the regression model was estimated using a Monte Carlo simulation procedure to capture uncertainty arising from the priors, the uncertainty in posterior estimates for survey countries (arising from the combined uncertainties of the priors and the surveys), and uncertainty in the regression model parameter estimates.

HALE uncertainty was estimated by drawing prevalences from the posterior prevalence distributions and combining these with the life table draws to generate an uncertainty distribution for HALE. In making the prevalence draws, allowance was made for correlation in prevalences across age groups, and for correlation between prevalences and mortality rates (arising from the country-level estimation process for GBD priors).

Results reported in this chapter include 95% uncertainty intervals for HALE and life expectancies for all member states. These uncertainty intervals will enable readers to compare HALE estimates, but allow them to avoid giving undue emphasis to small differences between countries.

RESULTS

Japanese women lead the world with an estimated average healthy life expectancy of 76.3 years at birth in the year 2000, 8.4 years lower than total life expectancy at birth (Table 17.2). HALE at birth for Japanese males is 5.1 years lower at 71.2 years. This is a narrower gap than for total life expectancy at birth of 7.2 years. After Japan, in second to sixth places, are Switzerland, San Marino, Andorra, Monaco and Australia with healthy life expectancies at birth (males and females combined) in the range 71.5 to 72.1 years, followed by a number of other industrialized countries of Western Europe. Note, however, that there is a considerable range of uncertainty in the ranks for countries other than Japan, with typical 95% uncertainty ranges of around 3 years for developed countries. Canada is in 17th place (70.0 years) and the USA in 28th place (67.2 years).

Other countries with reasonably high healthy life expectancies in the Americas include Chile (65.5 years), Costa Rica (65.3 years), Dominica (64.6 years), Mexico (64.2 years) and Uruguay (64.1 years). Brazil is split, with a high healthy life expectancy in its southern half, and a lower one in the north; the total average is a relatively low 57.1 years, at 54.9 for males and 59.2 for females.

China has a healthy life expectancy above the global average, at 62.1 years, 63.3 years for women and 60.9 for men. Other countries in the Asian region generally have lower HALE. Improving health in Vietnam has resulted in a healthy life expectancy of 58.9 years, while Thailand has not improved significantly over the past decade, though it is still ahead of Vietnam at 59.7 years. Healthy life expectancy in Myanmar (Burma) is just 49.1 years, substantially behind its Southeast Asian neighbors.

In Russia, healthy life expectancy is 60.6 for females, 5 years below the European average, but just 50.3 years for males, 9.6 years below the European average. This is one of the widest sex gaps in the world and reflects the sharp increase in adult male mortality in the early 1990s. The most common explanation is the high incidence of male alcohol abuse, which led to high rates of accidents, violence and cardiovascular disease. From 1987 to 1994, the risk of premature death increased by 70% for Russian males. Between 1994 and 1998, life expectancy improved for males, but has declined significantly again in the last three years. Similar rates exist for other countries of the former Soviet Union.

The bottom 10 countries for HALE are all in sub-Saharan Africa, where the HIV-AIDS epidemic is rampant. The lowest health expectancy in 2000 was estimated at 29.5 years in Sierra Leone. Life expectancy in several countries in southern Africa has been reduced 15–20 years in comparison to life expectancy without HIV. Other African countries have lost 5–10 years of life expectancy because of HIV (Salomon and Murray, 2001). AIDS is now the leading cause of death in sub-Saharan Africa, far surpassing the traditional deadly diseases of malaria, tuberculosis, pneumonia and diarrheal disease. AIDS killed 2.2 million Africans in 2000, as against 300 000 AIDS deaths 10 years previously.

Figure 17.1 shows average HALE at birth versus total life expectancy at birth for 191 countries. While lower life expectancies are generally associated with lower healthy life expectancy – the two indicators are correlated – there are large variations in healthy life expectancy for any given level of life expectancy. For example, for countries with a life expectancy of 70, healthy life expectancy varies from 57 to 61.5, a non-trivial variation. Full details of male and female HALE and total life expectancy at birth and at age 60, together with 95% uncertainty ranges, are also available by country in the World Health Report 2001 (WHO, 2001).

Overall, global healthy life expectancy at birth for males and females combined in 2000 is 56.0 years, 9.0 years lower than total life expectancy at birth. Global HALE at birth for females is just over 2 years greater than that for men (Table 17.3). In comparison, total life expectancy at birth is almost 4 years higher than that for men. HALE at birth ranges from a low of 39 years

Table 17.2. Healthy life expectancy and total life expectancy at birth, by sex, WHO member states, 2000

Rank	Member state	Healthy life expectancy (HALE) at birth			Life expectancy at birth	
		Persons	Males	Females	Males	Females
1	Japan	73.8	71.2 (69.9–72.5)	76.3 (74.6–77.8)	77.5 (77.4–77.7)	84.7 (84.4–85.1)
2	Switzerland	72.1	70.4 (68.7–72.1)	73.7 (71.3–75.7)	76.7 (76.3–77.0)	82.5 (82.1–82.9)
3	San Marino	72.0	69.7 (68.0–71.8)	74.3 (72.2–76.4)	76.1 (75.1–77.2)	83.8 (82.8–84.7)
4	Andorra	71.8	69.8 (67.4–73.0)	73.7 (70.7–77.9)	77.2 (74.4–81.7)	83.8 (80.2–89.5)
5	Monaco	71.7	69.4 (67.5–72.1)	73.9 (71.1–76.7)	76.8 (75.2–79.8)	84.4 (81.6–86.4)
6	Australia	71.5	69.6 (67.8–71.5)	73.3 (69.8–75.4)	76.6 (76.3–77.1)	82.1 (81.7–82.5)
7	Sweden	71.4	70.1 (68.7–71.6)	72.7 (70.6–74.6)	77.3 (77.0–77.6)	82.0 (81.7–82.4)
8	Iceland	71.2	69.8 (68.1–71.5)	72.6 (70.5–74.9)	77.1 (75.7–78.6)	81.8 (80.5–83.9)
9	Italy	71.2	69.5 (68.4–70.8)	72.8 (70.5–74.5)	76.0 (75.6–76.3)	82.4 (82.0–82.7)
10	Greece	71.0	69.7 (68.5–70.8)	72.3 (69.9–74.0)	75.4 (75.0–75.7)	80.8 (80.1–81.5)
11	New Zealand	70.8	69.5 (68.0–71.0)	72.1 (69.8–74.0)	75.9 (75.2–76.7)	80.9 (79.8–81.9)
12	France	70.7	68.5 (67.4–69.5)	72.9 (71.4–74.5)	75.2 (74.8–75.5)	83.1 (82.5–83.8)
13	Spain	70.6	68.7 (67.3–70.3)	72.5 (70.3–74.2)	75.4 (74.7–75.8)	82.3 (82.0–82.6)
14	Norway	70.5	68.8 (67.0–70.5)	72.3 (70.2–74.6)	75.7 (75.5–76.0)	81.4 (80.9–82.0)
15	Malta	70.4	68.7 (67.3–70.2)	72.1 (69.7–74.1)	75.4 (74.7–76.2)	80.7 (79.3–82.0)
16	Austria	70.3	68.1 (66.9–69.4)	72.5 (70.3–74.3)	74.9 (74.4–75.4)	81.4 (81.0–81.8)
17	Canada	70.0	68.3 (66.9–69.7)	71.7 (70.0–73.5)	76.0 (75.6–76.5)	81.5 (81.1–81.9)
18	Israel	69.9	69.3 (67.7–71.0)	70.6 (68.3–72.9)	76.6 (76.3–76.9)	80.6 (80.3–81.0)
19	United Kingdom	69.9	68.3 (66.8–69.7)	71.4 (69.2–73.1)	74.8 (74.6–75.0)	79.9 (79.7–80.2)
20	Luxembourg	69.8	67.6 (66.2–69.2)	72.0 (69.5–74.0)	73.9 (73.0–74.8)	80.8 (79.8–82.1)
21	Netherlands	69.7	68.2 (67.1–69.3)	71.2 (69.7–72.7)	75.4 (74.9–76.0)	81.0 (80.4–81.5)
22	Denmark	69.5	68.9 (67.5–70.3)	70.1 (68.2–72.0)	74.2 (73.8–74.5)	78.5 (78.2–79.0)
23	Germany	69.4	67.4 (66.0–68.7)	71.5 (69.4–73.3)	74.3 (74.0–74.8)	80.6 (80.2–80.9)
24	Belgium	69.4	67.7 (66.2–69.2)	71.0 (69.0–73.0)	74.6 (74.2–75.0)	80.9 (80.5–81.3)
25	Ireland	69.3	67.8 (66.3–69.1)	70.9 (68.6–72.7)	74.1 (73.6–74.5)	79.7 (79.3–80.0)
26	Finland	68.8	66.1 (64.9–67.2)	71.5 (69.9–73.0)	73.7 (73.5–74.0)	80.9 (80.5–81.3)
27	Singapore	67.8	66.8 (64.3–69.0)	68.9 (65.8–71.7)	75.4 (74.7–76.0)	80.2 (79.5–81.1)
28	United States of America	67.2	65.7 (63.8–67.5)	68.8 (66.5–71.0)	73.9 (73.7–74.2)	79.5 (79.3–79.6)

29	Slovenia	66.9	64.5 (62.1–66.7)	69.3 (66.5–71.9)	71.9 (71.5–72.3)	79.4 (78.9–80.2)
30	Cyprus	66.3	66.4 (64.6–68.7)	66.2 (63.4–68.8)	74.8 (74.3–75.6)	79.0 (78.3–79.8)
31	Portugal	66.3	63.9 (62.5–65.4)	68.6 (66.2–70.5)	71.7 (71.4–72.0)	79.3 (78.8–79.8)
32	Republic of Korea	66.0	63.2 (60.8–65.3)	68.8 (64.0–71.4)	70.5 (69.1–72.2)	78.3 (76.8–79.8)
33	Cuba	65.9	65.1 (63.0–67.2)	66.7 (64.4–68.8)	73.7 (73.3–74.0)	77.5 (77.1–77.8)
34	Czech Republic	65.6	62.9 (61.3–64.4)	68.3 (65.7–70.5)	71.5 (71.3–71.7)	78.2 (78.0–78.6)
35	Chile	65.5	63.5 (61.5–66.0)	67.4 (64.5–70.3)	72.5 (72.0–73.8)	79.5 (78.8–80.4)
36	Costa Rica	65.3	64.2 (61.9–66.9)	66.4 (63.1–69.2)	73.4 (72.7–74.5)	78.8 (78.1–79.8)
37	TFYR Macedonia[a]	64.9	63.9 (62.0–65.6)	65.9 (64.1–67.6)	70.2 (69.8–70.8)	74.8 (74.5–75.3)
38	Brunei Darussalam	64.9	63.8 (61.5–66.0)	65.9 (62.4–69.6)	73.4 (72.1–74.8)	78.7 (77.3–80.3)
39	Kuwait	64.7	64.6 (62.1–66.8)	64.8 (61.4–68.0)	74.2 (73.5–75.0)	76.8 (76.0–77.6)
40	Dominica	64.6	63.2 (59.7–66.1)	66.1 (63.3–69.3)	72.6 (71.5–73.6)	78.3 (77.0–79.7)
41	Yugoslavia	64.3	63.3 (62.1–64.7)	65.4 (63.2–67.3)	69.8 (69.6–70.1)	74.7 (74.5–75.0)
42	Mexico	64.2	63.1 (60.8–65.2)	65.3 (61.5–68.1)	71.0 (70.4–72.0)	76.2 (75.7–76.8)
43	Uruguay	64.1	61.7 (59.0–64.6)	66.5 (63.5–69.4)	70.0 (69.8–70.3)	77.9 (77.5–78.2)
44	Croatia	64.0	60.8 (59.5–62.0)	67.1 (64.7–69.2)	69.8 (69.5–70.1)	77.7 (77.3–78.1)
45	Jamaica	64.0	62.9 (59.8–65.8)	65.0 (62.1–68.1)	72.8 (72.0–74.7)	76.6 (75.3–78.3)
46	Panama	63.9	62.6 (60.1–65.1)	65.3 (62.6–68.0)	71.5 (70.7–72.2)	76.3 (75.8–76.7)
47	Argentina	63.9	61.8 (59.6–64.0)	65.9 (63.0–68.6)	70.2 (69.8–70.6)	77.8 (77.3–78.3)
48	Bosnia and Herzegovina	63.7	62.1 (60.3–64.3)	65.3 (62.8–67.9)	68.7 (67.4–70.7)	74.7 (73.3–76.0)
49	Bulgaria	63.4	61.0 (59.4–62.6)	65.8 (63.8–67.7)	67.4 (66.8–67.6)	74.9 (74.6–75.4)
50	Barbados	63.3	62.3 (59.7–65.0)	64.3 (60.9–67.7)	71.6 (70.4–72.8)	77.7 (76.6–78.9)
51	United Arab Emirates	63.1	62.3 (60.0–64.5)	63.9 (59.9–66.9)	72.3 (71.2–73.5)	76.4 (75.4–77.7)
52	Bahrain	62.7	63.0 (61.0–65.2)	62.3 (59.1–65.1)	72.7 (71.9–73.9)	74.7 (73.7–75.8)
53	Slovakia	62.4	59.6 (58.1–60.9)	65.2 (62.3–67.5)	69.2 (68.8–69.6)	77.5 (77.2–77.9)
54	Venezuela	62.3	60.4 (57.7–63.2)	64.2 (59.9–67.2)	70.6 (70.0–71.2)	76.5 (75.8–77.0)
55	China	62.1	60.9 (59.5–62.5)	63.3 (59.1–65.8)	68.9 (68.2–69.7)	73.0 (72.0–74.2)
56	Saint Lucia	62.0	60.7 (58.1–63.0)	63.3 (60.0–66.5)	69.2 (68.2–69.9)	74.2 (73.1–75.2)
57	Grenada	61.9	62.1 (59.5–65.1)	61.8 (57.8–65.7)	70.9 (69.5–72.1)	73.2 (72.1–74.6)
58	Antigua and Barbuda	61.9	61.7 (58.4–64.8)	62.1 (59.0–65.2)	71.8 (70.5–73.1)	76.6 (75.4–77.9)
59	Poland	61.8	59.3 (57.9–60.5)	64.3 (61.2–66.7)	69.2 (68.9–69.5)	77.7 (77.2–78.2)
60	Romania	61.7	59.5 (57.4–61.4)	64.0 (61.6–66.8)	66.2 (65.5–67.0)	73.5 (72.7–74.6)

(continued)

Table 17.2. (*continued*)

Rank	Member state	Healthy life expectancy (HALE) at birth			Life expectancy at birth	
		Persons	Males	Females	Males	Females
61	Trinidad and Tobago	61.7	60.3 (57.9–63.1)	63.0 (59.0–65.8)	68.5 (67.4–70.5)	73.8 (72.8–74.7)
62	Malaysia	61.6	59.7 (57.3–62.1)	63.4 (60.3–66.6)	68.3 (67.4–69.4)	74.1 (73.1–75.3)
63	Tunisia	61.4	61.0 (59.2–62.9)	61.7 (58.0–65.4)	69.2 (68.3–70.0)	73.4 (71.9–74.3)
64	Niue	61.1	60.8 (57.1–64.2)	61.4 (58.6–65.2)	69.5 (66.7–71.9)	72.8 (71.4–77.3)
65	Sri Lanka	61.1	58.6 (55.7–61.5)	63.6 (61.0–67.0)	67.6 (65.1–68.9)	75.3 (73.8–76.0)
66	Colombia	60.9	58.6 (56.2–61.0)	63.3 (59.8–66.2)	67.2 (66.3–68.1)	75.1 (74.3–75.8)
67	Paraguay	60.9	59.9 (56.7–63.4)	61.9 (58.8–65.5)	70.2 (69.0–71.5)	74.2 (72.4–75.7)
68	Saint Vincent and Grenadines	60.9	59.7 (57.1–62.2)	62.1 (59.1–65.0)	67.7 (66.5–68.7)	73.3 (72.2–74.8)
69	Estonia	60.8	56.2 (54.7–57.6)	65.4 (62.5–67.7)	65.4 (64.8–66.1)	76.5 (75.6–77.8)
70	Cook Islands	60.7	60.4 (58.1–62.8)	61.1 (57.7–64.9)	68.7 (67.8–69.4)	72.1 (71.2–73.0)
71	Lebanon	60.7	60.3 (57.6–63.1)	61.1 (57.4–65.1)	69.1 (67.7–70.7)	73.3 (72.2–74.7)
72	Tonga	60.7	59.3 (57.0–61.9)	62.0 (58.4–65.2)	67.4 (66.8–68.3)	72.9 (72.6–73.9)
73	Suriname	60.6	59.5 (57.0–61.9)	61.7 (58.5–64.6)	68.0 (66.6–69.6)	73.5 (71.8–75.3)
74	Qatar	60.6	59.3 (56.5–62.6)	61.8 (58.4–65.4)	70.4 (70.1–70.7)	75.0 (74.6–75.4)
75	Mauritius	60.5	58.6 (55.6–61.3)	62.5 (58.4–66.3)	67.6 (67.0–68.1)	74.6 (74.1–75.0)
76	Ecuador	60.3	58.4 (55.4–61.3)	62.2 (58.6–66.0)	68.2 (67.5–68.9)	74.2 (73.6–74.8)
77	Belarus	60.1	55.4 (53.4–57.5)	64.8 (62.7–66.9)	62.0 (61.0–62.9)	74.0 (73.2–74.9)
78	Hungary	59.9	55.3 (53.7–56.9)	64.5 (61.8–66.7)	66.3 (66.1–66.5)	75.2 (74.9–75.5)
79	Samoa	59.9	58.2 (55.6–60.6)	61.6 (59.0–64.4)	66.7 (65.5–67.7)	72.9 (71.8–74.0)
80	Thailand	59.7	57.7 (55.7–59.7)	61.8 (57.9–64.9)	66.0 (65.0–67.1)	72.4 (71.1–74.2)
81	Oman	59.7	59.2 (57.2–61.4)	60.3 (56.6–63.1)	69.5 (68.4–70.6)	73.5 (72.6–74.5)
82	Saint Kitts and Nevis	59.6	57.6 (54.7–60.7)	61.5 (57.8–65.6)	66.1 (65.3–67.3)	72.0 (70.8–73.3)
83	Fiji	59.6	58.7 (55.9–61.3)	60.5 (56.9–64.3)	66.9 (65.7–68.1)	71.2 (69.9–72.3)
84	Syrian Arab Republic	59.6	59.6 (55.3–60.9)	59.5 (54.9–62.2)	67.4 (66.5–68.0)	71.1 (70.4–71.8)
85	Saudi Arabia	59.5	58.3 (55.0–61.1)	60.7 (56.5–64.9)	68.1 (67.1–69.1)	73.5 (72.7–74.5)
86	Albania	59.4	56.5 (54.4–59.9)	62.3 (60.2–65.2)	64.3 (62.8–65.7)	72.9 (71.6–74.1)
87	Belize	59.2	58.0 (55.2–61.0)	60.4 (55.6–64.9)	69.1 (68.0–70.3)	74.7 (74.0–75.2)
88	Solomon Islands	59.0	58.0 (55.1–61.5)	60.1 (56.6–63.8)	66.6 (64.4–69.6)	71.4 (68.5–75.3)

89	Armenia	59.0	56.9 (55.0–58.6)	61.1 (58.1–64.1)	64.4 (63.8–65.0)	71.2 (70.2–72.2)
90	Philippines	59.0	57.0 (54.3–59.4)	60.9 (57.7–64.3)	64.6 (63.6–65.5)	71.1 (70.0–72.7)
91	Vietnam	58.9	58.2 (55.6–60.7)	59.7 (56.5–62.8)	66.7 (65.7–67.8)	71.0 (69.9–72.0)
92	Peru	58.8	57.8 (55.2–60.6)	59.8 (56.2–63.6)	66.7 (65.9–67.6)	71.6 (70.4–72.7)
93	Iran (Islamic Republic of)	58.8	59.0 (56.4–61.6)	58.6 (55.3–61.9)	68.1 (67.4–69.0)	69.9 (69.2–70.8)
94	Seychelles	58.7	57.0 (54.1–59.7)	60.4 (57.1–64.0)	66.5 (65.2–67.9)	74.2 (72.4–76.2)
95	Turkey	58.7	56.8 (55.4–58.2)	60.5 (57.4–63.2)	66.8 (66.6–68.0)	72.5 (71.9–74.0)
96	Jordan	58.5	58.2 (56.4–60.3)	58.8 (56.0–61.4)	68.5 (67.4–70.0)	72.5 (72.1–73.8)
97	Libyan Arab Jamahiriya	58.5	58.4 (55.7–61.4)	58.6 (55.2–62.5)	67.5 (66.4–68.7)	71.0 (70.0–72.2)
98	Republic of Moldova	58.4	55.4 (52.4–57.9)	61.5 (59.1–64.3)	63.1 (62.4–63.8)	70.5 (69.6–71.4)
99	Cape Verde	58.4	56.9 (53.7–60.2)	60.0 (56.3–63.8)	66.5 (64.4–67.9)	72.3 (71.1–73.3)
100	Lithuania	58.4	53.6 (51.6–55.5)	63.2 (60.2–65.9)	66.9 (66.1–67.8)	77.2 (76.7–78.2)
101	Algeria	58.4	58.4 (55.8–61.9)	58.3 (54.5–62.2)	68.1 (66.9–69.4)	71.2 (69.9–72.4)
102	Georgia	58.2	56.1 (54.1–58.3)	60.2 (57.3–62.8)	65.7 (64.0–67.7)	71.8 (70.3–74.2)
103	Bahamas	58.1	57.2 (54.0–60.5)	59.1 (54.2–64.0)	68.0 (67.1–68.9)	74.8 (73.9–75.6)
104	Palau	57.7	56.5 (54.3–58.6)	58.9 (55.7–62.4)	64.7 (63.6–65.2)	69.3 (68.4–70.3)
105	Latvia	57.7	51.4 (49.0–53.5)	63.9 (60.9–66.5)	64.2 (62.8–64.9)	75.5 (74.5–76.5)
106	Indonesia	57.4	56.5 (55.7–58.2)	58.4 (55.8–61.0)	63.4 (62.4–64.6)	67.4 (66.4–68.5)
107	El Salvador	57.3	55.3 (52.0–58.7)	59.4 (55.3–63.3)	66.3 (65.4–67.1)	73.3 (72.4–74.4)
108	Egypt	57.1	57.1 (55.4–58.8)	57.0 (54.1–59.3)	65.4 (64.8–66.0)	69.1 (68.5–69.7)
109	Brazil	57.1	54.9 (51.4–58.1)	59.2 (54.8–64.1)	64.5 (63.0–65.7)	71.9 (70.2–73.5)
110	Tuvalu	57.0	56.4 (54.0–58.9)	57.6 (54.0–61.0)	63.6 (62.0–64.8)	67.6 (65.7–68.7)
111	Nicaragua	56.9	55.8 (51.8–60.3)	58.0 (54.3–62.4)	66.4 (65.4–67.5)	71.1 (70.2–72.0)
112	Ukraine	56.8	52.3 (51.0–53.7)	61.3 (58.0–63.5)	62.6 (62.0–63.1)	73.3 (72.9–73.8)
113	Honduras	56.8	55.8 (52.5–59.6)	57.8 (53.6–62.0)	66.3 (64.5–67.9)	71.0 (69.2–72.5)
114	Vanuatu	56.7	56.0 (52.6–59.7)	57.4 (53.6–61.8)	64.2 (60.5–69.1)	68.1 (64.2–72.3)
115	Micronesia[b]	56.6	55.8 (52.8–58.8)	57.5 (54.0–61.0)	63.7 (61.6–66.1)	67.7 (65.8–69.9)
116	Dominican Republic	56.2	54.7 (50.9–58.2)	57.7 (53.4–61.9)	65.5 (64.5–66.4)	71.6 (70.5–72.6)
117	Marshall Islands	56.1	54.8 (51.9–57.9)	57.4 (54.3–60.3)	62.8 (61.4–64.3)	67.8 (66.6–69.0)
118	Russian Federation	55.5	50.3 (48.6–52.4)	60.6 (57.0–63.3)	59.4 (58.4–60.8)	72.0 (71.6–73.0)
119	DPR Korea[c]	55.4	54.9 (51.5–58.4)	56.0 (52.2–59.8)	64.5 (62.0–66.3)	67.2 (64.6–69.2)
120	Azerbaijan	55.4	53.3 (50.6–56.3)	57.5 (54.3–60.8)	61.7 (59.2–64.2)	68.9 (66.6–71.3)

(continued)

Table 17.2. *(continued)*

Rank	Member state	Healthy life expectancy (HALE) at birth			Life expectancy at birth	
		Persons	Males	Females	Males	Females
121	Morocco	54.9	55.3 (53.4–57.3)	54.5 (51.3–57.2)	66.1 (65.2–67.4)	70.4 (68.7–71.4)
122	Guatemala	54.7	53.5 (49.9–57.2)	56.0 (52.3–59.7)	63.5 (62.2–65.2)	68.6 (67.2–70.6)
123	Kazakhstan	54.3	50.5 (48.0–53.1)	58.1 (55.6–60.6)	58.0 (57.6–58.9)	68.4 (67.2–70.0)
124	Uzbekistan	54.3	52.7 (49.2–56.3)	55.8 (51.5–60.2)	62.1 (61.6–62.9)	68.0 (67.3–68.9)
125	Kiribati	53.6	52.8 (49.6–56.1)	54.4 (50.7–57.9)	60.4 (57.8–64.0)	64.5 (61.2–67.3)
126	Nauru	52.9	50.4 (47.0–54.4)	55.4 (51.0–60.2)	58.8 (55.3–62.9)	66.6 (62.5–71.3)
127	Kyrgyzstan	52.6	49.6 (46.5–53.1)	55.6 (51.2–60.1)	60.0 (58.5–61.7)	68.8 (66.8–70.8)
128	Iraq	52.6	52.6 (48.6–57.0)	52.5 (48.6–57.3)	61.7 (59.7–64.0)	64.7 (62.2–67.0)
129	Mongolia	52.4	50.3 (46.3–54.3)	54.5 (50.8–58.2)	61.2 (59.1–62.6)	66.9 (65.4–68.4)
130	Maldives	52.4	54.2 (50.3–58.2)	50.6 (46.4–55.9)	64.6 (62.9–66.2)	64.4 (62.4–66.7)
131	Turkmenistan	52.1	51.2 (48.3–54.3)	53.0 (50.1–56.7)	60.0 (59.3–60.8)	64.9 (64.3–66.0)
132	Guyana	52.1	51.4 (48.3–54.6)	52.8 (47.7–58.4)	61.5 (59.2–63.2)	67.0 (64.9–69.8)
133	India	52.0	52.2 (50.2–54.2)	51.7 (48.5–54.8)	59.8 (58.5–62.0)	62.7 (60.8–65.6)
134	Bolivia	51.4	51.4 (47.4–55.5)	51.4 (47.1–55.9)	60.9 (59.1–62.4)	63.6 (62.7–65.9)
135	Tajikistan	50.8	49.6 (46.2–53.2)	52.0 (47.8–56.1)	60.4 (59.0–62.3)	64.7 (63.0–66.9)
136	Sao Tome and Principe	50.0	50.3 (46.8–53.6)	49.7 (44.8–54.7)	60.3 (57.8–62.5)	61.9 (60.0–64.2)
137	Bangladesh	49.3	50.6 (47.4–54.1)	47.9 (43.6–52.6)	60.4 (58.6–62.3)	60.8 (59.1–62.6)
138	Bhutan	49.2	50.1 (44.8–55.1)	48.2 (43.5–53.7)	60.4 (57.0–64.4)	62.5 (58.9–66.3)
139	Yemen	49.1	48.9 (45.7–51.9)	49.3 (44.4–53.9)	59.3 (57.6–60.9)	62.0 (60.9–63.5)
140	Myanmar (Burma)	49.1	47.7 (43.8–51.6)	50.5 (45.7–54.3)	56.2 (53.5–58.0)	61.1 (57.6–62.8)
141	Pakistan	48.1	50.2 (46.6–54.2)	46.1 (41.5–51.1)	60.1 (58.6–62.5)	60.7 (58.6–63.1)
142	Cambodia	47.1	45.6 (43.1–48.0)	48.7 (45.4–52.4)	53.4 (52.7–54.2)	58.5 (57.9–59.5)
143	Gambia	46.9	47.3 (44.1–50.6)	46.6 (42.4–50.8)	55.9 (52.4–59.4)	58.7 (55.2–62.2)
144	Papua New Guinea	46.8	46.6 (42.8–50.5)	47.1 (43.6–50.9)	55.1 (52.8–57.7)	57.5 (54.8–60.0)
145	Ghana	46.7	46.5 (43.4–49.7)	46.9 (43.5–51.1)	55.0 (53.7–56.8)	57.9 (56.0–59.8)
146	Gabon	46.6	46.8 (42.9–50.0)	46.5 (42.6–49.9)	54.6 (50.3–59.0)	56.9 (51.9–60.2)
147	Comoros	46.0	46.2 (42.8–49.6)	45.8 (41.4–50.3)	55.3 (53.6–57.1)	58.1 (56.3–59.8)
148	Nepal	45.8	47.5 (44.4–51.1)	44.2 (39.1–49.8)	58.5 (56.8–60.5)	58.0 (56.5–59.7)

149	Sudan	45.1	45.7 (42.2–49.3)	44.4 (39.2–50.2)	55.4 (52.9–59.1)	57.8 (55.1–61.5)
150	Senegal	44.9	45.2 (42.1–48.0)	44.5 (40.9–48.4)	54.0 (52.6–56.0)	56.1 (54.7–58.1)
151	Equatorial Guinea	44.8	44.9 (40.6–48.7)	44.8 (40.2–49.4)	53.5 (49.0–57.0)	56.2 (52.4–59.6)
152	Laos[d]	44.7	43.7 (39.1–47.5)	45.7 (40.6–49.6)	52.2 (47.4–54.9)	56.1 (52.0–58.3)
153	South Africa	43.2	43.0 (41.1–45.0)	43.5 (40.5–46.4)	49.6 (48.8–50.6)	52.1 (51.0–53.0)
154	Haiti	43.1	41.3 (37.0–46.2)	44.9 (38.8–51.1)	49.7 (47.0–56.9)	56.1 (52.4–62.2)
155	Madagascar	42.9	43.2 (40.6–46.1)	42.6 (38.0–47.3)	51.7 (50.3–53.7)	54.6 (53.2–56.6)
156	Togo	42.7	42.7 (39.3–46.5)	42.7 (39.3–46.8)	50.5 (48.1–54.0)	53.0 (50.5–56.6)
157	Congo	42.6	42.5 (39.3–47.0)	42.8 (39.1–47.2)	50.1 (46.8–52.7)	52.9 (49.5–56.4)
158	Benin	42.5	43.1 (39.8–46.5)	41.9 (37.5–46.5)	51.7 (50.4–53.0)	53.8 (52.5–55.8)
159	Nigeria	41.6	42.1 (39.2–45.0)	41.1 (37.7–45.0)	49.8 (48.3–51.9)	51.4 (49.8–53.6)
160	Mauritania	41.5	42.1 (37.7–46.3)	40.8 (35.5–46.0)	51.7 (49.2–54.2)	53.5 (51.1–56.2)
161	Eritrea	41.0	41.4 (38.1–45.0)	40.5 (36.5–45.0)	49.1 (46.6–52.6)	51.0 (48.3–54.6)
162	Kenya	40.7	41.2 (38.7–44.4)	40.1 (36.7–43.8)	48.2 (46.2–50.3)	49.6 (47.5–51.8)
163	Cameroon	40.4	40.9 (37.6–44.0)	39.9 (36.7–43.2)	49.0 (47.6–50.4)	50.4 (48.9–51.9)
164	Guinea	40.3	40.4 (36.7–44.0)	40.1 (35.9–45.5)	49.0 (47.4–51.1)	52.0 (50.4–54.1)
165	Chad	39.3	38.6 (35.3–43.7)	39.9 (36.1–44.5)	47.4 (46.1–48.7)	51.1 (49.7–52.6)
166	Cote d'Ivoire	39.0	39.1 (36.7–42.6)	38.9 (35.9–42.1)	46.4 (44.9–48.5)	48.4 (46.8–50.6)
167	Zimbabwe	38.8	39.6 (37.4–41.9)	38.1 (34.7–41.3)	45.4 (44.7–46.5)	46.0 (44.9–47.1)
168	Swaziland	38.2	38.8 (34.1–44.2)	37.6 (32.6–42.7)	44.7 (39.4–50.7)	45.6 (40.8–52.0)
169	Tanzania[e]	38.1	38.6 (35.4–42.7)	37.5 (34.0–41.1)	45.8 (45.1–46.7)	47.2 (46.4–47.9)
170	Liberia	37.8	38.2 (34.0–42.4)	37.4 (33.5–41.5)	46.6 (43.3–51.3)	49.1 (45.7–53.9)
171	Botswana	37.3	38.1 (34.3–42.0)	36.5 (33.2–40.0)	44.6 (42.4–47.1)	44.4 (42.3–46.5)
172	Angola	36.9	36.2 (33.7–42.0)	37.6 (33.3–42.8)	44.3 (40.8–47.9)	48.3 (44.9–52.0)
173	Guinea-Bissau	36.6	36.7 (33.6–39.8)	36.4 (33.0–40.3)	44.5 (43.4–46.0)	46.9 (45.7–48.5)
174	Uganda	35.7	36.2 (33.4–39.8)	35.2 (31.1–39.6)	43.5 (40.8–47.3)	44.6 (41.7–48.7)
175	Namibia	35.6	36.5 (32.5–41.2)	34.7 (31.4–38.8)	42.8 (39.2–48.1)	42.6 (39.2–47.6)
176	Ethiopia	35.4	35.7 (32.2–40.9)	35.1 (30.4–40.9)	42.8 (39.0–48.3)	44.7 (40.5–50.5)
177	Lesotho	35.3	36.1 (33.1–39.7)	34.5 (31.2–38.7)	42.0 (38.8–45.7)	42.2 (38.6–47.3)
178	Djibouti	35.1	35.6 (31.3–40.4)	34.6 (30.1–39.6)	43.5 (39.9–48.2)	44.7 (40.1–49.3)
179	Somalia	35.1	35.5 (32.5–38.9)	34.7 (30.6–38.8)	43.8 (42.6–45.4)	45.9 (44.7–47.6)
180	Burkina Faso	34.8	35.4 (32.5–38.3)	34.1 (30.5–37.9)	42.6 (42.0–43.4)	43.6 (42.9–44.4)

(continued)

Table 17.2. (*continued*)

Rank	Member state	Healthy life expectancy (HALE) at birth			Life expectancy at birth	
		Persons	Males	Females	Males	Females
181	Mali	34.5	34.8 (31.5–39.3)	34.1 (29.5–38.9)	42.7 (40.3–45.2)	44.6 (42.2–47.3)
182	DR Congo[f]	34.4	34.4 (31.6–39.4)	34.4 (30.5–39.3)	41.6 (38.6–45.8)	44.0 (41.2–47.5)
183	Central African Republic	34.1	34.7 (31.6–38.2)	33.6 (30.3–37.3)	41.6 (40.3–43.1)	42.5 (41.1–44.4)
184	Afghanistan	33.8	35.1 (30.3–40.4)	32.5 (26.2–39.5)	44.2 (38.5–50.1)	45.1 (39.2–51.7)
185	Burundi	33.4	33.9 (30.4–37.5)	32.9 (29.3–36.9)	40.6 (37.7–43.7)	41.3 (38.2–45.5)
186	Niger	33.1	33.9 (30.9–37.7)	32.4 (27.1–37.6)	42.7 (40.5–46.1)	43.9 (42.1–46.7)
187	Zambia	33.0	33.7 (30.6–37.0)	32.3 (28.9–36.1)	39.2 (36.1–43.8)	39.5 (36.5–43.7)
188	Rwanda	31.9	32.0 (29.6–36.5)	31.8 (28.3–36.2)	38.5 (36.8–41.1)	40.5 (38.6–43.3)
189	Mozambique	31.3	31.5 (28.9–34.9)	31.1 (28.1–34.7)	37.9 (36.7–39.5)	39.5 (38.2–41.2)
190	Malawi	30.9	31.4 (28.2–34.6)	30.5 (26.8–34.4)	37.1 (33.6–41.1)	37.8 (34.0–42.2)
191	Sierra Leone	29.5	29.7 (26.4–36.0)	29.3 (25.2–35.1)	37.0 (32.9–43.3)	38.8 (35.3–44.7)

[a]The Former Yugoslav Republic of Macedonia.
[b]Federated States of Micronesia.
[c]Democratic People's Republic of Korea (North Korea).
[d]Lao People's Democratic Republic.
[e]United Republic of Tanzania.
[f]Democratic Republic of the Congo.

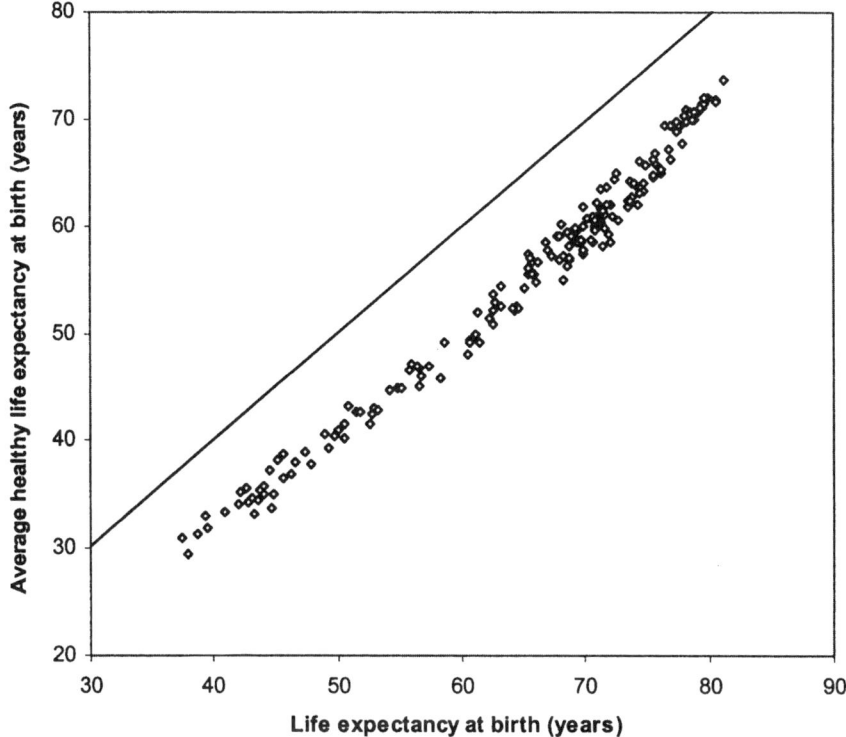

Figure 17.1. Healthy life expectancy at birth versus total life expectancy at birth, males and females combined, 191 countries, 2000

for African women to a high of 72 years in the low mortality countries of mainly Western Europe and North America. This is a 2-fold difference in healthy life expectancy between major regional populations of the world. The difference between HALE and total life expectancy is LHE (healthy life expectancy 'lost' due to disability). The equivalent 'lost' healthy years range from 20% (of total life expectancy at birth) in Africa to 11–12% in the European region and the Western Pacific region. The equivalent 'lost' healthy years at age 60 are a higher percentage of remaining life expectancy, due to the higher prevalence of disability at older ages. These range from around 40–50% in sub-Saharan Africa to around 25% in developed countries.

Figure 17.2 shows HALE at birth for women versus men for 191 countries in the year 2000. In the countries with HALE at birth of 45 years or lower, male and female HALE are almost the same. These countries are almost entirely African countries, but include the Lao People's Republic, Haiti and Nepal. There are a number of countries with HALE around 50 years where female

Table 17.3. Life expectancy (LE), healthy life expectancy (HALE), and lost healthy years as a percentage of total LE (LHE%), at birth and at age 60, by sex and region, 2000

Region[a]	Females			Males			Female–Male difference		
	HALE (years)	LE (years)	LHE% (%)	HALE (years)	LE (years)	LHE% (%)	HALE (years)	LE (years)	LHE% (%)
At birth									
Low mortality countries	72.0	81.2	11.4	68.0	75.1	9.5	4.0	6.1	1.9
Eastern Europe	61.0	72.2	15.5	54.0	62.9	14.2	7.0	9.3	1.3
Latin America	61.8	73.7	16.1	58.0	67.0	13.4	3.8	6.7	2.7
Eastern Mediterranean	55.9	69.4	19.5	56.4	66.1	14.7	−0.6	3.3	4.8
Asia/Pacific	57.5	67.6	15.0	56.2	63.9	12.2	1.3	3.6	2.8
Africa	38.9	48.8	20.3	39.5	47.0	15.9	−0.6	1.9	4.4
World	57.0	67.2	15.1	54.9	62.7	12.5	2.1	4.5	2.7
At age 60									
Low mortality countries	18.8	24.2	22.4	15.9	19.9	19.8	2.9	4.4	2.6
Eastern Europe	13.0	18.9	31.5	9.6	14.6	34.2	3.3	4.3	−2.7
Latin America	14.1	20.8	32.2	12.3	17.5	29.9	1.8	3.3	2.2
Eastern Mediterranean	10.3	18.0	42.4	10.4	16.1	35.5	0.0	1.9	6.9
Asia/Pacific	12.9	19.0	32.2	11.1	15.9	29.8	1.7	3.1	2.4
Africa	8.3	15.8	47.3	8.3	13.9	40.2	0.0	1.9	7.1
World	14.1	20.2	30.3	11.9	16.7	28.3	2.2	3.6	2.0

[a]*Low mortality countries* includes Western Europe, North America, Japan, Australia, New Zealand, Singapore and Brunei Darussalam; *Eastern Europe* includes Turkey and the former socialist countries of Eastern Europe and Central Asia; *Asia/Pacific* includes India, China and other Asian and Pacific countries apart from the five included in *low mortality countries*; *Africa* includes the countries of sub-Saharan Africa; North African countries are included in *Eastern Mediterranean*.

HALE at birth is actually lower than male HALE. These countries are mostly in Africa and the eastern Mediterranean region, but also include Afghanistan, Pakistan and Bangladesh. For other countries with HALE at birth of greater than 50 years, female HALE is generally higher than male HALE, though the gap is lower than for total life expectancy. In many countries of Eastern Europe, female HALE at birth is substantially higher than male, reflecting very high levels of adult mortality in men in the 1990s. Similar patterns are apparent for the male–female gap in healthy life expectancy at age 60, although the male–female reversal in eastern Mediterranean countries no longer occurs. In the countries with the longest healthy life expectancies, there is a trend to increasing female–male gap with increasing HALE, reflecting the greater

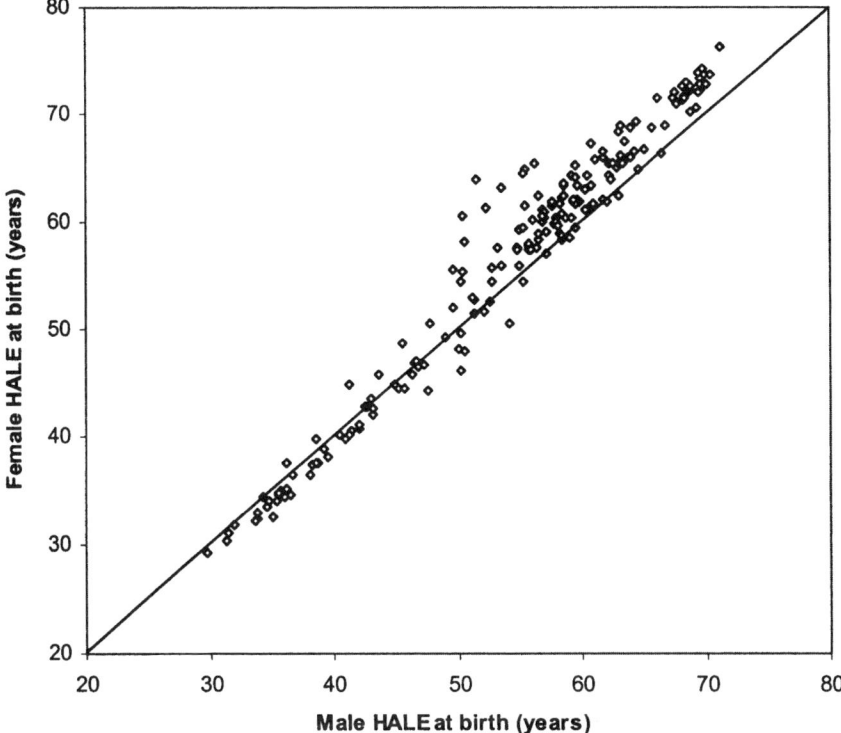

Figure 17.2. Healthy life expectancy at birth for females versus males, 191 countries, 2000

proportion of years of life lived at older ages by women aged 60 and over, where there are higher prevalences of disabling conditions such as dementia and musculoskeletal disorders.

Table 17.4 shows the top 10 disease and injury causes of death for developed countries (the low mortality countries plus Eastern Europe) and developing countries (the rest of the world). In developed countries, ischemic heart disease and cerebrovascular disease are together responsible for 36% of loss of healthy life, and death rates are higher for females than males. Lung cancer is the third leading cause of death, with a nearly 3-fold male excess.

Table 17.5 shows the top 10 disease and injury causes of disability (prevalence YLD) for developed and developing countries. In developed countries, depression is responsible for nearly 15% of loss of healthy life, and YLD rates are 40% higher for females than males. Alcohol dependence and harmful use is the second leading cause of YLD, with a large male excess, followed by dementia and hearing loss. In developing countries, in contrast,

Table 17.4. Ten leading causes of death, developed and developing countries, 2000

	% of total deaths	Male to female ratio
Developed countries[a]		
1 Ischemic heart disease	22.6	1.00
2 Cerebrovascular disease	13.8	0.65
3 Trachea, bronchus, lung cancers	4.5	2.79
4 Lower respiratory infections	3.7	0.97
5 Chronic obstructive pulmonary disease	3.0	1.58
6 Colon and rectum cancers	2.6	1.01
7 Stomach cancer	2.0	1.51
8 Self-inflicted injuries	1.9	3.67
9 Diabetes mellitus	1.8	0.73
10 Breast cancer	1.6	0.00
Developing countries		
1 Ischemic heart disease	9.1	1.21
2 Lower respiratory infections	8.0	1.20
3 Cerebrovascular disease	7.7	1.07
4 HIV/AIDS	6.9	1.02
5 Perinatal conditions	5.6	1.14
6 Diarrheal diseases	5.0	1.25
7 Chronic obstructive pulmonary disease	5.0	1.12
8 Tuberculosis	3.8	1.67
9 Malaria	2.6	0.92
10 Road traffic accidents	2.6	2.84

[a]Developed countries include European countries, former Soviet countries, Canada, USA, Japan, Australia, New Zealand.

depression is followed by iron-deficiency anemia, hearing loss, and then maternal conditions and chronic obstructive pulmonary disease. The latter reflects the impact of both smoking and indoor air pollution.

DISCUSSION AND CONCLUSIONS

Despite the fact that people live longer in the richer, more developed countries, and have greater opportunity to acquire non-fatal disabilities in older age, disability has a greater absolute (and relative) impact on healthy life expectancy in poorer countries. Separating life expectancy into equivalent years of good health and years of lost good health thus widens rather than narrows the difference in health status between the rich and the poor countries. At a global level, females live 4.5 years longer than men, but lose the equivalent of 2.4 extra years of good health to the non-fatal consequences of diseases and injuries. In other words, although females live longer, they spend a greater

Table 17.5. Ten leading causes of disability (YLD), developed and developing countries, 2000

	% of total YLD	Male to female ratio
Developed countries[a]		
1 Unipolar depressive disorders	14.9	0.60
2 Alcohol use disorders	8.0	4.12
3 Alzheimer and other dementias	5.7	0.65
4 Hearing loss, adult onset	4.9	1.10
5 Osteoarthritis	4.7	0.64
6 Cerebrovascular disease	3.3	0.85
7 Chronic obstructive pulmonary disease	2.6	1.68
8 Diabetes mellitus	2.6	0.91
9 Schizophrenia	2.3	1.08
10 Bipolar disorder	2.3	1.02
Developing countries		
1 Unipolar depressive disorders	23.0	0.68
2 Iron-deficiency anemia	10.8	0.81
3 Hearing loss, adult onset	9.4	1.19
4 Maternal conditions	8.4	–
5 Chronic obstructive pulmonary disease	7.2	1.18
6 Falls	6.1	1.33
7 Schizophrenia	6.0	1.04
8 Osteoarthritis	5.3	0.69
9 Bipolar disorder	5.2	1.02
10 Perinatal conditions	4.8	1.15

[a]Developed countries include European countries, former Soviet countries, Canada, USA, Japan, Australia, New Zealand.

amount of time with disability. However, this global average disguises enormous variations across the world in the sex difference in healthy life expectancy. The female–male difference in HALE at birth varies from a high of 10 years in some former Soviet Union countries to a low of −4 years for Pakistan.

People living in poor countries not only face lower life expectancies than those in richer countries but also live a higher proportion of their lives in poor health. Figure 17.3 shows average HALE at birth (with 95% uncertainty intervals), plotted against income per capita (gross domestic product measured in international dollars using purchasing power parity conversion rates). Richer countries should be much more active in seeking ways to improve the health of the world's poor. WHO has been a strong advocate for efforts to increase the resources available for this purpose. The recent report of its Commission on Macroeconomics and Health (2001) concluded that the bulk of the global disease burden is the result of a relatively small set of conditions,

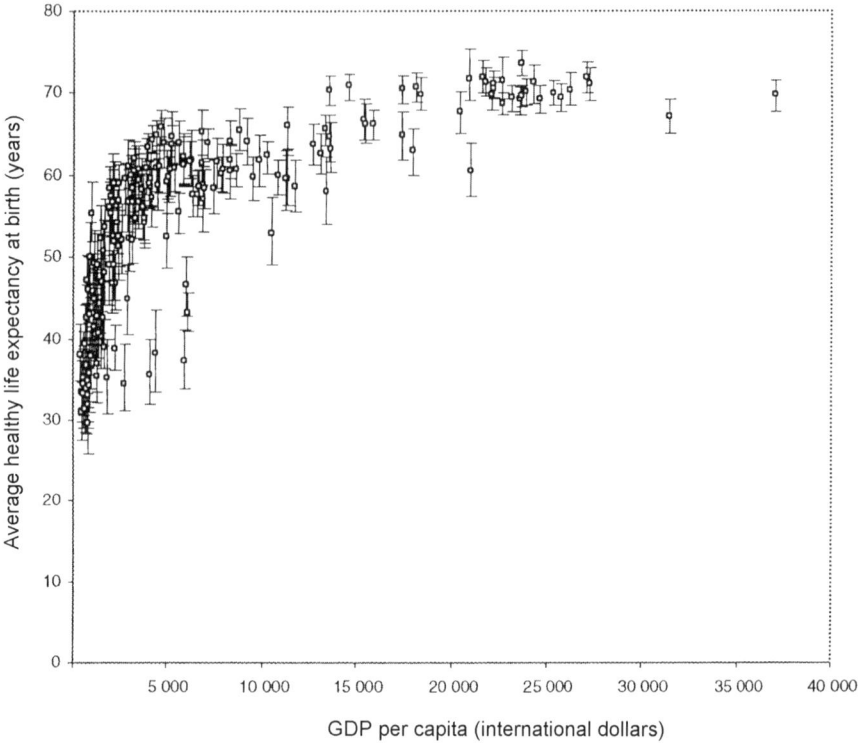

Figure 17.3. Healthy life expectancy at birth versus gross domestic product (GDP) per capita in international dollars (purchasing power parity conversion), 191 countries, 2000

each with an existing set of effective interventions. The main problems are the funding of these interventions and access of poor populations to these interventions. The Commission estimated that the essential interventions to target these problems could be provided for a per capita cost of around $34 per person per year.

Healthy life expectancy is a valuable tool for monitoring changes over time and differences between populations, but does not prevent policy-makers from considering the components separately – the fatal and non-fatal health outcomes, and the morbidity associated with different disease and injury causes. Although calculating HALEs is somewhat complex, complexity should not stand in the way of providing information critical to policy, together with estimates of the uncertainty in this information. As with any innovative approach, there are substantial limitations and gaps in the information base required for estimating healthy life expectancy for all countries of the world. We have attempted to maximize the comparability of the data derived from available nationally representative health surveys, and have used additional cross-population comparable information on health status derived from analysis of epidemiological data sources to improve comparability.

The WHO instrument has been used to collect population health data in over 55 countries at the time of writing, and this experience will be used to improve the health status measurement methods and to extend the surveys to more countries. In addition, WHO is investing considerable resources in the revision of the Global Burden of Disease estimates for the year 2000. These estimates will also contribute to improved estimation of healthy life expectancy, which will in turn assist in monitoring global health trends, and in particular, trends in the health and healthy life expectancy of populations around the world.

ACKNOWLEDGMENTS

The authors thank the many staff of the Global Program on Evidence for Health Policy who contributed to the development of life tables, burden of disease analysis and the development and conduct of the health surveys. These include Omar Ahmad, Lydia Bendib, Somnath Chatterji, Mie Inoue, Rafael Lozano, Doris Ma Fat, Claudia Stein, Bedirhan Üstün and Cao Yang.

REFERENCES

Commission on Macroeconomics and Health (2001) *Macroeconomics and Health: Investing in Health for Economic Development*. Geneva: World Health Organization.

Lopez, A.D., Ahmad, O., Guillot, M., Ferguson, B. Salomon, J.A., Murray, C.J.L. and Hill, K.H. (2002) *World Mortality in 2000; Life tables for 191 countries*. Geneva: World Health Organization.

Mathers, C.D., Murray, C.J.L., Salomon, J. and Lopez, A.D. (2001a) *Estimates of healthy life expectancy for 191 countries in the year 2000: methods and results*. GPE Discussion Paper No. 38. Geneva: World Health Organization. Also available on the worldwide web at www.who.int/evidence.

Mathers, C.D., Sadana, R., Salomon, J., Murray, C.J.L. and Lopez, A.D. (2001b) 'Healthy life expectancy in 191 countries, 1999', *Lancet* 357, 1685–1691.

Mathers, C.D., Stein, C., Tomijima, N., Ma Fat, D., Rao, C., Inoue, M., Lopez, A.D. and Murray, C.J.L. (2002) *Global Burden of Disease 2000: Version 2 methods and results*. Geneva: World Health Organization (GPE Discussion Paper No. 50).

Murray, C.J.L. and Lopez, A.D. (eds) (1996) 'The global burden of disease: a comprehensive assessment of mortality and disability from diseases, injuries and risk factors in 1990 and projected to 2020', *Global Burden of Disease and Injury Series*, vol. 1. Cambridge, MA: Harvard University Press.

Murray, C.J.L. and Frenk, J. (2000) *A framework for assessing the performance of Health Systems*. Bulletin of the World Health Organization 78(6): 717–731

Murray, C.J.L., Mathers, C.D., Lopez, A.D. and Stein, C. (2001) *The Global Burden of Disease 2000 project: aims, methods and data sources*. GPE Discussion Paper No. 36.

Geneva: World Health Organization. Also available on the worldwide web at www.who.int/evidence.

Murray, C.J.L., Tandon, A., Salomon, J. and Mathers, C.D. (2002) 'New approaches to enhance cross-population comparability of survey results', in Murray, C.J.L., Salomon, J.A., Mathers, C.D. and Lopez, A.D. (eds) *Summary Measures of Population Health: Concepts, Ethics, Measurement and Applications.* Geneva: World Health Organization.

Robine, J-M., Mathers, C.D. and Brouard, N. (1996) 'Trends and differentials in disability-free life expectancy: concepts, methods and findings', in Caselli, G. and Lopez, A. (eds) *Health and Mortality Among Elderly Populations.* Oxford: Clarendon Press, pp. 182–201.

Sadana, R., Mathers, C.D., Lopez, A., Murray, C. and Moesgaard-Iberg, K. (2002) 'Comparative analysis of more than 50 household surveys of health status', in Murray, C.J.L., Salomon, J.A., Mathers, C.D. and Lopez, A.D. (eds) *Summary Measures of Population Health: Concepts, Ethics, Measurement and Applications.* Geneva: World Health Organization.

Salomon, J. and Murray, C.J.L. (2000) *Compositional models for mortality by age, sex and cause.* GPE discussion Paper No. 11. Geneva: World Health Organization. Also available on the worldwide web at www.who.int/evidence.

Salomon, J.A. and Murray, C.J.L. (2001) 'Modelling HIV/AIDS epidemics in sub-Saharan Africa using seroprevalence data from antenatal clinics', *Bulletin of the World Health Organization,* 79(7), 596–607.

Salomon, J.S., Mathers, C.D., Murray, C.J.L. and Ferguson, B. (2001) *Methods for life expectancy and healthy life expectancy uncertainty analysis.* GPE discussion paper No. 10. Geneva, World Health Organization. Also available on the worldwide web at www.who.int/evidence.

Üstün, T.B., Chatterji, S., Villanueva, M., Bendib, L., Celik, C., Sadana, R., Valentine, N., Mathers, C., Ortiz, J., Tandon, A., Salomon, J., Yang, C., Xie Wan, J. and Murray, C.J.L. (2001) *WHO Multi-country Household Survey Study on Health and Responsiveness, 2000–2001.* GPE discussion paper No. 37. Geneva: World Health Organization. Also available on the worldwide web at www.who.int/evidence.

World Health Organization (2000) *World Health Report 2000. Health Systems: Improving Performance.* Geneva: World Health Organization. Also available on the worldwide web at www.who.int/whr.

World Health Organization (2001) *World Health Report 2001. Mental Health: New Understanding, New Hope.* Geneva: World Health Organization. Also available on the worldwide web at www.who.int/whr.

18

Health Expectancies in European Countries

ROM J.M. PERENBOOM, HERMAN VAN OYEN* and
MARGARETA MUTAFOVA[†]
TNO Prevention and Health, Leiden, The Netherlands, *Scientific Institute of Public
Health, Brussels, Belgium and [†]Medical Academy, Sofia, Bulgaria

INTRODUCTION

In the late 1980s the first health expectancies for three European countries were calculated: France (Robine *et al*, 1986), England and Wales (Bebbington, 1988) and the Netherlands (van Ginneken *et al*, 1989, 1991). One decade later health expectancies have been presented or published for 15 European countries.

In the early 1990s Europe comprised more than forty independent countries. Health expectancies have been calculated for almost all Western European countries with the exception of Portugal, Ireland, Greece, Iceland and Luxembourg and some of the smaller ones such as Andorra and Liechtenstein. Until now health expectancies have been calculated for only Bulgaria and Poland among the Central and Eastern European countries. Within some Western European countries, e.g. Belgium, Italy, Spain and the United Kingdom, calculations have also been made for specific regions.

Although health expectancy calculations are restricted to 15 European countries, this does not mean that there are only 15 health expectancy results. Most countries have calculated more than one type of health expectancy, all of which fit more or less within the classification system of health expectancies (Robine *et al*, 1995; Boshuizen *et al*, 1994; Robine and Romieu, 1998). This classification system, discussed in more detail in Chapter 14, classifies health expectancy indicators primarily in the framework of the ICIDH (International Classification of Impairments, Disabilities and Handicaps; World Health Organization, 1980), extended with disease-free life expectancy, life expectancy in good perceived health and a weighted version.

Determining Health Expectancies. Edited by J-M. Robine, C. Jagger, C.D. Mathers, E.M. Crimmins and R.M. Suzman.
© 2003 John Wiley & Sons, Ltd

In Table 18.1 the types of health expectancies are presented according to the classification system. In this table, one extra column is added, that of life expectancy in good mental health or mental health expectancy. This type of health expectancy, which is based on generic measurement instruments of mental health, is not yet part of the classification system.

As can be seen from Table 18.1, the most common health expectancy in Europe is disability-free life expectancy, although the methods of calculation are often different in the countries. In Sweden, a kind of disability-free life expectancy is calculated in combination with perceived health (Pettersson, 1990, 1995). Within this class, two subclasses are distinguished, functional limitation free and activity restriction free life expectancy.

Health expectancy based on perceived health is calculated in 10 different countries as 'life expectancy in good perceived health'. In Sweden, health expectancy is calculated using the combination of disabilities and perceived health (Pettersson, 1990, 1995).

Disease-free health expectancy is also a widely used health expectancy in Europe, although this class can be divided into two subtypes: generic disease free (without chronic diseases) and specific disease free. The latter is restricted to dementia-free life expectancy, calculated in four European countries. Because mental health is a growing problem and is more and more recognised as being so by public health policy makers, it can be expected that this type of health expectancy will be calculated more widely in the near future.

Handicap-free life expectancy is somewhat less common, being calculated in seven countries, although this type consists of very different subtypes, like mobility-handicap-free, independent life expectancy or occupational handicap-free. It should be noted here that active life expectancy (based on activities of daily living (ADL) and instrumental ADL (IADL) (Katz *et al*, 1983)), is classified as belonging to the subclass of independent life expectancy.

A different concept is that of health-adjusted life expectancy, in which weights are assigned to the levels of severity of ill health. Incorporating these weights in the calculation of health expectancy leads to a weighted version, called health-adjusted life expectancy (HALE), discussed in Chapter 12. In Europe, at the moment this has been done in the Netherlands only, using perceived health and disabilities.

In the Netherlands, examples of all classes of health expectancies are calculated. Most other countries have calculated three or four types of health expectancies. This is even the case in Bulgaria, where, despite its poor economic and social situation, a set of pilot studies as well as the first National Health Survey have been used to produce estimates of healthy life expectancy. Thus, for 15 different countries, over 40 different health expectancy results are available in total. But reality is even more complicated. Within each (sub) class of health expectancies, health is estimated with different measurement instruments, including factors like definition of the survey samples, interview

Table 18.1. Classes of health expectancy by country

Country		Classes of health expectancies				
Austria		Disability-free				
Belgium	Dementia free	Disability-free		Perceived health		
Bulgaria		Disability-free	Handicap-free	Perceived health	Generic mental health	
Denmark	Long-standing illness	Disability-free		Perceived health	Generic mental health	
Finland		Disability-free	Handicap-free	Perceived health		
France	Without chronic disease	Disability-free	Handicap-free			
	Dementia free					
Germany		Disability-free	Handicap-free	Perceived health		
Italy	Without major fatal diseases	Disability-free		Perceived health		
	Without fatal and chronic non-fatal diseases					
Netherlands	Dementia free Depression free	Disability-free	Handicap-free	Perceived health	Generic mental health	Health-adjusted life expectancies (different concepts)
Norway	Without chronic disease	Disability-free	Handicap-free	Perceived health		
Poland		Disability-free				
Spain		Disability-free		Perceived health	Generic mental health	
Sweden		Disability-free, combined with perceived health		Perceived health combined with Disability-free		
Switzerland	Dementia free	Disability-free				
United Kingdom		Disability-free	Handicap-free			

Table 18.2. Health expectancy results for European countries by class of health expectancies[a]

Country/source	Calendar year	Type	Males Total life expectancy	Males Health expectancy	Females Total life expectancy	Females Health expectancy
Disease-free						
Netherlands (1)	?	Depression (age 55)	22.6	19.4	27.8	22.4
Switzerland (2)	?	Dementia (age 65)	16.1 (Geneva)	15.0 (Geneva)	20.4 (Geneva)	18.6 (Geneva)
			16.9 (Zurich)	15.5 (Zurich)	21.0 (Zurich)	19.1 (Zurich)
Norway (3)	1985	Chronic disease (at birth)	71.9	38.9	78	37.9
Denmark (4, 5)	1986–1987	Long-standing illness (age 16)	56.7	40.4	62.4	42
France (6)	1988–1990	Dementia (age 65)	15.4	14.8	19.7	18.8
Italy (7)	1990	Fatal diseases (at birth)	74.1	70.8	80.7	77.0
Italy (7)	1990	Fatal and chronic non-fatal disease (at birth)	74.1	56.1	80.7	55.9
Belgium (8)	1991	Dementia (age 65)	14.0	13.1	18.3	16.1
France (9)	1991	Chronic disease (at birth)	72.9	48.7	81.2	49.0
Netherlands (10)	1993	Dementia (age 65)	14.5	14.0	19.0	17.7
Disability-free						
Finland (11)	?	Functional limitations (age 25)	47.1	31.3	54.6	33.2
France (12)	1982	At birth	70.7	61.9	78.9	67.1
Norway (3)	1985	Functional limitations (age 15)	58.8	50.2	65.2	51.4
United Kingdom (13)	1985	Functional limitations (at birth)	71.7	63.6	77.5	66.5
Denmark (4, 5)	1986–1987	Functional limitation (age 16)	56.7	49.8	62.4	52
Spain (14, 15)	1986	Functional limitations (at birth)	73.2	61.6	79.6	63.6
Sweden (16, 17)	1986–1990	Combination of disabilities and perceived health (age 16–84 years)	57.6	33	62.2	33.1
Poland (18)	1988	Unclassified (at birth)	67.1	59.8	75.7	62.6
Belgium (19)	1989–1990	Unclassified (KUL-study, age 55)	20.0	18.0	25.1	21.7
Switzerland (20)	1989	At birth	74.0	67.1	80.9	72.9
Italy (21)	1990	At birth	73.5	68.0	80.0	72.3
Austria (22)	1992	Activity restrictions (at birth)	72.9	69.0	79.4	72.4
Bulgaria (23, 24, 25)	1992	Unclassified (age 60)	16.0	8.0	19.2	7.3
Netherlands (26)	1994	At birth	74.6	62.7	80.3	60.8
Germany (27)	1995	Unclassified (at birth)	73.8	68.9	80.0	74

(continued)

Table 18.2. *(continued)*

Country/source	Calendar year	Type	Males Total life expectancy	Males Health expectancy	Females Total life expectancy	Females Health expectancy
Handicap-free						
Norway (3)	1985	Independent life (age 65)	14.4	13.3	18.2	16.9
Denmark (4, 5, 28)	1986–1987	Age 16	56.7	54.3	62.4	59
Finland (29)	1986	General (age 65)	13.4	4.3	17.4	5.6
Finland (29)	1986	Independent life (age 65)	13.4	2.5	17.4	2.4
France (30)	1991	General (at birth)	72.9	63.8	81.1	68.5
France (30)	1991	Mobility (at birth)	72.9	71.7	81.1	78.8
Netherlands (31)	1991–1992	General (at birth)	74.2	61.4	80.2	63.5
Bulgaria (24, 25)	1992	Mobility (age 60)	16	14.1	19.2	15.4
Bulgaria (32)	1992	Occupational (age 16–59)	41.2	40.5	42.8	42.2
United Kingdom (33)	1994	Independent life (age 65)	14.8	13.5	18.6	15.6
Germany (27)	1995	Occupational (at birth)	73.8	64.2	80.0	73.2
Perceived health						
Norway (3)	1985	At birth	72.6	69.0	79.0	74.1
Denmark (4, 5)	1986–1987	Age 16	56.7	53	62.4	57.1
Finland (34)	1986	Age 25	47.1	41.5	54.6	46.9
Sweden (16, 17)	1986–1990	Combination of disabilities and perceived health (age 16–84 years)	57.6	33	62.2	33.1
Belgium (19, 35)	1989–1990	Age 15	58.3	54.6	64.9	60.2
Italy (36)	1990	At birth	73.5	58.6	80.0	58.4
Spain (14, 37)	1991	At birth	72.6	54.5	80.5	53.3
Bulgaria (24, 25)	1992	Age 60	16	6.9	19.2	6.2
Netherlands (26)	1994	At birth	74.6	60.1	80.3	60.3
Germany (27)	1995	At birth	73.8	62.4	80.0	64.2
Mental health						
Denmark (38)	1994	SF-36 (age 16)	57.3	54.7	62.5	57.4
Netherlands (39)	1995	ABS (age 16)	59.3	52.6	64.9	54.6
Spain (40)	1995	GHQ-12 (age 65)	16.4	14.1	20.5	16.5
Bulgaria (41, 42)	1996	GHQ-12 (age 65)	12.7	5.1	15.3	4.3
Netherlands (43)	1996	MHI-5 (age 16)	59.3	54.4	64.9	54.1

[a]Further details and other age groups can be found in Robine and Romieu (1998) and in Robine *et al* (1998).
Sources: 1: Deeg and Beekman, 1996; 2: Herrmann and Michel, 1996; 3: Grotvedt and Viksand, 1994; 4: Rasmussen and Brønnum-Hansen, 1990; 5: Brønnum-Hansen, 1991; 6: Ritchie *et al*, 1994; 7: Egidi and Frova, 1997; 8: Roelands *et al*, 1994; 9: Robine *et al*, 1996; 10: Perenboom *et al*, 1996; 11: Valkonen *et al*, 1997; 12: Robine *et al*, 1986; 13: Bebbington, 1992; 14: Gispert and Gutiérrez Fisac, 1995; 15: Ministerio de Sanidad y Consumo, 1993; 16: Egidi and Frova, 1997; 17: Grotvedt and Viksand, 1994; 18: Haber and Dowd, 1994; 19: Van Oyen and Roelands, 1994; 20: Bisig and Gutzwiller, 1994; 21: Egidi and Buratta, 1995; 22: Kytir, 1994; 23: Mutafova *et al*, 1994; 24: Mutafova *et al*, 1997; 25: Mutafova and Maleshkov, 1995; 26: Perenboom *et al*, 1997; 27: Brückner, 1997; 28: Brønnum-Hansen and Rasmussen, 1990; 29: Valkonen, 1994; 30: Robine and Mormiche, 1993; 31: Boshuizen and van de Water, 1994; 32: Mutafova *et al*, 1996; 33: Bebbington and Darton, 1996; 34: Valkonen *et al*, 1997; 35: Van Oyen *et al*, 1995; 36: Buratta and Crialesi, 1993; 37: Regidor Poyatos *et al*, 1995; 38: Brønnum-Hansen and Rasmussen, 1996; 39: Perenboom and van de Water, 1997a; 40: Gispert *et al*, 1998; 41: Mutafova *et al*, 1999a; 42: Mutafova *et al*, 1999b; 43: Perenboom and van Herten, 1999.

methods etc. So even within the (sub) classes comparison between countries is not easy. Later in this chapter European initiatives to deal with this complication are discussed, and in Chapter 14 this problem is discussed in more detail. Another complication in comparing the results of health expectancies is that they refer to certain calendar years. Some countries have calculated health expectancies for only one year, or by pooling the data from different calendar years, and other countries have calculated them in chronological series and present trends. For some countries the most recent health expectancies are almost 10 years old or older.

Health expectancies can be calculated for each year of age, for males and females separately or for the combination of sexes. In most European countries the results refer to age at birth for males and females separately, but for some countries results are also or even only published for the age of 65 years. Dementia-free life expectancy is only presented for the older age groups (65 or even 85 years).

As discussed elsewhere in this book, comparison between countries is almost impossible, even within the different classes of the classification system (Boshuizen and van de Water, 1994). Nevertheless, in the sections following we give an overview of some results by class of health expectancy for the different countries. However, this chapter would not be complete if we look only at the results of calculations of health expectancies, presented in summary in Table 18.2. At the end of this chapter we briefly discuss the policy relevance and usage of health expectancies in Europe and some of the European initiatives to harmonise the calculations of health expectancies in the European Union and in other European countries.

DISEASE-FREE HEALTH EXPECTANCY

In four countries a more or less generic disease-free life expectancy is calculated: Denmark (Rasmussen and Brønnum-Hansen, 1990; Brønnum-Hansen, 1991), France (Robine et al, 1996), Italy (Egidi and Frova, 1997) and Norway (Grotvedt and Viksand, 1994). Although all these disease-free life expectancies refer to diseases in general, results cannot easily be compared. Denmark, France and Norway all use the concept of longstanding or chronic diseases; the Italian results, however, refer to the combination of fatal and non-fatal chronic diseases. So it is not surprising that the results differ greatly between the countries, ranging from about 38 years of disease-free life expectancy for females in Norway to 77 years for females in Italy.

For four countries dementia-free life expectancy is calculated as an example of the disease-specific free life expectancy: Belgium (Roelands et al, 1994), France (Ritchie et al, 1994), the Netherlands (Perenboom et al, 1996) and Switzerland (Herrmann and Michel, 1996). Although different ways are used to diagnose dementia, in all four countries, diagnosis is based on the DSM-III-R or DSM-IV (Diagnostic and Statistical Manual of Mental Disorders) criteria, thereby allowing comparison between the countries. The results for each country are very similar. At the age of 65 males can expect to have a life expectancy with dementia of 0.5 to 1 year, females about 1.5 to 2.0 years.

A final example of life expectancy free of a specific disease is depression-free life expectancy for the Netherlands based on the Center for Epidemiological Studies Depression Scale (CES-D) (Deeg and Beekman, 1996). At the age of 55, males can expect to have 3.2 years with depression, females 5.4 years.

For France and Norway, chronological series of data exist for disease-free life expectancies. In France between 1981 and 1991 the number of years without chronic diseases seems to remain stable for both males and females (Robine and Romieu, 1998). In Norway the situation for males and females differs. Between 1975 and 1985 for males the number of years without chronic diseases has not changed, while for females there is a decrease of almost 2 years (Grotvedt and Viksand, 1994).

DISABILITY-FREE LIFE EXPECTANCY

As in other regions of the world, the most common class of health expectancy calculated is disability-free life expectancy. This is the type of health expectancy that Sullivan calculated in 1971 (Sullivan, 1971a, 1971b) and with which he laid the basis of the work of today. Within the class of disability-free life expectancy, two subclasses can be distinguished: functional limitation free life expectancy and activity restriction free life expectancy. Functional limitation refers to restrictions in bending and picking up things, walking etc. Activity restrictions refer to problems in more complex human activities like cooking and dressing. A third type of disability-free life expectancy is that of 'unclassified disability-free life expectancy' (Robine et al, 1995).

In European countries, health expectancies of both subclasses are present. Denmark (Brønnum-Hansen, 1998), the Netherlands (van Ginneken et al, 1992), Norway (Grotvedt and Viksand, 1994), Spain (SESPAS, 1993; Gispert and Gutiérrez Fisac, 1995; Ministerio de Sanidad and Consumo, 1993) and the United Kingdom (Bebbington, 1992, 1995; Bone et al, 1995) have calculated functional limitation free life expectancy while Austria (Kytir, 1994), Italy (Buratta and Crialesi, 1993), the Netherlands (Boshuizen and van de Water, 1994) and Switzerland (Bisig et al, 1992; Spuhler and Bisig, 1991) have calculated activity restriction free life expectancy. In the Central European countries Poland (Haber and Dowd, 1994) and Bulgaria (Mutafova, 1993) (for the age of 65 only), the 'unclassified disability-free life expectancy' has been calculated (Robine and Romieu, 1998). Although also in Germany (Brückner, 1997), Belgium (van Oyen and Roelands, 1994) and in the Netherlands

(Perenboom *et al*, 1997), a kind of unclassified disability-free life expectancy is calculated.

Within each subclass, different measurement instruments are used, so that comparison between the countries is impossible. Results for functional limitation free life expectancy range from 61.6 years for males in Spain to 66.5 years for females in the United Kingdom. For activity restriction free life expectancy, results range from 59.9 years for Dutch females in 1990 to 76.2 years for Italian females, also in 1990. These differences can hardly be due to real differences in healthy years, but refer mainly to differences in the items used to measure this health concept.

In the group of unclassified disability-free life expectancies, differences range from 60.8 years for females in the Netherlands to almost 74 years for females in Germany in 1995. In the Netherlands and in Belgium this disability-free life expectancy is based on a combination of questions aiming at activity restrictions and functional limitations. In Germany, however, this disability-free life expectancy is based on a kind of global disability indicator, 'the days persons report to be unable to fulfil their usual tasks or perform their usual activities due to ill health or injury'. In this sense and in terms of the former version of the ICIDH, the German disability-free life expectancy is close to a general handicap-free life expectancy.

For some countries chronological series of health expectancies are available within the class of disability-free life expectancy. Denmark (Brønnum-Hansen, 1998), the Netherlands (Perenboom *et al*, 1993, 1997) and the UK (Bebbington and Darton, 1996) have chronological series, allowing investigation of developments over time. The overall picture for males is clear: in all chronological series disability-free life expectancy appears to increase. For females, however, the results are not as clear. Some results point to a stabilisation, other results even to a decrease in the number of years without disabilities. Only in the UK between the years 1980 and 1994 does there seem to be an increase in disability-free life expectancy for females at the age of 65.

HANDICAP-FREE LIFE EXPECTANCY

In the REVES classification system, handicap-free life expectancy is divided into three subclasses: independent life expectancy, mobility handicap-free life expectancy and occupational handicap-free life expectancy. A frequently used type of health expectancy, active life expectancy, based on a complete set of ADL activities can be classified as a form of independent life expectancy (Robine *et al*, 1995; Robine and Romieu, 1998). In addition to these subclasses, there is one other type, general handicap-free life expectancy. This type refers to those handicap-free life expectancies that cannot be assigned to the other three subclasses or when handicap is assessed in a global manner.

In four countries a general handicap-free life expectancy is calculated: Finland (Valkonen, 1994), France (Robine and Mormiche, 1993), the Netherlands (Boshuizen and van de Water, 1994) and the UK (Bebbington and Darton, 1996). Independent life expectancy is calculated in three countries: Finland (Valkonen, 1994), Norway (Grotvedt and Viksand, 1994) and the UK (Bebbington and Darton, 1996). Mobility handicap-free life expectancy, referring to the ability to go outdoors without help from other persons or assistive devices, is calculated in three countries: Bulgaria, where the recommended instruments of the WHO are used (Mutafova *et al*, 1994), France (Robine and Mormiche, 1993) and again the UK (Bebbington and Darton, 1996). Finally occupational handicap-free life expectancy is calculated in two countries. Firstly in Bulgaria, where data from medical expert commissions are used to estimate the number of occupationally handicapped and the handicapped years with a distinction made in the levels of severity (Mutafova *et al*, 1996). However, data were only available for the age groups 16 to 59 years, so results are restricted to these ages (using a partial life table). In Germany occupational handicap-free life expectancy is based on self-reported 'certified handicap levels'. These levels are defined in documents to those whose health conditions meet certain predefined conditions and make them eligible for certain benefits, ranging from social security to special work contracts (Brückner, 1997).

As is the case with disability-free life expectancy, handicap-free life expectancy chronological series also exist for some European countries. Finland, France, Germany, Norway and the UK all have such series for one or more subclasses of the handicap-free life expectancy. With some exceptions the number of years that are handicap-free seems to increase over the years, although this is not always the case when the changes in total life expectancy are taken into account. In the UK, for males and females the number of handicap-free life years increased between 1976 and 1991, but there seems to be a downward trend between 1991 and 1994 (Robine and Romieu, 1998).

LIFE EXPECTANCY IN GOOD PERCEIVED HEALTH

The second most popular health concept for the calculation of health expectancies is perceived health, this being used in 10 different countries to calculate life expectancies in good perceived health. Perceived health refers to the single item question where people are asked how they perceive or judge their own health state: (very) good, fair, poor or very poor/bad. The use of this concept as an indicator of health status and also in the calculation of health expectancy is a subject of discussion, because it is not always clear whether the concept is understood in the same way in different countries, different age groups or at different times (Deeg, 1999; Hoeymans, 1997). Although this question is asked in almost every health survey, the wording and the response categories differ between surveys, years and countries. Even when the same question is used with the same response categories, comparison of the presented or published results is not always possible because the cut-off point between health and ill health can differ (Boshuizen and van de Water, 1994). For instance, although in Denmark (Rasmussen and Brønnum-Hansen, 1990), Belgium (van Oyen and Roelands, 1994), Bulgaria (Mutafova *et al*, 1997), Norway (Grotvedt and Viksand, 1994), Finland (Valkonen, 1994), Germany (Brückner, 1997) and the Netherlands (Perenboom *et al*, 1993) almost the same question was used to measure perceived health, the published results cannot be compared due to the use of different cut-off points. In Denmark, Belgium, Norway and Finland the response category 'fair' is classified as healthy, while in the Netherlands and Bulgaria it is classified as unhealthy. Moreover, in Germany (Egidi, 1990) and in Italy (Egidi, 1988) the questions differ in the way they ask the questions about perceived health in the previous weeks.

To compare life expectancy in good perceived health between Denmark and the Netherlands, Boshuizen recalculated the Danish results to make them comparable with the Dutch (and vice versa) (Boshuizen and van de Water, 1994). The results show that total life expectancy in Denmark is substantially lower than in the Netherlands. If the response categories 'very good' and 'good' are classified as in good health, life expectancy in perceived good health does not differ significantly between the two countries. For females in Denmark, the percentage of life expectancy spent in good health is slightly higher than in the Netherlands. When the response category 'fair' is also classified as good health, the differences become more apparent, in favour of the Danish population.

In some countries, chronological series of life expectancy in good perceived health exist, for instance for Finland for the years 1978 and 1986 (Valkonen, 1994), for Germany for some years between 1986 and 1995 (Brückner, 1997), for the Netherlands for the years between 1983 and 1994 (Perenboom *et al*, 1997) and for Spain for the years 1986 and 1991 (Regidor Poyatos *et al*, 1995). In Finland and Spain there seems to be an upward trend for both males and females in life expectancy in good perceived health. This is in contrast to Germany where, despite an increase in total life expectancy, a downward trend can be viewed in healthy life expectancy. In the Netherlands, for males there seems to be an upward trend, for females a downward or stable situation.

MENTAL HEALTH EXPECTANCY

In four European countries life expectancy in good mental health or mental health expectancy has been calculated, albeit all countries used different instruments or methods. In Spain (Gispert *et al*, 1998; Jagger *et al*, 1998) and Bulgaria (Mutafova *et al*, 1999a, 1999b), the General Health Questionnaire

(12-item version, GHQ-12) was used, but in Spain (to be more specific in Catalonia) the prevalence of ill health was calculated using the probability of each GHQ-12 score to be healthy while in Bulgaria a cut-off point was used to differentiate between health and ill health. In Denmark the 5-item Mental Health Inventory (a subscale of the SF-36, MHI-5) was used (Jagger *et al*, 1998; Brønnum-Hansen and Rasmussen, 1996), while in the Netherlands results based on two different instruments are available: a chronological series for the years 1989 until 1995, based on the Bradburn Affect Balance Scale (ABS), and results for one year, based on the MHI-5 (Perenboom and van de Water, 1997a; Perenboom and van Herten, 1999).

Most comparable are the results from Denmark and the Netherlands, where the MHI-5 was used. Although the total life expectancy in the Netherlands is significantly higher for both males and females than in Denmark, for males good mental health expectancy is almost equal, while the mental health expectancy for Dutch females is almost three years less than that of Danish females.

The results for Bulgaria require special attention. Good mental health expectancy at the age of 65 is very low, and when expressed as a percentage of total life expectancy for males is only 40%, and for females not even 30% (Mutafova *et al*, 1999a). One explanation may be the current economic and social situation in Bulgaria. On the other hand it could be that for Bulgaria the wrong cut-off point between health and ill health has been chosen. A study in the Netherlands (Perenboom and van de Water, 1997a) reveals that to have comparable results for the overall prevalence of mental ill health between the GHQ-12 and other instruments (ABS and the MHI-5), a cut-off point in the GHQ-12 between 4 and 5 or even between 5 and 6 has to be chosen, instead of between 1 and 2, as is recommended (Goldberg and Williams, 1988; Koeter and Ormel, 1991).

The chronological series in the Netherlands allows us to look at developments in mental health expectancy between 1989 and 1995. Results show that for both males and females at the age of 16 mental health expectancy does not change significantly.

HEALTH-ADJUSTED LIFE EXPECTANCY

The last class of health expectancies is a special one, not based on a specific health concept, but on the weighting of different health states. Most work in this type of health expectancy is done outside Europe (Canada), but in the Netherlands, health-adjusted life expectancies (HALEs) are calculated, assigning weights to different states of perceived health (Perenboom and van de Water, 1997a). For the weighting of the states of perceived health, the results of a kind of visual analogue scale for perceived health were used. Between 1983 and 1994 the HALEs for males increased from 67.8 years to 69.4 years; the HALEs for females remained almost the same at 73.1 years. Further examination showed that the number of years in mild ill health increased, while the number of years in moderate or severe ill health remained the same or decreased over this period.

Although HALEs can provide a more realistic view of the health expectancy because of the way different levels of severity of ill health are assigned different weights, it does not provide insight into the dynamics within the years in ill health. Presenting the results for the different levels independently, on the other hand, gives a clear view of the dynamics in health status, especially when relating to trends in time.

USAGE AND POLICY RELEVANCE OF HEALTH EXPECTANCY IN EUROPE

This chapter on health expectancies in Europe would not be complete if we do not look at the usage and policy relevance of the health expectancy results in Europe. In the framework of Euro-REVES 1 (see 'Conclusions' section, below), an inventory has been carried out among the countries of the European Union to gain more insight into the indicator's policy relevance and usage (van de Water *et al*, 1996). This study showed that in several European countries health expectancies play a role in health policy documents. In Denmark, both the 'public health, health behaviour, prevention programme, 1991' (DIKE, 1991) and the 'Health promotion programme of the government of Denmark' 1992 (Ministry of Health, 1992) are based on health expectancies. In England and Wales, although not explicitly mentioned, health expectancy is an indicator for 'Health of the Nation' targets. In France, health expectancy plays an important role in the report of the High Commission on Public Health 'Health in France, 1994' (Haut Comité de la Santé Publique, 1994). In the Netherlands, health expectancy is a key indicator for the policy document 'Public Health Status and Forecasts, 1993 and 1997' (Volksgezondheid Toekomst Verkenning, 1993; Ruwaard and Kramers, 1997). A health plan was published in Spain for the Catalan region (1991) and for the Basque region (1994), both choosing disability-free life expectancy as one of the indicators, and results on health expectancies are published by the Spanish Ministry of Health (Regidor Poyatos *et al*, 1995). Finally in Sweden, health expectancies form important background information for considerations about health (Socialstyrelsen, 1995). It should also be mentioned that the European Office of the World Health Organization has included health expectancy in its 'Health for All by the year 2000' programme with health expectancies being chosen to be indicators for monitoring the progress of two of the targets.

CONCLUSIONS

One of the advantages of health expectancy as an indicator of population health is that it allows comparison between different groups and countries, especially because health expectancy is independent of the age structure of the populations (Jagger, 1997). Our European tour reveals that comparability is a goal still to be achieved. In the 10 years since REVES began and since health expectancies for European countries have been calculated, it is still almost impossible to compare them, due to varying instruments and cut-off points. In Europe, several initiatives have been started to harmonise instruments and methods and in Chapter 14, these initiatives are presented in more detail. We will briefly mention here the initiatives that relate directly to health expectancy, Euro-REVES 1 and 2.

Euro-REVES 1 was initiated as a concerted action, aimed at building a European network of researchers, statisticians and policy makers to create awareness of the advantages of health expectancies. It resulted in recommendations for calculation, for more attention to mental health and for the policy relevance, as mentioned previously (Jagger *et al*, 1998; Jagger, 1997; van de Water and Perenboom, 1995; van de Water *et al*, 1995; Robine *et al*, 1997). Euro-REVES 2 is a research programme in the framework of the Health Monitoring Programme, funded by the European Union, to set up a coherent set of health expectancy indicators to be used in surveys in the member states of the European Union.

If the same instruments and methods are used, the results and differences can be surprising. As we can see at this moment, for dementia, where the same criteria for diagnosis are used, it appears that life expectancy with dementia in several European countries is almost the same. On the other hand, comparing Denmark and the Netherlands on perceived health or on mental health, using the same instrument and cut-off point, the Danish situation seems better.

But comparisons can also be made on a more aggregated level. In this case some conclusions can be drawn for all the European countries, which are not dealt with in detail in this chapter. For instance, in every European country, females have a higher total life expectancy than males, but their health expectancy is the same or even lower than that of males. So the gain in life years is lost in ill health. A look at the chronological series available shows that total life expectancy is increasing in the European countries, but this is not always accompanied by an increase in health expectancy. Health expectancies seem to stabilise or even decrease. A closer look shows that there seems to be an increase in the number of years in mild ill health and a decreasing or stable situation for the number of years in moderate or severe ill health (Robine and Romieu, 1998; Perenboom *et al*, 1997).

A final conclusion is that in the few Eastern European countries that have calculated health expectancies the health situation is poor. The situation of mental health in Bulgaria is a striking example of this inequity between countries. More insight into the health situation in Eastern European countries by means of health expectancies is necessary. Next to the harmonisation of the instruments, this should be a major topic to be reached in the second decade of REVES and the first decade of the third millennium.

REFERENCES

Bebbington, A.C. (1988) 'The expectation of life without disability in England and Wales', *Social Science and Medicine* 27, 321–326 [published erratum appears in *Social Science and Medicine* 1993, 36(5), 713–714].

Bebbington, A.C. (1992) 'Expectation of life without disability measured from the OPCS disability surveys', in Robine, J-M., Blanchet, M. and Dowd, J.E. (eds) *Health Expectancy*. London: HMSO.

Bebbington, A.C. (1995) 'Health expectancies and health policies in the UK', in van de Water, H.P.A. and Perenboom, R.J.M. (eds) *Report of the First Meeting of the Euro-REVES subcommittee Policy Relevance and Conceptual Harmonization*. Leiden: TNO Prevention and Health.

Bebbington, A.C. and Darton, R.A. (1996) *Healthy Life Expectancy in England and Wales: Recent Evidence*. London: PSSRU.

Bisig, B. and Gutzwiller, F. (1994) 'Konzept des Indikators behinderungsfreie Lebenserwartung und Illustration am Beispiel Schweiz', in Imhof, A.E. and Weinknecht, R. (eds) *Erfüllt leben-in Gelassenheit sterben*. Berlin: Verlag Duncker & Humblot.

Bisig, B., Michel, J-P., Minder, C.M., Paccaud, F., Santos-Eggimann, B. and Spuhler, T. (1992) 'Disability-free life expectancy (DFLE): available data in Switzerland', in Robine, J-M., Blanchet, M. and Dowd, J.E. (eds) *Health Expectancy*. London: HMSO.

Bone, M.R., Bebbington, A.C., Jagger, C., Morgan, K. and Nicolaas, G. (1995) *Health Expectancy and its Uses*. London: HMSO.

Boshuizen, H.C. and van de Water, H.P.A. (1994) *An International Comparison of Health Expectancies*. Leiden: TNO Prevention and Health.

Boshuizen, H.C. and van de Water, H.P.A. and Perenboom, R.J.M. (1994) 'International comparison of health expectancy: preliminary results', in Mathers, C.D., McCallum, J. and Robine, J-M. (eds) *Advances in Health Expectancies*. Canberra: Australian Institute of Health and Welfare.

Brønnum-Hansen, H. (1991) *Loss of Healthy Years in Denmark: an English Summary of a Danish Report*. Copenhagen: DICE.

Brønnum-Hansen, H. (1998) 'Trends in health expectancy in Denmark, 1987–1994', *Danish Medical Bulletin* 45(2), 217–221.

Brønnum-Hansen, H. and Rasmussen, N. K. (1990) *Years of Disability in the Danish population: Calculations Based on Data from the National Health Interview Survey 1986/87*. Copenhagen: DICE.

Brønnum-Hansen, H. and Rasmussen, N. K. (1996) 'Mental health expectancy in Denmark 1994', Paper presented at the 2nd annual meeting of Euro-REVES, London.

Brückner, G. (1997) 'Health expectancy in Germany: what do we learn from the reunification process?', Paper presented at REVES 10, Tokyo.

Buratta, V. and Crialesi, R. (1993) 'Salute e speranza di vita', in *Studi di Popolazione. Nuovi approcci per la descrizione e l'interpretazione. Convegno dei Giovani studiosi dei problemi di Popolazione*. Rome: Universita 'la Sapienza', dip. Scienze Demografiche.

Dansk Institut for Klinisk Epidemiologi (DIKE) (1991) *Sundhedstilstand, sundhedsadfaerd, forebyggelseprogram* (Public health, health behaviour, prevention program). Copenhagen: DIKE.

Deeg, D.J.H. (1999) 'Self rated health: does it measure health as well as we think it does?', Paper presented at the 11th REVES meeting, London.

Deeg, D.J.H. and Beekman, A.T.F. (1996) 'Depression-free life expectancy in the Netherlands', Paper presented at the 2nd Euro-REVES meeting, London.

Egidi, V. (1988) 'Stato di salute e morbosita della popolazione', in *The Second Report on the Italian Demographic Situation*. Rome: Istituto di ricerche sulla popolazione.

Egidi, V. (1990) 'Life expectancy in good health. Population aging and changing lifestyles in Europe', in *Fourth Sitting of the Seminar on Present Demographic Trends and Lifestyles in Europe*. Strasbourg.

Egidi, V. and Buratta, V. (1995) 'Country report: Italy', in van de Water, H.P.A. and Perenboom, R.J.M. (eds) *Report of the First Meeting of the Euro-REVES Subcommittee Policy Relevance and Conceptual Harmonization*. Leiden: TNO Prevention and Health.

Egidi, V. and Frova, L. (1997) 'Mortality, morbidity and health related quality of life in developed countries: concepts, methods and indicators', Paper presented at the International Population Conference, Beijing.

Gispert, R. and Gutiérrez Fisac, J.L. (1995) 'Health Expectancy indicators: the report from Spain', in van de Water, H.P.A. and Perenboom, R.J.M. (eds) *Report of the First Meeting of the Euro-REVES subcommittee Policy Relevance and Conceptual Harmonization*. Leiden: TNO Prevention and Health.

Gispert, R., Rajmil, L., Rué, M., Glutting, J.P. and Roset, M. (1998) 'Mental health expectancy: an indicator to bridge the gap between psychiatric and public health perspectives about the population's health', *Acta Psychiatrica Scandinavica*, 98, 182–186.

Goldberg, D.P. and Williams, P.A. (1988) *User's Guide to the General Health Questionnaire*. Windsor, Berkshire: NFER-Nelson Publishing.

Grotvedt, L. and Viksand, G. (1994) 'Life expectancy without disease and disability in Norway', in Mathers, C.D., McCallum, J. and Robine, J-M. (eds) *Advances in Health Expectancies*. Canberra: Australian Institute of Health and Welfare.

Haber, L.D. and Dowd, J.E. (1994) 'A human development agenda for disability: statistical considerations. A report prepared for the United Nations Statistical Division', unpublished.

Haut Comité de la Santé Publique (1994) *La santé en France: rapport général* (Health in France: general report). Paris: Haut Comité de la Santé Publique.

Herrmann, F.R. and Michel, J-P. (1996) 'Dementia free life expectancy in Switzerland: comparison between expected and observed estimates', Paper presented at the 9th meeting of REVES, Rome.

Hoeymans, F.H.G.M. (1997) *Functional status and self-rated health in elderly men: the role of aging and chronic diseases*. Amsterdam: University of Amsterdam.

Jagger, C. (1997) *Health Expectancy Calculation by the Sullivan Method: A Practical Guide*. Montpellier, France: Euro-REVES.

Jagger, C., Ritchie, K, Brønnum-Hansen, H., Deeg, D., Gispert, R., Grimley Evans J., Hibbett, M., Lawlor, B., the MRCCFAS group, Perenboom, R., Polge, C. and Van Oyen, H. (1998) 'Mental health expectancy – the European perspective: a synopsis of results presented at the conference of the European network for the calculation of health expectancies (Euro-REVES)', *Acta Psychiatrica Scandinavica* 98, 85–91.

Katz, S., Branch, L.G., Branson, M.H., Papsidero, J.A., Beck, J.C. and Greer, D.S. (1983) 'Active life expectancy', *New England Journal of Medicine* 309, 1218–1224.

Koeter, M.W.J. and Ormel, J. (1991) *General Health Questionnaire*. Nederlandse bewerking/Handleiding.

Kytir, J. (1994) 'Lebenserwartung frei von Behinderung', *Statistische Nachrichten* 8, 650–657.

Ministerio de Sanidad y Consumo (1993) *Health Indicators (Period 1990–1991). Evaluation in Spain of European regional program Health for All*. Madrid: Ministerio de Sanidad y Consumo.

Ministry of Health (1992) *The Health Promotion Programme of the Government of Denmark*. Copenhagen: Ministry of Health.

Mutafova, M. (1993) 'Disability-free life expectancy in Bulgaria', in Robine, J-M., Mathers, C.D., Bone, M.R. and Romieu, I. (eds) *Calculation of Health Expectancy: Harmonization, Consensus Achieved and Future Perspectives*. Montrouge: John Libbey Eurotext.

Mutafova, M. and Maleshkov, C. (1995) 'Healthy life expectancy in Bulgaria', in van de Water, H.P.A. and Perenboom, R.J.M. (eds) *Report of the First Meeting of the Euro-REVES Subcommittee Policy Relevance and Conceptual Harmonization*. Leiden: TNO Prevention and Health.

Mutafova, M., Maleshkov, C. and Tonkova, S. (1994) Disability-free life expectancy in Bulgaria – a pilot investigation', in Mathers, C.D., McCallum, J. and Robine, J-M. (eds) *Advances in Health Expectancies*. Canberra: Australian Institute of Health and Welfare.

Mutafova, M., van de Water, H.P.A., Perenboom, R.J.M., Boshuizen, H.C. and Maleshkov, C. (1996) 'Occupational handicap-free life expectancy in Bulgaria 1976–1992 based on data of the medical expert commissions', *Social Science and Medicine* 43, 537–542.

Mutafova, M., van de Water, H.P.A., Perenboom, R.J.M., Boshuizen, H.C. and Maleshkov, C. (1997) 'Health expectancy calculations: a novel approach to studying population health in Bulgaria', *Bulletin of the World Health Organization* 75, 147–153.

Mutafova, M., van de Water, H.P.A., Maleshkov, C., Perenboom, R.J.M. and Tonkova, S. (1999a) 'Additional study for assessment of the mental health expectancy in Bulgaria', Paper presented at the 11th meeting of REVES, London.

Mutafova, M., van de Water, H.P.A., Maleshkov, C., Tonkova, S., Perenboom, R.J.M. and Boshuizen, H.C. (1999b) 'Attempt for the assessment of the mental health of the population in Bulgaria', in Egidi, V. (ed.) *Towards an Integrated System of Indicators to Assess the Health Status of the Population*. Rome: ISTAT [Essays no. 4].

Perenboom, R.J.M. and van Herten, L.M. (1999) 'Mental health expectancy in the Netherlands, a new approach, based on the MHI-5 of the SF-36', Paper presented at the 11th meeting of REVES, London.

Perenboom, R.J.M. and van de Water, H.P.A. (1997a) 'Levensverwachting in goede geestelijke gezondheid in Nederland, 1989–1995: een eerste proeve', in van der Maas, P.J. and Kramers, P.G.N. (eds) *Volksgezondheid Toekomst Verkenning 1997: deel III: Gezondheid en Levensverwachting gewogen*. Maarssen: Elsevier/de Tijdstroom, pp. 139–152.

Perenboom, R.J.M. and van de Water, H.P.A. (1997b) 'Mental Health Expectancy (MHE) in the Netherlands 1989–1994', in *Book of Abstracts of the 8th Congress of the International Psychogeriatric Association (IPA)*. Jerusalem: IPA.

Perenboom, R.J.M. and van de Water, H.P.A. (1997c) *Trends in gezonde levensjaar equivalenten.* Leiden: TNO Preventie en Gezondheid.

Perenboom, R.J.M., Boshuizen, H.C. and van de Water, H.P.A. (1993) 'Trends in health expectancies in the Netherlands 1981–1990', in Robine, J-M., Mathers, C.D., Bone, M.R. and Romieu, I. (eds) *Calculation of Health Expectancy: Harmonization, Consensus Achieved and Future Perspectives.* Montrouge: John Libbey Eurotext.

Perenboom, R.J.M., Boshuizen, H.C., Breteler, M.M.B., Ott, A. and van de Water, H.P.A. (1996) 'Dementia-free life expectancy (DemFLE) in the Netherlands', *Social Science and Medicine* 43, 1703–1707.

Perenboom, R.J.M., van Herten, L.M., Boshuizen, H.C. and van de Water, H.P.A. (1997) 'Trends in de gezonde levensverwachting in Nederland 1983–1994, met een verdeling naar ernst van ongezondheid', in van der Maas, P.J. and Kramers, P.G.N. (eds) *Volksgezondheid Toekomst Verkenning 1997; deel III: Gezondheid en Levensverwachting gewogen.* Maarssen: Elsevier de Tijdstroom, pp. 53–77.

Pettersson, H.A. (1990) 'Swedish population health index', Paper presented at the 4th meeting of REVES, Leiden.

Pettersson, H. (1995) 'Use of health expectancies in Sweden', in van de Water H.P.A. and Perenboom R.J.M., (eds) *Report of the First Meeting of the Euro-REVES subcommittee Policy Relevance and Conceptual Harmonization.* Leiden: TNO Prevention and Health.

Rasmussen, N.K. and Brønnum-Hansen, H. (1990) 'The expectation of life without disability in Denmark', Paper presented at the 12th scientific meeting of the International Epidemiological Association, Los Angeles, USA.

Regidor Poyatos, E., Rodriguez, C. and Gutiérrez Fisac, J.L. (1995) *Indicadores de salud: tercera evaluacion en Espana del programa regional europea Salud para Todos.* Madrid: Ministerio de Sanidad y Consumo.

Ritchie, K., Robine, J-M., Letenneur, L. and Dartigues, J-F. (1994) 'Dementia-free life expectancy in France', *American Journal of Public Health* 84, 232–236.

Robine, J-M. and Mormiche, P. (1993) 'L'espérance de vie sans incapacité augmente', *INSEE Première* 281, 1–4.

Robine, J-M. and Romieu, I. (1998) *Health Expectancy in the European Union; Progress achieved.* Montpellier: Euro-REVES.

Robine J-M., Colvez, A., Bucquet, D., Hatton, F., Morel, B. and Lelaidier, S. (1986) 'l'Espérance de vie sans incapacité en France en 1982', *Population* 41, 1025–1042.

Robine, J-M., Romieu, I., Cambois, E., van de Water, H.P.A., Boshuizen, H.C. and Jagger, C. (1995) *Global Assessment in Positive Health: Contribution of the Network on Health Expectancy and the Disability Process to World Health Report 1995 (WHR95) by World Health Organization (WHO).* Montpellier: Euro-REVES.

Robine, J-M., Mormiche, P. and Cambois, E. (1996) 'Evolution des courbes de survie totale, sans maladie chronique et sans incapacité en France de 1981 à 1991: application d'un modèle de l'OMS', *Annales de Démographie Historique* 99–115.

Robine, J-M., Brouard, N., Jagger, C., Ritchie, K. and van de Water, H.P.A. (1997) *Euro-REVES: a Concerted Action in Support of Harmonization of Health Expectancy Calculations in Europe.* Montpellier: Euro-REVES.

Robine, J-M., Romieu, I. and Jee, M. (1998) *Health Expectancy in OECD Countries.* Montpellier: REVES.

Roelands, M., van Oyen, H. and Baro, F. (1994) 'Dementia-free life expectancy in Belgium', *European Journal of Public Health* 4, 33–37.

Ruwaard, D. and Kramers, P.G.N. (1997) *Volksgezondheid Toekomst verkenning 1997: De som der delen.* Bilthoven/Utrecht: RIVM/Elsevier/De Tijdstroom.

Socialstyrelsen (National Board of Health and Welfare) (1995) *Welfare and Public Health in Sweden 1994*. Stockholm: Socialstyrelsen.

Sociedad Espanola de Salud Publica y Administracion Sanitaria (SESPAS) (1993) *Informe SESPAS 1993: La salud y el sistema sanitario en Espana*. Barcelona: SG Editores.

Spuhler, T. and Bisig, B. (1991) 'Disability-free life expectancy in Switzerland 1991', Paper presented at the 4th REVES meeting, Leiden.

Sullivan, D.F. (1971a) 'A single index of mortality and morbidity', *HSMHA Health Reports* 86, 347–354.

Sullivan, D.F. (1971b) *Disability components for an index of health – a methodological study of an aggregative measure of several forms of disability intended for use as one component of a joint mortality-morbidity index*. Rockville: National Center for Health Statistics (US Department of Health, Education, and Welfare – Public Health Service).

Valkonen, T. (1994) 'Country report', in Mathers, C.D., McCallum, J. and Robine, J-M. (eds) *Advances in Health Expectancies*. Canberra: Australian Institute of Health and Welfare.

Valkonen, T., Sihvonen, A.P. and Lahelma, E. (1997) 'Health expectancy by level of education in Finland', *Social Science and Medicine* 44, 801–808.

van de Water, H.P.A. and Perenboom, R.J.M. (1995) *Report of the First Meeting of the Euro-REVES subcommittee Policy Relevance and Conceptual Harmonization*. Leiden: TNO Prevention and Health/Euro-REVES.

van de Water, H.P.A., Perenboom, R.J.M. and Boshuizen, H.C. (1995) 'Health expectancy: policy relevance, classification and present use in European countries', in van de Water, H.P.A. and Perenboom, R.J.M. (eds) *Report of the First Meeting of the Euro-REVES Subcommittee Policy Relevance and Conceptual Harmonization*. Leiden: TNO Prevention and Health.

van de Water, H.P.A., Perenboom, R.J.M. and Boshuizen, H.C. (1996) 'Policy relevance of the health expectancy indicator; an inventory in European Union countries', *Health Policy* 36, 117–129.

van Ginneken, J.K.S., Bannenberg, A.F.I. and Dissevelt, A.G. (1989) *Gezondheidsverlies ten gevolge van een aantal belangrijke ziektecategorieën in 1981–1985 – methodologische aspecten en resultaten*. Leiden: NIPG-TNO/CBS.

van Ginneken, J.K.S., Dissevelt, A.G., van de Water, H.P.A. and van Sonsbeek, J.L.A. (1991) 'Results of two methods to determine health expectancy in the Netherlands in 1981–1985', *Social Science and Medicine* 32, 1129–1136.

van Ginneken, J.K.S, van de Water, H.P.A. and van Sonsbeek, J.L.A. (1992) 'Gezonde levensverwachting: betekenis en resultaten', in Gunning-Schepers, L.J. and Mootz, M. (eds) *Gezondheidsmeting*. Houten: Bohn Stafleu Van Loghum.

van Oyen, H. and Roelands M. (1994) 'Estimates of health expectancy in Belgium', in Mathers, C.D., McCallum, J. and Robine, J-M. (eds) *Advances in Health Expectancies*. Canberra: Australian Institute of Health and Welfare.

van Oyen, H., Tafforeau, J. and Roelands, M. (1995) 'Health expectancy indicators in Belgium', in van de Water, H.P.A. and Perenboom, R.J.M. (eds) *Report of the First Meeting of the Euro-REVES Subcommittee Policy Relevance and Conceptual Harmonization*. Leiden: TNO Prevention and Health.

Volksgezondheid Toekomst Verkenning (1993) *Volksgezondheid toekomst verkenning. De gezondheidstoestand van de Nederlandse bevolking in de periode 1950–2010*. The Hague: Sdu Publishers.

World Health Organization (1980) *International Classification of Impairments, Disabilities, and Handicaps*. Geneva: World Health Organization.

19

Health Expectancy Research in North American Countries

VICKI L. LAMB
Duke University, Durham, NC, USA

INTRODUCTION

Systematic research on the measurement of health expectancy began in North America. In 1971 Sullivan presented the primary technique for cross-sectional estimates of health expectancy in a US government publication. An important contribution on the use of health expectancy measures in disability research was the book by Wilkins and Adams (1983), *Healthfulness of Life: A Unified View of Mortality, Institutionalization, and Non-institutionalized Disability in Canada, 1978.* There continues to be fruitful research in the US and Canada by members of the REVES network and others, leading to the development and use of varied techniques for modeling and estimating health expectancy. Other chapters in this book examine innovative methods to estimate dynamic models (Chapter 11), weighted or adjusted models (Chapters 12 and 13), as well as trends and changes in health expectancy (Chapter 4), for countries including Canada and the US. Therefore, the purposes of the current chapter are: (1) to present a brief historical overview of health expectancy research in North American countries prior to the first REVES working group meeting, and (2) to discuss the cross-sectional healthy life expectancy research for Canada and the US presented at REVES meetings and/or recently published. Attention will focus on the ways disability is conceptualized and measured in the studies of health expectancy. At the end, a short discussion of some of the longitudinally based research will be provided.

THE DEVELOPMENT OF A HEALTH EXPECTANCY MEASURE

In a paper entitled 'Measuring community health levels', Sanders (1964) first proposed a measure of community health levels, which combined morbidity and

Determining Health Expectancies. Edited by J-M. Robine, C. Jagger, C.D. Mathers, E.M. Crimmins and R.M. Suzman.
© 2003 John Wiley & Sons, Ltd

mortality measures. Sanders suggested the use of a 'modified life table method of analysis in measuring comparative adequacy of health services for different population groups' (1964, p. 1067). At the end of the paper Sanders indicated that persons within the Public Health Service, US Department of Health, Education, and Welfare, were working towards estimating such models.

   The method for estimating healthy life expectancy was outlined in a US government publication by Sullivan (1971). The so-called 'Sullivan method' makes use of population prevalence rates of disability and current mortality rates in life table models. The estimates are a reflection of the health levels of a population at a particular point in time adjusted for age-specific mortality levels. Using two measures of disability, Sullivan calculated life expectancy, disability-free life expectancy, and disabled life expectancy at birth and at age 65 years. Such estimates were made for the total US population, as well as by sex and race.

GLOBAL ACTIVITY LIMITATION MEASURES OF DISABILITY

The early North American studies of health expectancy typically used global activity limitation measures to model disability. The National Health Interview Survey (NHIS) series in the US and the 1978–1979 Canadian Health Survey (CHS) included such measures. In these surveys the respondent's major activity was determined: play (for preschoolers), going to school, keeping house, working, retired and other. The respondent was asked about activity limitations due to ill-health. This information was used to define 'long-term' limitation or disability. In a number of the early studies information also was gathered on 'short-term' disability through questions about the number of days in the previous two weeks the respondent had to restrict activity and/or stay in bed due to ill-health. The early publications of US time-series trends of healthy life expectancy (HLE) tended to present population-based estimates. Later studies of Canadian or US data have presented separate male and female estimates to contrast sex differences in the total expected years of life and in expected years of healthy life.

US ESTIMATES OF POPULATION HLE USING GLOBAL ACTIVITY LIMITATION MEASURES

In 1970 the US Department of Health, Education and Welfare published *Toward a Social Report*, a monograph of social indicators. The first chapter, on health and illness indicators, presented estimates of expectation of healthy life at birth, and at age 65, for the years 1958 to 1966. The estimates of ill-health, or disability, were based upon global limitation measures of bed-disability days and institutional confinement drawn from annual US National Health

Table 19.1. Estimated national trends in healthy life expectancy at birth and at age 65 in the US

A. Life and health expectancy measures at birth, based upon bed-disability and institutional confinement

Year	LE	HLE	I/BLE
1958	69.5	67.2	2.3
1959	69.6	67.8	1.8
1960	69.9	67.9	2.0
1961	69.9	68.0	1.9
1962	70.2	68.1	2.1
1963	70.0	67.9	2.1
1964	69.9	67.9	2.0
1965	70.2	68.2	2.0
1966	70.2	68.2	2.0

B. Life and health expectancy measures at age 65, based upon bed-disability and institutional confinement

Year	LE	HLE	I/BLE
1958	14.2	13.1	1.1
1959	14.3	13.3	1.0
1960	14.5	13.4	1.1
1961	14.4	13.3	1.1
1962	14.6	13.5	1.1
1963	14.4	13.3	1.1
1964	14.3	13.2	1.1
1965	14.6	13.5	1.1
1966	14.6	13.5	1.1

C. Life and health expectancy measures at birth, based upon bed-disability, limitations in major, short-term, and other activities

Year	LE	HLE	SLE	OLE
1966	70.0	56.5	3.4	10.1
1969	70.4	57.8	4.1	8.5
1972	71.0	56.4	4.3	10.3
1974	71.9	55.8	4.8	11.3
1976	72.7	56.0	5.1	11.6

LE = Total life expectancy; HLE = Healthy life expectancy; I/BLE = Institution or bed-days disabled life expectancy; SLE = Severely disabled life expectancy; OLE = Other disabled life expectancy.
Sources: Panels A and B: US Dept of Health, Education and Welfare (1970). Reproduced with permission Panel C: Colvez and Blanchet (1983). 'Potential gains in life expectancy free of disability a tool for Health planning'. International Journal of Epidemiology **12**, 224–229, by permission of Oxford University Press.

Interview Surveys. As Panels A and B in Table 19.1 indicate, for the period 1958–1966 there was little change in life expectancy and healthy life expectancy at birth, or at age 65. Life expectancy at birth increased from 69.5 to 70.2 years, of which 2 years were to be spent in ill-health. Life expectancy at age 65 ranged from 14.2 to 14.6 years, of which 1.1 years were to be spent in ill-health.

At the first REVES meeting Colvez (1992) presented an overview of his earlier research (Colvez and Blanchet, 1983) that extended the population time-series of US trends in disability. Overall, between the years 1966 and 1976, there was a 2.7-year increase in total life expectancy at birth, as indicated in Panel C of Table 19.1. In terms of years lost by restricted activities, there was a 1.7-year increase for severe disabilities (bed disability and inability to do main activity), and a 1.5-year increase in other disabilities (short-term and other limitations). The result was a net loss of 0.5 years of disability-free life expectancy between 1966 and 1976.

In 1991 Stoto and Durch used 1987 morbidity and mortality estimates to consider the US goals associated with the *Healthy People 2000* (US Department of HHS, 1990) objectives. The authors estimated population-based healthy life expectancy at birth and at age 65, using 'limitations in major activities' to operationalize disability. Stoto and Durch (1991) estimated that in 1987, life expectancy at birth was 66.8 years, of which 75.1 years, or 89%, were to be spent in good health. For age 65, life expectancy was estimated to be 17.2 years, of which 13.2 years, or 77%, were to be spent disability-free.

CANADIAN ESTIMATES OF MALE AND FEMALE HLE USING GLOBAL ACTIVITY LIMITATION MEASURES

Wilkins and Adams (1983) calculated disability-free life expectancy for Canada using the 1978–1979 Canadian Health Survey data. The definition of disability was based upon: (1) persons who answered positively to any of the three long-term limitation questions (inability to perform, or restricted or limited in the ability to perform the major activity, and restricted or limited in performing secondary, non-major activities), (2) persons who had no long-term limitations, but experienced short-term disability (i.e., bed and/or disability days within the past two weeks), and (3) the proportion of the Canadian population who were institutionalized in long-term facilities for mental and physical disabilities. The institutionalization calculations excluded units or facilities that provided short-stay beds. Wilkins and Adams (1983) estimated that at age 65 years, males would have a life expectancy of 14.4 years and a healthy life expectancy of 8.4 years. For females, the estimates were 18.7 and 10.6, respectively. These estimates indicate that, on average, 58.3% of a 65-year-old Canadian male's expected life will be spent in good health. A 65-year-old Canadian female would expect 57.2% of her life to be in good health.

At the first REVES working group meeting, Wilkins (1992) presented calculations of healthy life expectancy for the province of Quebec. The Quebec Health Survey (QHS) of 1987 had only one question regarding activity limitation: 'Compared to other (persons) of the same age in good health, is ____ limited in the kind or amount of activity he (she) can do because of a long-term physical or mental condition or health problem?' Questions about disability and/or bed days in the past two weeks were comparable to those of the NHIS and the CHS. Wilkins (1992) presented calculations of healthy life expectancy for Quebec, based upon: (1) long-term limitations, (2) short-term limitations, and (3) proportion of the Quebec population in long-term care facilities (homes for the aged, nursing homes and chronic care hospitals). The results indicated that at age 65, females have 18.9 years of remaining life, of which 13.2 years would be healthy. At the same age, males can expect to have 14.2 years of life, with 10.6 disability-free years.

US ESTIMATES OF MALE AND FEMALE HLE USING GLOBAL ACTIVITY LIMITATION MEASURES

Sex-based estimates of US healthy life expectancy using data from the US National Health Interview Survey (NHIS) series were calculated by Crimmins *et al* (1989, 1992a, 1992b) for the years 1970 and 1980 and by McKinlay *et al* (1989) for the years 1964, 1974 and 1985. Later, Crimmins *et al* (1997) updated their time series to include 1990 estimates. The techniques for determining prevalences of population disability, however, were not identical for the two research teams.

The 1970 and 1980 results by Crimmins and her associates were presented at the first REVES meeting (1992a, 1992b). Their definition of 'disabled' included: (1) persons who answered positively to any degree of long-term activity limitation (unable to perform, are limited in performing major activity, are limited in performing secondary activity) due to health; (2) persons who had no long-term limitations, but who experienced short-term limitations (i.e., bed and/or disability days within the past two weeks); and (3) the proportion of the US population who were institutionalized for mental and physical disabilities. The latter group included persons in: (a) all mental hospitals and residential treatment centers, (b) total tuberculosis hospitals, (c) chronic disease hospitals, (d) all homes for the aged, (e) all homes and schools for the mentally handicapped and (f) all homes and schools for the physically handicapped. An attempt was made to include all persons who would not be included in the NHIS sampling frame (see Appendix A of Crimmins *et al* (1989) for an extended discussion of the estimation of the institutionalized population). The 1990 estimates by Crimmins *et al* (1997) used the same analytic strategy to conceptualize disability. The definition of the disabled used by McKinlay and associates (1989) was more limited. It included only: (1) persons who were limited or unable to do their major

Table 19.2. Estimated trends in healthy life expectancy by sex for age 65 in the US

Year	Males			Females		
	LE	HLE	% HLE	LE	HLE	% HLE
A. Global activity limitation (as reported)						
1964	12.8	6.6	51.56	16.2	10.2	62.96
1970	13.0	6.4	49.23	16.8	8.7	51.78
1974	13.4	7.2	53.73	17.5	10.7	61.14
1980	14.2	6.6	46.47	18.4	8.9	48.36
1985	14.6	10.5	71.91	18.6	13.4	72.04
1990	15.1	7.4	49.00	18.9	9.8	51.85
B. Major activity limitation						
1964	12.8	6.6	51.56	16.2	10.2	62.96
1970[a]	13.0	7.2	55.38	16.8	10.2	60.71
1974	13.4	7.2	53.73	17.5	10.7	61.14
1980[a]	14.2	8.4	58.33	18.7	10.7	58.15
1985	14.6	10.5	71.91	18.6	13.4	72.04

LE = Total life expectancy; HLE = Healthy life expectancy; % HLE = Proportion of life expectancy in health.
[a]Indicates recalculation of HLE estimates to eliminate short-term disability measures.
Sources: 1964, 1974, 1985: McKinlay *et al* (1989); 1970, 1980: Crimmins *et al* (1989); 1990: Crimmins *et al* (1997).

activity and (2) estimates of persons age 65 years and older residing in nursing homes, based upon Nursing Home Survey data estimates.

Panel A of Table 19.2 reports the life expectancy (LE), healthy life expectancy (HLE) and proportion of life expectancy that is healthy (% HLE), for males and females, as reported by Crimmins *et al* (1989, 1997), and McKinlay *et al* (1989). The McKinlay estimates show great gains in both the years of HLE and the proportion of HLE for elderly males and females in 1985. Interestingly, such trends were not noted at birth or at age 45 in 1985 (see McKinlay *et al*, Table 3, p. 203).

Because the McKinlay calculations did not include the less severe forms of disability, or types of institutionalization for mental and emotional disabilities for persons of all ages (other than nursing homes for persons aged 65 years and older), their estimated years of HLE and proportions of years expected to be spent in health are larger than those calculated by Crimmins *et al* (1989). However, Crimmins and her associates did present a detailed table of the determination of healthy life expectancy in 1970 and 1980 (Crimmins *et al*, 1989, Table 4, p. 245). Therefore, it is possible to recalculate their results by excluding persons limited in secondary activities for those two years. The incompatible definitions of institutionalization remain, nonetheless.

The recalculations (marked with superscript[a]) are included in Table 19.2, Panel B ('Major activity limitations'). There appears to be a trend in the increase of years of life expectancy and healthy life expectancy for both males and females. Also, compared to males, females can expect more total years of expected life as well as more years of disabled life. What remains unclear is whether there is a trend in the proportion of expected life to be lived in a healthy state for persons aged 65.

MULTIPLE MEASURES OF DISABILITY LIMITATIONS

There has been a general shift away from measuring disability based upon global assessments of limitation in major activities. Clearly, these questions are unsuitable for portions of the population who do not engage in the designated activities, such as the elderly. Thus, many of the REVES and other research papers have utilized a number of specific personal care activities of daily living (ADL) items to estimate population-based measures of healthy life expectancy, based on the early work by Katz *et al* (1983). For the US, the majority of the HLE work based upon ADL measures of disability have used longitudinal data to measure disability transitions with dynamic multistate life tables, and are discussed in Chapter 11.

It should be noted that studies using only the ADL items are measuring quite severe disability, i.e., the difficulty or inability to attend to basic personal care and hygiene matters that are performed routinely by most persons. There have been other research efforts, using cross-sectional data for Canada or the US, which have attempted to examine multiple measures of personal limitations to get a broader view of the disabled population. Unfortunately, such studies use different combinations of disability measures, which yield results that are not completely comparable.

At the first REVES working group meeting, Wilkins and Adams (1992) presented estimates of healthy life expectancy in Canada based upon multiple measures of functional limitations from the 1986 Health and Activity Limitation Survey (HALS) in Canada. Wilkins and Adams (1992) created a composite score of disability based upon the 23 HALS limitation items, and used the Sullivan technique to estimate healthy life expectancy values. The disability measures included three ADL items, five instrumental activities of daily living (IADLs) items, four physical performance items, seven sensory items, three cognitive/mental disability items, plus a global measure of limitations in one's major activity. At birth, males were expected to live 73.0 years, of which 61.3 will be healthy years. The expected years of life for females at birth was 79.8 years with 64.9 years to be disability-free. The estimates at age 65 for males were 14.9 years of remaining life with 8.1 years of healthy life. For females at age 65, the expected years of life was 19.2 years and 9.4 years of disability-free life.

For the US, Manton and Stallard (1991) calculated healthy life expectancy using multiple measures of disability limitations using data collected in the National Long Term Care Surveys (NLTCS) of 1982 and 1984. The NLTCS is a nationally representative sample of all persons aged 65 years and older in the US, both community and institutional residents. Disability was measured using 27 items, which included nine ADL items, thirteen IADL items, four physical performance limitations, as well as one sensory item, the ability to see well enough to read a newspaper. Manton and Stallard used the Grade of Membership technique (a multivariate clustering technique based on fuzzy-set mathematics: Manton *et al*, 1994) to develop profiles of disability. They then calculated age-sex prevalence rates for the disability profiles to estimate life expectancy in each disability state (including non-disabled). The results indicated that at age 65 males could expect 14.4 years of total life and 11.9 years of healthy life. For 65-year-old females, the estimates are 18.6 and 13.6 years, respectively.

RACE/SEX COMPARISONS OF HLE

The 1990 US census contained questions regarding the performance of everyday activities. Hayward and Heron (1999) used the 1990 5% Public Use Microdata Sample (PUMS) of the US census to estimate racial differentials in disability-free life expectancy for the US adult population. Individuals aged 20 and older are classified as having a disability if they had 'a physical, mental or other health condition that lasted six or more months' and the condition (a) limited the kind or amount of work they could do at a job or (b) prevented them from working at a job' (Hayward and Heron, 1999, p. 80). The researchers constructed disability prevalence rates for five-year age cohorts by sex for whites, African Americans, Asian Americans, Native Americans and Hispanics.

An important finding from this research is that for all US racial groups having a longer life does not always translate into having better health. Whites and Asian Americans were found to have both longer life and better health. However, Native Americans were shown to have longer life and worse health. African Americans were found to be the most disadvantaged racial group with both lower years of expected life and a greater proportion of years in poor health. Hispanics also have fewer years of life expectancy; however, unlike African Americans, 'the period of life Hispanics live with a health impairment is relatively compressed' (Hayward and Heron, 1999, p. 88). Regarding gender differences, Hayward and Heron consistently found that across all racial groups, women live longer years and spend more years in ill-health.

Geronimus *et al* (2001) used the 1990 US census data to estimate African American and white differences in healthy life expectancy at age 16 for women and men. Disability was measured using the census questions that asked about health-related difficulties in working, in getting around outside, and in performing personal activities, such as bathing, dressing, or getting around inside the home. The nationwide estimates indicated that African Americans have fewer years of healthy life expectancy compared to whites for both sexes, and that African Americans have a greater proportion of expected life to be spent disabled.

In addition to presenting national estimates of healthy life expectancy by race and sex, the authors also calculated such estimates for specific local populations in the US. Geronimus and her colleagues matched local death certificate data with local disability data from the 1990 US census PUMS files to estimate local survival curves and healthy life expectancy estimates. Such estimates indicated large differences in healthy life expectancy for poverty areas as compared to non-poverty areas for both races. Living in poor locations has a negative effect on years of healthy life expectancy, and the effect is particularly negative for African Americans living in poor urban locations.

The research by Hayward and Heron (1999) and Geronimus *et al* (2001) is important for a number of reasons. First, they show that census data are useful for estimating healthy life expectancy. Second, the data can be used to estimate disparities in healthy life expectancy for a number of racial groups beyond African Americans and whites (Hayward and Heron, 1999). Third, census data linked to local death certificate data make it possible to estimate healthy life expectancy by local area to consider the effect of the relative wealth of an area on population health and well-being (Geronimus *et al*, 2001).

Crimmins *et al* (1996; Crimmins and Saito, 2001) have examined changes over two decades in healthy life expectancy for African Americans and whites by level of education. They find that racial differences in healthy life expectancy are greater among persons with lower education and that over the two decades increase in healthy life expectancy is concentrated among those with the highest levels of education. These studies contribute to a better understanding of the effects of regional variations (see Chapter 6) and social inequities (see Chapter 5) on healthy life expectancy.

ESTIMATES OF UNMET OR RESIDUAL DISABILITY

REVES researchers have extended healthy life expectancy estimates to include estimates of unmet needs (Carrière and Légaré, 2000), or residual disabilities (Agree, 1999). Unmet need or residual disability has been characterized as the need for more help or assistance than is currently being received. This type of research has important policy implications in planning future long-term care needs.

In the 1995 Chicago REVES working group meeting, Carrière and Légaré called for a redefinition of health expectancy to include a measure of the need

Table 19.3. Estimates of health expectancy and unmet disability needs in Canada and the US

	Total	Men	Women
A. Canada for age 65			
Total life expectancy	17.13	14.89	19.12
Without disability	8.96	8.26	9.58
Without handicap	1.69	2.13	1.29
Without net handicap	3.55	2.44	4.54
in private household	1.94	1.52	2.32
in institution	1.61	0.92	2.22
With net handicap	2.93	2.06	3.71
B. United States for age 70			
Total life expectancy	13.91	12.08	15.28
Without disability	9.43	8.93	9.81
With disability and sufficient care	1.47	1.07	1.76
With residual disability	3.02	2.08	3.71

The disability and/or handicap estimates are based on different sets of indicators, and therefore the estimates are not comparable between countries.
Sources: Panel A: Carrière and Légaré (2000); Panel B: Agree (1999) reprinted from *Social Science and Medicine* **48** 'The influence of personal care and assistive devices on the measurement of disability' 427–443 (1999) with permission from Elsevier Science.

for assistance. Their subsequent publication, Carrière and Légaré (2000), outlined the concept using a decision tree for coding disability and handicap states, based upon the ICIDH (WHO, 1980) classification, and to model 'unmet needs with handicaps'. Disability was based upon 'questions on agility and mobility, vision, hearing impairment, speech impairment, and mental and other disabilities' (Carrière and Légaré, 2000, p. 111). Persons were considered to have a handicap if they required assistance in performing ADLs, IADLs, or mobility functions. If the assistance was reported to be inadequate, the person was assessed as having a 'net handicap' due to unmet assistance needs. The authors used data on persons aged 65 years and older from the 1986 Health and Activity Limitation Survey (HALS) in Canada to estimate life expectancy measures for each of the disability/handicap states. Data from the 1986 Canadian census were used to represent the institutionalized Canadian population, who were classified as 'handicapped with needs met'. Panel A in Table 19.3 reproduces the results from this study. The results are significant in identifying the years of unmet needs for assistance with handicaps. For example, females are expected to experience 4.5 years of handicaps in which their assistance needs are being met (2.2 years to be spent in institutions), and an additional 3.7 years in which their handicap needs are not met. Men are expected to have 2.4 years with assistance needs met, and 2.1 years in which such needs will not be met. The researchers also presented regional estimates of unmet handicap needs in Canada.

In 1999 Agree published a framework for defining disability based upon care received. In this framework, 'underlying disability' refers to 'the amount of functional disability that would be experienced in the absence of any modifications or adjustments' and 'residual disability' refers to 'the degree of disablement that remains after personal care or assistive devices have ameliorated some part of the total underlying need' (Agree, 1999, p. 429). Agree estimated health expectancy measures for US elderly using data from the first wave of the Survey of Asset and Health Dynamics of the Oldest Old (AHEAD), a survey conducted in 1993–1994 on community dwelling persons aged 70 years and older, and their spouses. The measure of underlying disability is based upon responses to questions about difficulties in performing six activities of daily living. Residual disability occurs when the respondent indicated that she or he continues to have difficulty with the ADL task after accounting for the assistance already received. Panel B of Table 19.3 reports the health expectancy estimates for this study. The results indicate that years of residual disability are twice as long as years receiving sufficient care for ADL difficulties for both males and females.

The results from the two studies cannot be directly compared because the Canadian study used ADL and IADL tasks to measure disability and handicap, whereas the US study only used ADL tasks to measure underlying and residual disabilities. One would expect that for the US, years without disability would be slightly lower and years of 'sufficient care' would be greater if IADL tasks were included. It is interesting to note the similarity in predicted years of unmet needs for both studies. These studies point to the importance of considering demand for long-term care that is unmet in the community, and represent an important extension of HLE research.

LONGITUDINALLY BASED ESTIMATES OF HEALTHY LIFE EXPECTANCY

A number of US research teams have made estimates of healthy life expectancy for the older population based on the longitudinal data available for this age group (Branch et al, 1991; Crimmins et al, 1994, 1996; Guralnik et al, 1993; Land et al, 1994; Laditka and Wolf, 1998; Manton and Land, 2000; A. Rogers et al, 1989, 1990; R. Rogers et al, 1989, 1992). These estimates have generally been made with the aim of exploring a theoretical or methodological issue rather than to provide estimates for measuring population health. Theoretical issues include the compression of morbidity (Crimmins et al, 1994; R. Rogers et al, 1989) and population differentials in healthy life (Branch et al, 1991, Crimmins et al, 1996; Guralnik et al, 1993). Much of this work has also been devoted to developing and contrasting methods of estimation (Laditka and Wolf, 1998; Manton and Land, 2000). Because of the differences in methodological approaches and numerous analytic variations, it is difficult to compare the point estimates from these studies.

CONCLUSIONS

Cross-sectional studies of Canadian and US healthy life expectancy continue to be useful to show the state of population health at a particular point in time, as well as to show the differences among subgroups of a population. This chapter has presented only the more basic cross-sectional HLE studies using data from Canada and the US. Overall, HLE research in North America has a number of distinctive characteristics that are covered here and in other chapters in this book, which include trend estimates of HLE, the inclusion of institutional populations in national estimates, multiple ways of measuring disability, the use of weighted or adjusted models, the use of longitudinal and simulation data to estimate dynamic models, the estimation of racial, economic and regional variations in HLE, and the estimation of unmet or residual disability needs (see Wilkins, 2001 on the contributions from Canada). Such productive research will continue as REVES moves into the 21st century. Longitudinally based estimates will continue to evolve as methods and data continue to develop.

REFERENCES

Agree, E.M. (1999) 'The influence of personal care and assistive devices on the measurement of disability', *Social Science and Medicine* 48, 427–443.

Branch, L.G., Guralnik, D.J., Foley, D.J., Kohout, F.J., Wetle, T.T., Ostfeld, A. and Katz, S. (1991) 'Active life expectancy for 10 000 caucasian men and women in three communities', *Journal of Gerontology*, 46, M145–150.

Carrière, Y. and Légaré, J. (2000) 'Unmet needs for assistance with ADLs and IADLs: a measure of healthy life expectancy', *Social Indicators Research* 51, 107–123.

Colvez, A. (1992) 'Changes in disability-free life expectancy in the USA between 1966 and 1976', in Robine, J-M., Blanchet, M. and Dowd, J.E. (eds) *Health Expectancy.* London: HMSO.

Colvez, A. and Blanchet, M. (1983) 'Potential gains in life expectancy free of disability: a tool for health planning', *International Journal of Epidemiology* 12, 224–229.

Crimmins, E.M. and Saito, Y. (2001) 'Trends in healthy life expectancy in the United States, 1970–1990: gender, racial, and educational differences', *Social Science and Medicine* 52, 1629–1641.

Crimmins, E.M., Saito, Y. and Ingegneri, D. (1989) 'Changes in life expectancy and disability-free life expectancy in the United States', *Population and Development Review* 15, 235–267.

Crimmins, E.M., Saito, Y. and Ingegneri, D. (1992a) 'Recent values of disability-free life expectancy in the United States', in Robine, J-M., Blanchet, M. and Dowd, J.E. (eds) *Health Expectancy.* London: HMSO.

Crimmins, E.M., Saito, Y. and Ingegneri, D. (1992b) 'Changes in life expectancy and disability-free life expectancy in the United States', in Robine, J-M., Blanchet, M. and Dowd, J.E. (eds) *Health Expectancy*. London: HMSO.

Crimmins, E.M., Hayward, M.D. and Saito, Y. (1994) 'Changing mortality and morbidity rates and the health status and life expectancy of the older population', *Demography* 31, 159–175.

Crimmins, E.M., Hayward, M.D. and Saito, Y. (1996) 'Differentials in active life expectancy in the older population of the United States', *Journal of Gerontology* 51B, S111–S120.

Crimmins, E.M., Saito, Y. and Ingegneri, D. (1997) 'Trends in disability-free life expectancy in the United States, 1970–90', *Population and Development Review* 23, 555–572.

Geronimus, A.T., Bound, J., Waidmann, T.A., Colen, C.G. and Steffick, D. (2001) 'Inequalities in life expectancy, functional status, and active life expectancy across selected black and white populations in the United States', *Demography* 38, 227–251.

Guralnik, J.M., Land, K.C., Blazer, D.G., Fillenbaum, G.C. and Branch, L.G. (1993) 'Educational status and active life expectancy among older blacks and whites', *New England Journal of Medicine* 329, 110–116.

Hayward, M.D. and Heron, M. (1999) 'Racial inequality in active life among adult Americans', *Demography* 36(1), 77–91.

Katz, S., Branch, L.G., Branson, M.H., Papsidero, J.A., Beck, J.C. and Greer, D.S. (1983) 'Active life expectancy', *New England Journal of Medicine* 309, 1218–1224.

Laditka, S.B. and Wolf, D.A. (1998) 'New methods for analyzing active life expectancy', *Journal of Aging and Health* 10, 214–241.

Land, K.C. and Guralnik, J.M. and Blazer, D.G. (1994) 'Estimating increment–decrement life tables with multiple covariates from panel data: The case of active life expectancy', *Demography* 31, 297–319.

Manton, K.G. and Land, K.C. (2000) 'Active life expectancy estimates for the US elderly population: A multidimensional continuous-mixture model of functional change applied to completed cohorts, 1982–1996', *Demography* 37, 253–265.

Manton, K.G. and Stallard, E. (1991) 'Cross-sectional estimates of active life expectancy for the US elderly and oldest-old populations', *Journal of Gerontology* 46(3), S170–182.

Manton, K.G., Woodbury, M.A. and Tolley, H.D. (1994) *Statistical Applications Using Fuzzy Sets*. New York: Wiley.

McKinlay, J.B., McKinlay, S.M. and Beaglehole, R. (1989) 'A review of the evidence concerning the impact of medical measures on recent mortality and morbidity in the United States', *International Journal of Health Services* 19, 181–208.

Rogers, A., Rogers, R. and Branch, L.G. (1989) 'A multistate analysis of active life expectancy', *Public Health Reports* 104, 222–226.

Rogers, A., Rogers, R. and Branch, L.G. (1990) 'Longer life but worse health? Measurement and dynamics', *The Gerontologist* 30, 640–649.

Rogers, R., Rogers, A. and Belanger, A. (1989) 'Active life among the elderly in the United States: Multistate life table estimates and population projections', *Milbank Quarterly* 67, 370–411.

Rogers, R., Rogers, A. and Belanger, A. (1992) 'Disability-free life among the elderly in the United States', *Journal of Aging and Health* 4, 19–42.

Sanders, B.S. (1964) 'Measuring community health levels', *American Journal of Public Health* 54, 1063–1070.

Stoto, M.A. and Durch, J.S. (1991) 'National health objectives for the year 2000: The demographic impact of health promotion and disease prevention', *American Journal of Public Health* 81, 1456–1465.

Sullivan, D.F. (1971) 'A single index of mortality and morbidity', *HSMHA Health Report*, 86, 347–354.

US Department of Health, Education and Welfare (1970) *Toward a Social Report*. Washington, DC: US Department of Health, Education and Welfare.

US Department of Health and Human Services (1990) *Health People 2000: National Health Promotion and Disease Prevention Objectives*. Washington, DC: Public Health Service.

Wilkins, R. (1992) 'Health expectancy in Quebec, 1987', in Robine, J-M., Blanchet, M. and Dowd, J.E. (eds) *Health Expectancy*. London: HMSO.

Wilkins, R. (2001) 'Healthy life expectancy in low mortality countries: the Canadian experience', Paper presented at the IUSSP Second Seminar on Longevity and Health, Beijing, China.

Wilkins, R. and Adams, O. (1983) *Healthfulness of Life: A Unified View of Mortality, Institutionalization, and Non-institutionalized Disability in Canada, 1978*. Montreal: Institute for Research on Public Policy.

Wilkins, R. and Adams, O. (1992) 'Health expectancy in Canada, 1986', in Robine, J-M., Blanchet, M. and Dowd, J.E. (eds) *Health Expectancy*. London: HMSO.

World Health Organization (1980) *International Classification of Impairments, Disabilities, and Handicaps*. Geneva: WHO.

20

Health Expectancy in Australia and New Zealand

PETER DAVIS, COLIN D. MATHERS* and PATRICK GRAHAM†

*Christchurch School of Medicine, Christchurch, New Zealand and †WHO, Geneva, Switzerland

INTRODUCTION

The distinctive features of health expectancy research in this region have been the early initiative taken by official agencies in Australia and the contribution of important international, scientific collaborations. This chapter will first review the data sources available for health expectancy research, and then outline key findings for national estimates over time and for special populations. Finally, conclusions will be drawn about the future of health expectancy research in this region and its significance for theory and policy.

DATA SOURCES

One aspect of health expectancy research in this region has been the willingness of official statistical agencies – more especially in Australia – to experiment with new, disability-based measures of health status. The principal data collections derived from official collections and used in time series analyses for the two countries are presented in Table 20.1.

An important difference between the two countries is evident from the review of data sources in the table. While Australia has mounted nationally representative surveys tailored to the assessment of handicap and disability for all three collections, in New Zealand the first such collection specifically designed for this purpose was available only following the 1996 census. This means that data definitions required for the calculation of health expectancies and for tracking trends over time have been collected in a consistent fashion only in Australia.

Determining Health Expectancies. Edited by J-M. Robine, C. Jagger, C.D. Mathers, E.M. Crimmins and R.M. Suzman.
© 2003 John Wiley & Sons, Ltd

Table 20.1. Health expectancy in Australia and New Zealand: data sources

	Australia		New Zealand
1981	ABS Survey of Handicapped Persons (33 000 households and 5300 patients in institutions)	1981	Social Indicators Survey: sample of 6891 (15 and older)
1988	ABS Survey of Disabled and Aged Persons: samples of approximately 67 000 (households) and 6700 (health establishments)	1991/92	Household Health Survey: sample of 5873 (15 and older)
1993	ABS Survey of Disability, Ageing and Carers: samples of 42 000 (households) and 4800 (health establishments)		
1998	ABS Survey of Disability, Ageing and Carers: samples of 36 951 (households) and 5176 (health establishments)	1996/97	New Zealand Disability Surveys: samples of 20 848 (households) and 1016 (residential facilities)

ABS (1982, 1990, 1993, 1999).

This is confirmed in the review of data definitions. In Table 20.2 the definitions of disability and handicap adopted in the Australian data collections are outlined. The Australian surveys used definitions of disability and handicap based on a late 1970s draft conceptual framework for the first version of the World Health Organization's International Classification of Impairments, Disabilities and Handicaps. Essentially a disabled person was a person with any one of a range of disabilities or impairments that had lasted, or were likely to last, six months or more. Handicap was defined according to the ability to perform in one of a number of task areas, with the level of severity defined in relation to the number of tasks and the amount of assistance required. The Australian definitions of disability and handicap are discussed in more detail below.

In New Zealand, by contrast, a functional limitation definition of disability has been adopted, with no clear and separate identification of handicap (Table 20.3). Thus, for the first two data collections in New Zealand the definitions used were relatively ad hoc. These drew on concepts of functional disability, with a mixture of difficulty and severity providing further levels of discrimination. In the most recent set of surveys a large number of disability screening questions were used – 28 for adults, and 12 for children – with two levels of the severity of functional limitation defined by the amount and frequency of assistance required.

In both Australia and New Zealand the Sullivan (1971) method has been employed for calculating health expectancy estimates, reflecting the difficulty in

Table 20.2. Data definition: Australia

Concept	1981	1988	1993	1999
I	One or more of 12 conditions[a]	15 conditions[b]	17 conditions[c]
II	No personal help or supervision required, no difficulty in performing 5 tasks, but uses aid or has difficulty walking 200 metres or up and down stairs			
III	No personal help or supervision required, but difficulty in performing one or more of 5 identified tasks			
IV	Personal help or supervision required or unable perform one or more tasks		Includes profound handicap	Includes profound handicap

Disability levels: I = disability (or impairment); II = mild handicap; III = moderate handicap; IV = severe handicap.
[a] Mathers (1991).
[b] Mathers (1996).
[c] Australian Institute of Health and Welfare (1999).

Table 20.3. Data definition: New Zealand

Concept	1980/81[a]	1992/93[b]	1996/97[c]
I	12 functional limitations	8 functional limitations	10 functional limitations (no assistance need)
II	Level of difficulty experienced	Use of help with daily activities	Requiring some assistance
III	Not defined	Not defined	Requiring daily or continuous assistance

Disability levels: I = disability (or functional limitation); II = mild to moderate handicap (or dependency); III = moderate to severe handicap (or dependency).
[a] Department of Statistics (1984).
[b] Statistics New Zealand, Ministry of Health (1993).
[c] Health Funding Authority, Ministry of Health (1998).

assembling the large-scale longitudinal data sets required for the application of multistate methods.

TRENDS IN HEALTH EXPECTANCIES FOR AUSTRALIA

Mathers (1991, 1994, 1996) has published estimates of disability-free life expectancy, handicap-free life expectancy and severe handicap-free life expectancy for Australia in 1981, 1988 and 1993. Unlike other countries for which recent health expectancy time series are available, the time series for Australia indicate that the expectation of years with disability has increased for both males and females during the 1980s and 1990s. Data from the 1998 Survey of Disability, Ageing and Carers became available in early 1999 (Australian Bureau of Statistics, 1999) and this section examines the latest Australian estimates of trends in health expectancies over the period of the late 1980s through to the late 1990s.

DISABILITY AND HANDICAP PREVALENCE DATA

All four Australian population surveys have included a reasonably large household sample (around 0.25% of the population living in households) and an institutional sample (around 3% of residents of hospitals, nursing homes, hostels and retirement homes).

The 1981 and 1988 Australian Bureau of Statistics (ABS) surveys on disability defined a person with a disability as having one or more of the following conditions which had lasted or were likely to last for six months or more:

- loss of sight, not corrected by glasses or contact lenses
- loss of hearing, with difficulty communicating or use of aids
- loss of speech
- blackouts, fits or loss of consciousness
- slowness at learning or understanding
- incomplete use of arms or fingers
- incomplete use of feet or legs
- a nervous or emotional condition that restricts everyday activities
- restrictions in physical activities or physical work
- disfigurement or deformity
- need for help or supervision because of a mental illness or condition
- treatment or medication for any other long-term condition or ailment and still restricted (Australian Bureau of Statistics, 1990).

These conditions include impairments, disabilities, and a handicap, as defined in the WHO International Classification of Impairments, Disabilities and Handicaps framework, and even some health conditions, and should perhaps be viewed as defining a wider population likely to contain those persons with a disability.

In the 1993 Australian Bureau of Statistics Survey of Disability, Ageing and Carers, the list of screening questions for disability was expanded to include:

- difficulty gripping and holding small objects
- head injury, stroke or any other brain damage with long-term effects that restrict everyday activities
- any other long-term condition that restricts everyday activities

The 1998 survey added two further additional screening questions:

- chronic or recurring pain that restricts everyday activities
- breathing difficulties that restrict everyday activities

For the analyses presented in this chapter, estimates have been derived from the 1993 and 1998 survey data using definitions consistent with the 1981 and 1988 survey screening questions.

The Australian Bureau of Statistics surveys defined a handicapped person as 'a disabled person aged five years or over who was further identified as being limited to some degree in his/her ability to perform tasks in relation to one or more of the following five areas: self care, mobility, verbal communication, schooling, and/or employment'. Severity of handicap for persons aged five years or over was assessed, for self-care, mobility and verbal communication, as follows:

(a) *Severe handicap* – personal help or supervision required or the person is unable to perform one or more of the tasks; in the 1993 and 1998 surveys this category was further divided into severe and profound handicap. In this section, the term 'severe handicap' refers to severe and profound handicap combined.

(b) *Moderate handicap* – no personal help or supervision required, but the person has difficulty in performing one or more of the tasks.

(c) *Mild handicap* – no personal help or supervision required and no difficulty in performing the tasks, but the person uses an aid, or has difficulty walking 200 metres or up and down stairs.

All disabled children under the age of five years were regarded as being handicapped; the severity of their handicap was not assessed.

CHANGES IN PREVALENCE OF DISABILITY AND HANDICAP FROM 1981 TO 1998

The age-standardised prevalence of disability increased substantially between 1981 and 1988, from 14.9 to 16.8% for males, and from 12.8 to 14.4% for females (Mathers, 1996). The increase in the reported prevalence of handicap was much greater, from 9.4 to 13.7% for males and from 8.7 to 12.2% for females. In contrast, the prevalence of severe handicap did not increase for men between 1981 and 1988, and increased by only a small amount for women (Figure 20.1).

For both sexes, the age-standardised prevalence of disability increased slightly between 1988 and 1993. In contrast, the age-standardised prevalence of handicap declined slightly, from 13.7% to 13.3% for males and from 12.2% to 11.7% for females. The prevalence of severe handicap also declined slightly, to become very close to its levels in 1981 (Figure 20.2). For both sexes, the

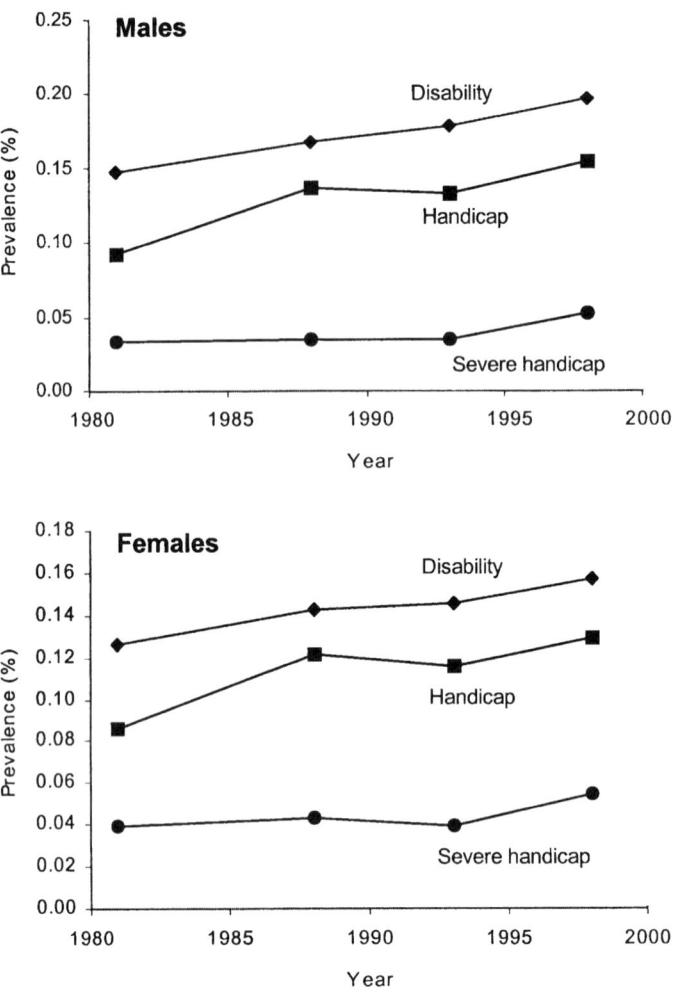

Figure 20.1. Trends in age-standardised prevalence of disability and handicap, Australia, 1981 to 1998

prevalence of severe handicap increased between 1988 and 1993 for people aged less than 40 years, but decreased slightly for people of 40 years and over.

From 1993 to 1998, prevalence of disability, handicap and severe handicap increased significantly for both sexes. Age-standardised prevalence of disability rose to 19.6% for males and 15.7% for females. These increases occurred broadly across all age groups and were not confined to the old. Unlike previous periods, where the increases in disability and handicap prevalence were largely confined to the mild severity levels, between 1993 and 1998 the most substantial

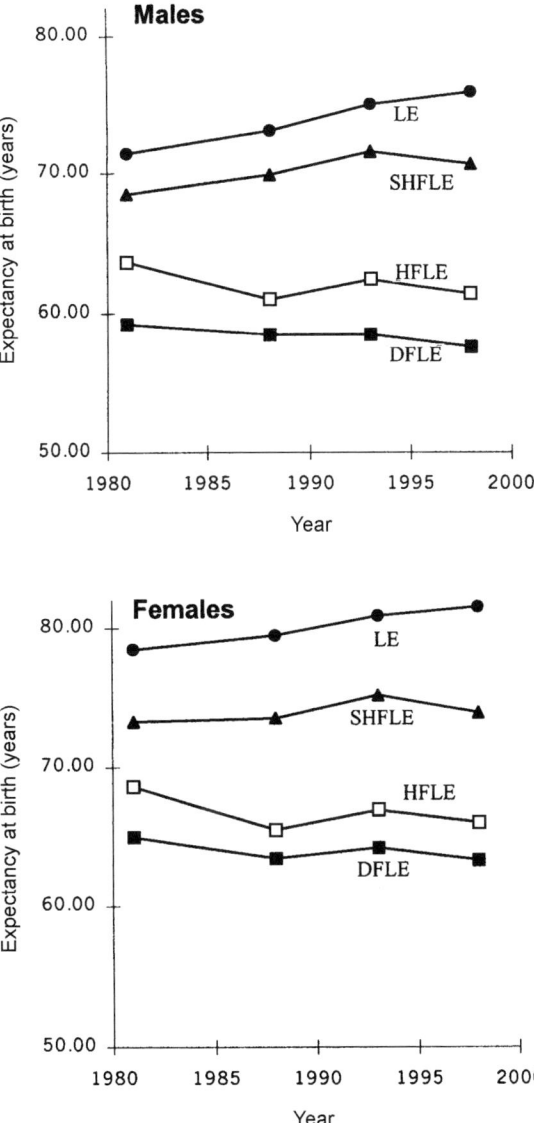

Figure 20.2. Trends in disability-free life expectancy (DFLE), handicap-free life expectancy (HFLE), severe handicap-free life expectancy (SHFLE) and total life expectancy (LE) at birth, by sex, Australia, 1981 to 1998.

increase occurred for severe and profound handicap, which rose from under 4% from 1981 to 1993 to around 5.5% in 1998.

Mathers (1991) has discussed in detail possible factors involved in the substantial increase in reported disability and handicap prevalence levels in Australia during the 1980s. Self-assessment of limitations or need for assistance in relation to specified activities may have changed in line with changing community perceptions of disability and handicap during the 1980s. Changing attitudes may have resulted in people being more aware of disabling conditions, or more willing to report such conditions and may also have affected how people interpreted 'need' and 'difficulty', concepts used to determine presence and severity of handicap. Another factor may have been changes in the availability of aids for disabled people, as use of an aid is a determinant of mild handicap. Government programmes for provision of aids expanded during the 1980s and may have contributed to the increase in self-reported prevalence of handicap.

The substantial increase in the prevalence of severe handicap between 1993 and 1998 is more difficult to understand. There were a number of changes in the 1998 survey design and interviewing methods (ABS, 1999; AIHW, 1999), including:

- the use of a computer-assisted instrument for interviews;
- a re-ordering of the questions on core activities which were used to identify profound or severe handicap;
- inclusion of the SF-12 health status instrument (which included questions on activity) inserted before the questions on handicap;
- persons in institutional care were classified as having severe or profound handicap using the same criteria as the household sample in 1998 whereas in 1993 the profound but not the severe criteria were applied.

It is possible that the majority of the apparent increase in disability rates may be due to increased identification of people with disabilities rather than an actual increase in the proportion of people with disabilities in each age group. There are indications that this could be the case. First, in the 1998 survey there were fewer people than in previous surveys who stated they needed assistance but who did not have a disability (as determined by the screening questions). Second, most of the increase appears to be in the 'severe' category rather than the 'profound' category, suggesting that the new methodology has drawn in some of those previously classified as having 'moderate' core activity restrictions (AIHW, 1999).

Further investigation and analysis are needed to understand the significance of the increase in the profound or severe rates of handicap between 1993 and 1998. The most striking increase is for boys aged 5–14 years, from 7.3% to 10.6% for people with any handicap, and from 2.7% to 4.9% for those with a profound or severe handicap. This may reflect an increased labelling and recognition of particular disabilities for this group, such as specific learning disabilities, attention deficit disorder or autism, but this needs further investigation (AIHW, 1999).

HEALTH EXPECTANCIES IN 1998

The 1998 survey data and projected life tables for 1998 have been used to estimate health expectancies for Australia for 1998. The 1998 life tables have been constructed by projecting forwards recent trends in age-sex specific mortality rates from the most recently published official life table for 1995–1997 (Australian Bureau of Statistics, 1999). Total life expectancy at birth was 75.9 years for Australian males and 81.5 years for Australian females in 1993. Disability-free life expectancy at birth was 57.5 years for males and 63.3 years for females (Table 20.4). The difference between these two sets of figures is the expectation at birth of years of disability: 18.4 years for men and 18.2 years for women. In other words, for both men and women, around 76% of life will be lived without disability on average, if death rates and disability prevalence rates at all ages remain constant at their 1998 levels, respectively.

Of the years of disability, 14.6 are years of handicap and 5.2 are years of severe or profound handicap for males. Females experience more years of handicap from birth (15.5) and 7.6 of these are years of severe handicap, almost double that for males. Men have a lower life expectancy at birth than women and also a lower expectation of years of disability, handicap and severe handicap.

Table 20.4. Australia: health expectancies at birth and at age 65, by gender, 1998

	HE (years)		HE/LE (%)	
	Males	Females	Males	Females
Expectation of life at birth:				
with severe handicap	5.2	7.6	6.9	9.3
with handicap, not severe	9.4	7.8	12.4	9.6
with disability, but not handicapped	3.8	2.7	5.0	3.3
free of disability	57.5	63.3	75.8	77.7
Total life expectancy at birth (LE)	*75.9*	*81.5*		
Expectation of life at age 65:				
with severe handicap	3.0	5.5	18.6	27.9
with handicap, not severe	4.7	4.1	28.9	20.6
with disability, but not handicapped	1.9	1.2	11.9	6.3
free of disability	6.6	9.0	40.6	45.2
Total life expectancy at age 65	*16.1*	*19.8*		

Table 20.5. Australia: trends in health expectancies at birth, by gender, 1981, 1988, 1993 and 1998

	1981	1988	1993	1998	1981–1998
Males					
Life expectancy	71.4	73.1	75.0	75.9	+4.5
Severe handicap expectancy	2.9	3.2	3.4	5.2	+2.3
Handicap expectancy	7.8	12.1	12.6	14.6	+6.8
Disability expectancy	12.2	14.7	16.6	18.4	+6.2
Disability-free expectancy	59.2	58.4	58.4	57.5	−1.7
Females					
Life expectancy	78.4	79.5	80.9	81.5	+3.1
Severe handicap expectancy	5.2	6.0	5.7	7.6	+2.4
Handicap expectancy	9.8	14.0	14.0	15.5	+5.7
Disability expectancy	13.4	16.0	16.7	18.2	+4.8
Disability-free expectancy	65.0	63.4	64.0	63.3	−1.7

Similar patterns are evident for health expectancies at age 65, although the proportion of remaining life spent free of disability is much lower at 41% for men and 45% for women (see lower panel of Table 20.4). Although total life expectancies of females significantly exceed those of males at all ages, the sex differentials for health expectancies are much lower and decrease more rapidly with age. Indeed, life expectancy free of severe handicap is only 1.2 years greater for women at age 65.

TRENDS IN HEALTH EXPECTANCIES FROM 1981 TO 1998

Between 1988 and 1998, life expectancy at birth increased from 73.1 to 75.9 years for males and 79.5 to 81.5 years for females (Table 20.5). Over the same period, disability-free life expectancy dropped by around 1.5 years for both males and females. Most of this decrease was concentrated in levels of handicap and disability below the severe level in the 1980s, but between 1993 and 1998 there was a significant expansion in the years lived with severe handicap for both males and females.

A similar pattern was found for health expectancies at age 65 (Table 20.6). The proportion of remaining life at age 65 which is free of disability remained almost constant for women at around 46%, whereas that for men declined from 45% in 1988 to 41% in 1993. Unlike other countries for which health expectancy time series are available, Australian health expectancies do not yet provide any evidence for the occurrence of compression of morbidity, when that is defined in terms of a fairly wide definition of disability. Instead, they suggest a continuing expansion in expected years with disability at milder and more severe levels.

Table 20.6. Australia: trends in health expectancies at age 65, by gender, 1981, 1988, 1993 and 1998

	1981	1988	1993	1998	1981–1998
Males					
Life expectancy	13.9	14.8	15.7	16.1	+ 2.3
Severe handicap expectancy	2.0	2.2	2.4	3.0	+ 1.0
Handicap expectancy	2.3	4.4	5.0	4.7	+ 2.4
Disability expectancy	1.7	1.4	1.9	1.9	+ 0.2
Disability-free expectancy	7.9	6.7	6.5	6.6	− 1.4
Females					
Life expectancy	18.1	18.7	19.5	19.8	+ 1.8
Severe handicap expectancy	4.3	5.0	4.7	5.5	+ 1.3
Handicap expectancy	2.4	4.1	4.6	4.1	+ 1.7
Disability expectancy	1.4	1.1	1.2	1.3	− 0.1
Disability-free expectancy	10.0	8.6	9.1	9.0	− 1.1

TRENDS AND DIFFERENTIALS IN HEALTH EXPECTANCIES IN NEW ZEALAND

The data available in the New Zealand case are much less complete and follow less consistent definitions between collections (see Table 20.3 above). The first collection was part of a social indicators survey, the second a component of a health survey, and third more closely linked to disability. Achieving consistency across these surveys has been difficult. Hence to date, for example, it has only been possible to achieve comparability between the first two collections on a single mobility-based measure of disability, the ability to climb stairs. Therefore the New Zealand results on trends in health expectancy reported below are restricted to the expectation of life able to climb stairs. Details of the exact question wording are given in Davis *et al* (1999).

HEALTH EXPECTANCIES IN 1996/97

The most comprehensive set of information on disability and health expectancy in New Zealand is provided in the 1996/97 New Zealand Disability surveys (Tobias and Cheung, 1999). The two main sources of data were the 1996 Household Disability Survey and the 1997 Disability Survey of Residential Facilities (HFA/MOH, 1998). Both surveys used the functional concept of disability defined as limitation in activity resulting from a long-term condition or health problem. Classification of disability status proceeded via an initial screening questionnaire which asked about difficulties performing a range of tasks (28 items for adults, 12 items for children), with those reporting disability further classified according to their need for assistance with daily activities. The areas of disability addressed by the screening questionnaire were:

- hearing (three items)
- speaking (two items)
- sight (four items)
- mobility (five items)
- agility (seven items)
- learning (one item)
- remembering (one item)
- intellectual disability (two items)
- psychiatric and psychological disability (two items)
- residual category (one item)

Respondents who responded positively to any of these items were considered to have a disability. However, respondents were not considered to have a disability if they used a device that completely eliminated their limitation (such as an effective hearing aid). Furthermore, the limitation had to have lasted, or be expected to last, six months or more at the time of interview.

This information was used in a major review of the health status of the New Zealand population (Ministry of Health, 1999). This also included an analysis of the elasticity of the health expectancy measure – its sensitivity to small changes in mortality and/or disability – and its population dynamics (for example, the potential gain in health expectancy that would result from eliminating death or disability risk in a particular age group).

Table 20.7 reports gender- and ethnic-specific estimates of disability-free and disabled life expectancy at birth and at age 65 for varying levels of disability severity. With respect to gender differences, the results reported in the table exhibit the standard pattern of smaller differences in disability-free life expectancy than for total life expectancy. However, the ethnic group differences in disability-free life expectancy are of about the same magnitude as differences in total life expectancy. This contrasts with earlier results suggesting markedly greater ethnic differentials in health expectancy than for total life expectancy, a result that has been shown to hold for three distinct types of health expectancy measures (Davis *et al*, 1999).

Despite the shorter total life expectancy of Maori compared to non-Maori, the expectation of life with disability requiring assistance is similar or slightly greater for Maori. Thus for Maori men disability requiring assistance accounts for 14.7% of the total life expectation, whereas the comparable figure for non-Maori men is 12.7%. Similarly the expectation of life with a disability requiring assistance accounts for 18.0% of the life span for Maori women, while the comparable figure for non-Maori is 14.4%.

Table 20.7. New Zealand: health expectancies at birth and at age 65 by gender and ethnicity 1996/7

	Total		Maori		Non-Maori	
	Male	Female	Male	Female	Male	Female
Expectation of life at birth (years):						
with disability requiring daily assistance	2.3	3.7	2.4	4.0	2.2	3.7
with disability requiring non-daily assistance	7.5	8.0	7.5	8.9	7.4	8.0
with disability, not requiring assistance	6.8	7.0	5.7	5.8	7.0	6.9
free of disability	57.7	60.9	51.6	52.9	58.7	62.0
Total life expectancy at birth	*74.3*	*79.6*	*67.2*	*71.6*	*75.3*	*80.6*
Expectation of life at age 65 (years):						
with disability requiring daily assistance	1.5	2.5	1.1	2.5	1.5	2.6
with disability requiring non-daily assistance	4.3	4.8	3.7	4.5	4.4	4.8
with disability, not requiring assistance	2.2	2.5	1.7	1.0	2.3	2.6
free of disability	7.5	9.2	5.7	6.5	7.6	9.3
Total life expectancy at age 65	*15.5*	*19.0*	*12.2*	*14.5*	*15.8*	*19.3*

Source: Health Funding Authority, and Ministry of Health (1998, p. 108).

TRENDS IN DISABILITY PREVALENCE AND HEALTH EXPECTANCY FROM 1981 TO 1991

As noted previously the only measures available for studying changes in health expectancy in New Zealand are based on the ability to climb stairs and this information is available for only two time points, 1980/81 and 1992/93. Using the relevant gender-specific age distribution at the 1991 census as the standard, age-standardised prevalences of stair climbing problems for men increased from 4.9% in 1980/81 to 7.1% in 1992/93 for men and from 8.6% to 10.2% for women. Age-specific rates for the two years are shown in Figure 20.3. The rates increase across the age range, as expected, and for most age groups show a small increase between 1980/81 and 1992/3.

Table 20.8 reports changes in health expectancy at age 15 and at age 65 between 1980/81 and 1992/93. While life expectancy at age 15 improved by about two years for both men and women over this period, the expectation of life able to climb stairs remained unchanged. A similar pattern holds for life expectancy at age 65. Thus, although the definition of health expectancy used

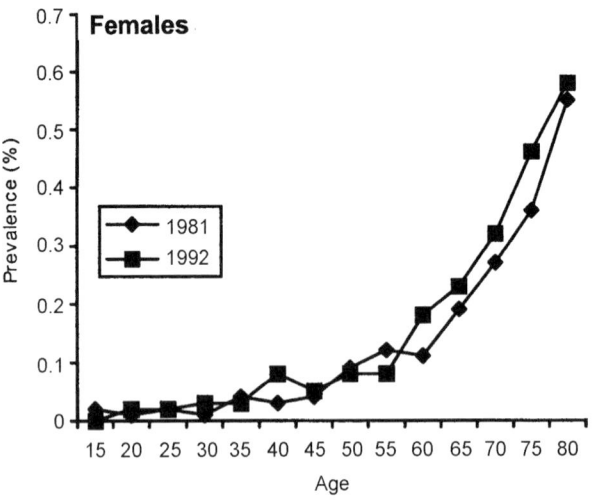

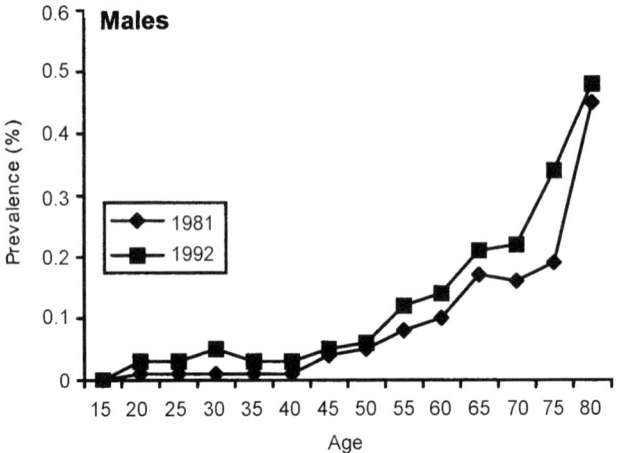

Figure 20.3. Age-specific prevalence of stair climbing problems, 1981 and 1992

in New Zealand is not strictly comparable to Australia, a similar pattern has emerged – namely, an improvement in longevity over the 1980s, but little or no increase in disability-free life expectancy over the same period.

DIFFERENTIALS IN PARTIAL HEALTH EXPECTANCY FROM 1981 TO 1991

While the Australian collections have concentrated on achieving a consistent, representative and comprehensive data series, the New Zealand data have

Table 20.8. New Zealand: trends in health expectancies between 1980/81 and 1992/93 at ages 15 and 65 by gender

	Male			Female		
	1980/81	1992/93	Change	1980/81	1992/93	Change
Age 15						
Able to climb stairs	52.5	52.6	+ 0.1	54.5	54.5	0.0
Total life expectancy	56.7	58.8	+ 2.1	62.5	64.4	+ 1.9
Age 65						
Able to climb stairs	9.9	10.0	+ 0.1	10.5	10.2	− 0.3
Total life expectancy	13.3	14.8	+ 1.5	17.1	18.4	+ 1.3

permitted the study of sub-national and special populations defined by socioeconomic status (SES) and ethnicity. Because of data limitations, these analyses have to date been restricted to the 15 to 64 age group, necessitating the use of the concepts of partial life and health expectancy (Graham and Davis, 1990; Davis *et al*, 1999).

Table 20.9 documents changes in partial health expectancy between ages 15 and 64 over the period 1980/81 and 1992/93, separately for Maori and non-Maori. While the pattern for Maori and non-Maori men is similar – with a small increase in partial life expectancy and a small decline in partial health expectancy – there is a suggestion that, although health expectancy improved slightly for non-Maori women, it declined by 1.6 years for Maori women. The temporal changes are small, however, and 95% confidence intervals for the change over time include zero (that is, no significant change).

The ethnic group differences in partial health expectancy are substantial at both time points. Non-Maori–Maori differences in partial health expectancy range from approximately three to five years, whereas differences in total life

Table 20.9. New Zealand: changes in partial health expectancy between ages 15 and 64, over the period 1980/81 to 1992/93, by gender and ethnicity

	Male			Female		
	1980/81	1992/93	Change	1980/81	1992/93	Change
Maori						
Able to climb stairs	40.6	40.1	− 0.5	42.6	41.0	− 1.6
Total life expectancy	45.1	45.8	+ 0.7	46.5	47.3	+ 0.8
Non-Maori						
Able to climb stairs	45.3	44.9	− 0.4	45.8	46.0	+ 0.2
Total life expectancy	47.0	47.3	+ 0.3	48.2	48.5	+ 0.3

expectancy range from one to two years. For women, the ethnic group differential in partial expectancy widened from 3.2 years in 1980/81 to 5.0 years in 1992/93.

Variation in health expectancy according to an occupationally based measure of SES has also been studied in New Zealand. The available evidence points to a possible widening of socioeconomic inequalities in health expectancy. Over the period 1980/81 to 1992/93 the only group to sustain an increase in health expectancy was the highest SES group (Davis *et al*, 1999).

CONCLUSIONS

Unlike other developed countries (see Chapters 4, 18, 19), health expectancies for Australia suggest that expansion of morbidity is occurring at all levels of disability. Possible factors involved in the substantial increase in expected years of disability during the 1980s have been discussed in detail by Mathers (1991). Self-assessment of limitations or need for assistance in relation to specified activities may have changed in line with changing community perceptions of disability and handicap. Changing attitudes may have resulted in people being more aware of disabling conditions, or more willing to report such conditions and may also have affected how people interpreted 'need' and 'difficulty', concepts used to determine presence and severity of handicap. Another factor may have been changes in the availability of aids for disabled people, as use of an aid is a determinant of mild handicap. Government programmes for provision of aids expanded during the 1980s and may have contributed to the increase in self-reported prevalence of handicap.

The most recent Australian population survey of disability suggests that the overall prevalence of disability is continuing to increase in Australia, but for the first time there is a significant expansion in the expected years with severe handicap (these were very stable from 1981 to 1993). A number of factors suggest that this increase may be due to changes in survey methodology and represent predominantly a shift in classification from moderate to severe handicap rather than a real increase in handicap severity. The data suggest that there is an increasing prevalence of severe and profound handicap among boys and that this may reflect an increased labelling and recognition of particular disabilities for this group, such as specific learning disabilities, attention deficit disorder or autism, but this needs further investigation. There have been increases in the rates of autism in Europe and North America, which are possibly due to changes in diagnostic criteria and a wider recognition of its expression (AIHW, 1999).

The conclusions with regard to trends in health expectancy in New Zealand are necessarily more tentative, because of the more limited data available. The one comparable health expectancy measure available suggests that, while small gains in life expectancy were made over the decade of the 1980s, most of the additional life expectation is accounted for by an increase in the expectation of life with some mobility limitation.

The New Zealand results also highlight important ethnic and social variation in health expectancy and suggest that these differentials may have widened over the 1980s, a decade of major social and economic change in New Zealand. These findings point to a need for a more elaborated version of the compression/expansion of morbidity hypothesis that recognises the potential for social variation in the evolution of population health.

Australia has been a pioneer in the adoption, development and application of the health expectancy concept: its official agencies have shown a readiness to commit resources to fund the collection of a representative, comprehensive and consistent data series; key scientific collaborations have established the intellectual leadership of the country in the wider health expectancy movement; and to an important extent health expectancy measures have been integrated into the country's established statistical system of indicators. New Zealand, by contrast, has been slower to adopt and adapt the health expectancy concept, and it has not been afforded the required resources or consistency of support to provide it with an established place in the country's statistical system. Nevertheless, the prominence given to health expectancy in a recent census-based disability survey is indicative of the growing acceptance of the concept in New Zealand's statistical framework, although this is showing a trend towards a health-adjusted life expectancy concept. Future progress in both countries will depend on adequate resources, continuing scientific development, and demonstrated utility and application to the pertinent issues in public policy.

ACKNOWLEDGEMENTS

We thank Martin Tobias, of the New Zealand Ministry of Health, for his helpful contributions to this chapter.

REFERENCES

Australian Bureau of Statistics (ABS) (1982) *Handicapped Persons Australia 1981*. ABS Cat. No. 4343.0. Canberra, ACT: ABS.

Australian Bureau of Statistics (ABS) (1990) *Disability and Handicap in Australia 1988*. ABS Cat. No. 4120.0. Canberra, ACT: ABS.

Australian Bureau of Statistics (ABS) (1993) *Disability, Ageing and Carers: Summary of Findings Australia 1993*. ABS Cat. No. 4430.0. Canberra, ACT: ABS.

Australian Bureau of Statistics (ABS) (1999) *Disability, Ageing and Carers: Summary of Findings Australia 1998*. ABS Cat. No. 4430.0. Canberra, ACT: ABS.

Australian Institute of Health and Welfare (AIHW) (1999). *Australia's Welfare 1999*. Canberra, ACT: AIHW.

Davis, P., Graham, P. and Pearce, N. (1999) 'Health expectancy in New Zealand 1981–1991: Social variation and trends in a period of social and economic change', *Journal of Epidemiology and Community Health* 53(9), 519–527.

Department of Statistics (1984) *Report on the Social Indicators Survey*. Wellington, NZ: Department of Statistics.

Graham, P. and Davis, P. (1990). 'Life expectancy free of disability: A composite measure of population health status', *Community Health Studies* XIV, 138–145.

Health Funding Authority, Ministry of Health (1998) *Disability in New Zealand. Overview of the 1996/97 Surveys*. Wellington, NZ: Health Funding Authority and Ministry of Health.

Mathers, C.D. (1991) *Health Expectancies in Australia, 1981 and 1988*. Canberra, ACT: Australian Institute of Health.

Mathers, C. (1994) 'Health expectancies in Australia 1993: preliminary results', in Mathers, C., McCallum, J. and Robine, J.-M. (eds) *Advances in Health Expectancies*. Canberra: Australian Institute of Health and Welfare.

Mathers, C.D. (1996) 'Trends in health expectancies in Australia 1981–1993', *Journal of the Australian Population Association* 13(1), 1–16.

Ministry of Health (1999) *Our Health, Our Future. Hauora Pakari, Koiora Roa. The Health of New Zealanders 1999*. Wellington, NZ: Ministry of Health.

Statistics New Zealand, Ministry of Health (1993) *A Picture of Health*. Wellington, NZ: Statistics New Zealand and Ministry of Health.

Sullivan, D. (1971) 'A single index of mortality and morbidity', *Health Services and Mental Health Administration (HSMHA) Health Reports* 86, 347–354.

Tobias, M. and Cheung, J. (1999) 'Independent life expectancy in New Zealand 1996–97', *Australian Health Review* 22, 78–91.

Index

NOTE: abbreviations used in subheadings: ADLs = activities of daily living; DALY = disability-adjusted life year; DFLE = disability-free life expectancy; EC = European Community; HALE = health-adjusted life expectancy; IADLs = instrumental activities of daily living; ICIDH = International Classification of Impairments, Disabilities and Handicaps; OECD = Organisation for Economic Cooperation and Development; REVES = Réseau Espérance de Vie en Santé; WHO = World Health Organization.